T0331907

Musculoskeletal Imaging: Radiographic/MRI Correlation

Editor

ANNE COTTEN

MAGNETIC RESONANCE IMAGING CLINICS OF NORTH AMERICA

www.mri.theclinics.com

Consulting Editors
SURESH K. MUKHERJI
LYNNE S. STEINBACH

November 2019 • Volume 27 • Number 4

ELSEVIER

1600 John F. Kennedy Boulevard • Suite 1800 • Philadelphia, Pennsylvania, 19103-2899

http://www.mri.theclinics.com

MRI CLINICS OF NORTH AMERICA Volume 27, Number 4
November 2019 ISSN 1064-9689, ISBN 13: 978-0-323-70872-2

Editor: John Vassallo (j.vassallo@elsevier.com)
Developmental Editor: Kristen Helm

Magnetic Resonance Imaging Clinics of North America (ISSN 1064-9689) is published quarterly by Elsevier Inc., 360 Park Avenue South, New York, NY 10010-1710. Months of issue are February, May, August, and November. Business and Editorial Offices: 1600 John F. Kennedy Blvd., Ste. 1800, Philadelphia, PA 19103-2899. Customer Service Office: 3251 Riverport Lane, Maryland Heights, MO 63043. Periodicals postage paid at New York, NY and additional mailing offices. Subscription prices are $404.00 per year (domestic individuals), $736.00 per year (domestic institutions), $100.00 per year (domestic students/residents), $437.00 per year (Canadian individuals), $959.00 per year (Canadian institutions), $545.00 per year (international individuals), $959.00 per year (international institutions), and $275.00 per year (international and Canadian students/residents). International air speed delivery is included in all *Clinics* subscription prices. All prices are subject to change without notice. **POSTMASTER:** Send address changes to *Magnetic Resonance Imaging Clinics*, Elsevier Health Sciences Division, Subscription Customer Service, 3251 Riverport Lane, Maryland Heights, MO 63043. Customer Service (orders, claims, online, change of address): Elsevier Health Sciences Division, Subscription **Customer Service, 3251 Riverport Lane, Maryland Heights, MO 63043. Tel:1-800-654-2452 (U.S. and Canada); 314-447-8871 (outside U.S. and Canada). Fax: 314-447-8029. E-mail: journalscustomer service-usa@elsevier.com (for print support); journalsonlinesupport-usa@elsevier.com (for online support).**

Reprints. For copies of 100 or more of articles in this publication, please contact the Commercial Reprints Department, Elsevier Inc., 360 Park Avenue South, New York, NY 10010-1710. Tel.: 212-633-3874; Fax: 212-633-3820; E-mail: reprints@elsevier.com.

Magnetic Resonance Imaging Clinics of North America is covered in the *RSNA Index of Imaging Literature, MEDLINE/PubMed (Index Medicus),* and *EMBASE/Excerpta Medica.*

Contributors

CONSULTING EDITORS

SURESH K. MUKHERJI, MD, MBA, FACR
Professor, Department of Radiology, Michigan
State University, East Lansing, Michigan, USA

LYNNE S. STEINBACH, MD, FACR
Emeritus Professor of Radiology on Full Recall,
Department of Radiology and Biomedical
Imaging, University of California, San
Francisco, San Francisco, California, USA

EDITOR

ANNE COTTEN, MD, PhD
Service de Radiologie et Imagerie
Musculosquelettique, Centre de Consultations
et d'Imagerie de l'Appareil Locomoteur, Lille
Cedex, France

AUTHORS

ERIN F. ALAIA, MD
Assistant Professor, Department of Radiology,
Division of Musculoskeletal Radiology, NYU
Langone Health, New York, New York, USA

**GINA M. ALLEN, BM, MRCGP, MRCP,
FRCR, MFSEM, MScSEM**
St Luke's Radiology Oxford Ltd, St Luke's
Hospital, The University of Oxford, Oxford,
United Kingdom

SOOHEIB ANDOULSI, MD
Department of Radiology, Centre Hospitalier
de l'Université de Montréal, Montréal, Québec,
Canada

SAMMY BADR, MD, MSc
Department of Musculoskeletal Radiology, Lille
University Hospital, Lille University School of
Medicine, Service de Radiologie et Imagerie
Musculosquelettique, Centre de Consultations
et d'Imagerie de l'Appareil Locomoteur
(C.C.I.A.L.), Lille, France

SARAH D. BIXBY, MD
Associate Professor, Department of Radiology,
Boston Children's Hospital, Harvard Medical
School, Boston, Massachusetts, USA

FREDERIK BOSMANS, MD
Department of Radiology, AZ Sint-Maarten
Mechelen, University Hospital Antwerp,
Mechelen, Belgium

NATHALIE BOUTRY, MD, PhD
Head of Pediatric Imaging Department, Hôpital
Jeanne de Flandre, CHU Lille, Lille, France

FRANCESCO PIO CAFARELLI, MD
Department of Clinical and Experimental
Medicine, Foggia University School of
Medicine, Foggia, Italy

ÉTIENNE CARDINAL, MD
Medvue, Montréal, Québec, Canada

**VICTOR CASSAR-PULLICINO, LRCP,
MRCS, DMRD, FRCR, MD**
Department of Radiology, Robert Jones and
Agnes Hunt Orthopaedic Hospital NHS
Foundation Trust, Oswestry, United Kingdom

ANNE COTTEN, MD, PhD
Department of Musculoskeletal Radiology, Lille
University Hospital, Lille University School of
Medicine, Service de Radiologie et Imagerie
Musculosquelettique, Centre de Consultations

et d'Imagerie de l'Appareil Locomoteur (C.C.I.A.L.), Lille, France

JULIEN DARTUS, MD
Lille University School of Medicine, Department of Orthopedic Surgery, Lille University Hospital, Service d'Orthopédie D, Hôpital Roger Salengro, CHRU de Lille, Lille, France

IOAN N. GEMESCU, MD
Department of Radiology and Medical Imaging, University Emergency Hospital Bucharest, Bucharest, Romania

PAOLA CECY KUENZER GOES, MD
Division of Musculoskeletal Radiology, Laboratorio Delboni Auriemo, DASA, São Paulo, Brazil

GIUSEPPE GUGLIELMI, MD
Department of Clinical and Experimental Medicine, Foggia University School of Medicine, Foggia, Italy; Department of Radiology, Scientific Institute Hospital "Casa Sollievo della Sofferenza", San Giovanni Rotondo, Italy

THIBAUT JACQUES, MD, MSc
Department of Musculoskeletal Radiology, Lille University Hospital, Lille University School of Medicine, Service de Radiologie et Imagerie Musculosquelettique, Centre de Consultations et d'Imagerie de l'Appareil Locomoteur (C.C.I.A.L.), Lille, France

JÉRÉMY JEANTROUX, MD
Service d'Imagerie Médicale, Clinique St-François, Haguenau, France

ROWENA JOHNSON, MB ChB, FRCR
Nuffield Orthopaedic Centre, Oxford University Hospitals, Oxford, United Kingdom

GUILLAUME LEFEBVRE, MD
Department of Musculoskeletal Radiology, Lille University Hospital, Service de Radiologie et Imagerie Musculosquelettique, Centre de Consultations et d'Imagerie de l'Appareil Locomoteur (C.C.I.A.L.), Lille, France

ANTONELLO LEONE, MD
Institute of Radiology, Catholic University, School of Medicine, Fondazione Policlinico Universitario A. Gemelli, IRCSS, Rome, Italy

HÉLOÏSE LERISSON, MD
Department of Pediatric Imaging, Hôpital Jeanne de Flandre, CHU Lille, Lille, France

DANA J. LIN, MD
Clinical Assistant Professor, Department of Radiology, Division of Musculoskeletal Radiology, NYU Langone Health, New York, New York, USA

JACQUES MALGHEM, MD
Professor Emeritus, Department of Radiology, Cliniques Universitaires Saint Luc, Brussels, Belgium

ADRIANA P. MARTINEZ, MD, MSc, FRCSC
Department of Orthopedic Surgery, University of Ottawa, The Ottawa Hospital Civic Campus, Ottawa, Ontario, Canada

PAUL MICHELIN, MD, MSc
Department of Radiology, Rouen University Hospital, Imagerie de l'Appareil Locomoteur, CHU Rouen Normandie, Rouen, France

THOMAS P. MOSER, MD, MSc
Department of Radiology, Centre Hospitalier de l'Université de Montréal, Montréal, Québec, Canada

CHARBEL MOURAD, MD
Musculoskeletal Radiologist, Department of Radiology, Hôpital Libanais Geitaoui HLG-CHU, Beyrouth, Lebanon; Institut de Recherche Expérimentale et Clinique (IREC), Université Catholique de Louvain, Brussels, Belgium

PATRICK OMOUMI, MD, PhD
Head of Musculoskeletal Radiology, Department of Diagnostic and Interventional Radiology, Lausanne University Hospital, Centre Hospitalier Universitaire, Lausanne, Switzerland

MINI N. PATHRIA, MD
Professor of Clinical Radiology, University of California San Diego Health System, San Diego, California, USA

CHRISTOPH REHNITZ, MD
Department of Diagnostic and Interventional Radiology, Heidelberg University Hospital, Heidelberg, Germany

MONIQUE REIJNIERSE, MD, PhD
Head of Musculoskeletal Radiology,
Department of Radiology, Leiden University
Medical Centre, Leiden, The Netherlands

ZEHAVA SADKA ROSENBERG, MD
Professor, Department of Radiology,
Professor, Department of Orthopaedic
Surgery, Division of Musculoskeletal
Radiology, NYU Langone Health, New York,
New York, USA

IGNACIO MARTÍN ROSSI, MD
Centro Rossi, Buenos Aires, Argentina

KOLJA M. THIERFELDER, MD, MSc
Institute of Diagnostic and Interventional
Radiology, Pediatric Radiology and
Neuroradiology, Rostock University Medical
Centre, Rostock, Germany

CÉLINE TILLAUX, MD
Department of Pediatric Imaging, Hôpital
Jeanne de Flandre, CHU Lille, Lille, France

**PRUDENCIA N.M. TYRRELL, MBBCh, BAO,
FRCR**
Department of Radiology, Robert Jones and
Agnes Hunt Orthopaedic Hospital NHS
Foundation Trust, Oswestry, United Kingdom

BRUNO C. VANDE BERG, MD, PhD
Institut de Recherche Expérimentale et
Clinique (IREC), Université Catholique de
Louvain, Head of Musculoskeletal Radiology,
Department of Radiology, Cliniques
Universitaires Saint Luc, Brussels,
Belgium

FILIP M. VANHOENACKER, MD, PhD
Department of Radiology, AZ Sint-Maarten
Mechelen, University Hospital Antwerp,
Ghent University, Mechelen,
Belgium

MARC-ANDRÉ WEBER, MD, MSc
Institute of Diagnostic and Interventional
Radiology, Pediatric Radiology and
Neuroradiology, Rostock University Medical
Centre, Rostock, Germany

TIMOTHY WOO, MBChB, MA, FRCR
Department of Radiology, Robert Jones and
Agnes Hunt Orthopaedic Hospital NHS
Foundation Trust, Oswestry,
United Kingdom

JONATHAN ZEMBER, MD
Assistant Professor of Pediatrics and
Radiology, Childrens National Medical Center,
DC, Washington, DC, USA

Contents

imaging. Radiographs can provide fine bony detail, but lack soft tissue definition and can be complicated by overlying structures. MR imaging allow(s) excellent soft tissue contrast, but some bony abnormalities can be difficult to discern. This makes the 2 modalities highly complementary. In this article, the authors discuss the correlation between radiographic and MR imaging appearances focusing first on disease affecting the vertebral body itself, its surrounding structures, and finally global spinal alignment.

This article focuses on the variety of imaging features of paravertebral ossifications that are of practical interest in the diagnosis of diseases. The spinal anatomy is reviewed and correlated to paravertebral ligamentous ossifications and their potential clinical impact. A vertebral bony outgrowth is secondary to inflammation or degeneration and can be characterized based on its origin and growth direction, in addition to appreciation of intervertebral disc space preservation or loss. Imaging in rheumatology patients is highlighted because early detection of disease is of increasing importance. A correlation between radiographs and MR imaging is made.

This review proposes a structured approach to analyzing conventional radiographs of adult hips by focusing on alterations of radiological bone density, femoral head contours, and the joint space. Conventional radiography enables detecting subtle changes in cortical contours and joint space width due to its high spatial resolution. It is limited to the detection of cortical changes in areas to which the x-ray beam is tangent. It has reduced sensitivity for the detection of trabecular bone and medullary changes. Radiographic findings in common hip disorders, such as osteoarthritis, osteonecrosis, transient osteoporosis, and subchondral insufficiency fractures, are correlated to changes on MR imaging and computed tomography.

Knee radiographs are widely used in clinical practice. Many features can be depicted when a systematic analysis of the different views is performed. This article focuses on different types of joint effusion and on the analysis of the bone outlines of the knee, particularly on the lateral view. Systematic analysis of these bone outlines and knowledge of several key points are particularly useful for the depiction of abnormal bone morphology or positioning, and of several conditions, such as trochlear dysplasia, patellar dislocation, impaction fractures, or ligament injuries and avulsion fractures.

The focus of this article is to illustrate various pathologic entities and variants, heralding disease about the ankle, based on scrutiny of AP radiographs of the ankle, with correlative findings on cross-sectional imaging. Many of these entities can only be detected on the AP ankle radiograph and, if not recognized, may lead to delayed diagnosis and persistent morbidity to the patient. However, a vigilant radiologist, equipped with the knowledge of the characteristic appearance and typical locations of the imaging findings, should be able to make the crucial initial diagnosis and surmise additional findings to be confirmed on cross-sectional imaging.

Fractures are common in children, although accurate diagnosis is confounded by mimics of fractures some of which are unique to the pediatric population. Such fracture mimics include developmental variations of the growth plates, normal anatomic structures that simulate fracture lines, and/or metabolic disorders that alter the pattern of ossification. Although subtle clues on plain radiographs may help to discriminate between a true fracture or injury and a fracture mimic, MR imaging may be helpful to eliminate uncertainty or expedite diagnosis.

Normal bone growth of the pediatric knee as well as normal variants of ossification result in different appearances that can be identified on imaging (radiography/MR imaging). Familiarity with these changes is important to avoid confusing normal growth with pathology. This article illustrates the main features related to normal bone growth (growth arrest lines, physeal changes, ossification centers within the epiphysis, hematopoietic marrow within the metaphysis) and physis disappearance (« FOPE »). Variants in femur (epiphyseal irregularities, subchondral anomalies of posterior condyles, periosteal desmoid), tibia (tibial tuberosity ossification), and patella (dorsal defect, bipartite patella, lower pole fragmentation) are also described.

Imaging bone tumors often causes uncertainty, especially outside dedicated sarcoma treatment centers. Conventional radiography remains the backbone of bone tumor diagnostics, but MR imaging has a role. Radiographs are crucial for assessing the tumor matrix and aggressiveness. MR imaging is the best modality for local staging. This article reviews semiological aspects of bone tumors: patient age, tumor localization, pattern of bone destruction/margins, aggressiveness, growth speed, matrix formation, periosteal reaction, cortical involvement, size, and number of lesions. All aspects are discussed in terms of their appearance on radiographs and MR imaging, with a focus on the correlation between the 2 modalities.

MR imaging is nowadays regarded as the preferred imaging modality for evaluation of soft tissue lesions. As plain radiographs are often the first step in evaluation of musculoskeletal disorders, identification of subtle soft tissue signs may be helpful to select patients who need to be referred for subsequent MR imaging. Although not very sensitive, certain plain film findings, such as intralesional calcification or gas, may allow one to make to a more specific tissue diagnosis and may obviate the need for invasive diagnostic procedures and potential harmful treatment.

MAGNETIC RESONANCE IMAGING CLINICS OF NORTH AMERICA

PROGRAM OBJECTIVE

The goal of *Magnetic Resonance Imaging Clinics of North America* is to keep practicing physicians up to date with current clinical practice by providing timely articles reviewing the state of the art in patient care.

TARGET AUDIENCE

All practicing physicians and healthcare professionals who provide patient care utilizing findings from Magnetic Resonance Imaging.

LEARNING OBJECTIVES

Upon completion of this activity, participants will be able to:
1. Review semiological aspects in the imaging of bone tumors and their appearance on both radiographs and on MRI
2. Discuss a structured approach to analyze conventional radiographs of normal and abnormal adult hips.
3. Recognize the role of MRI during the diagnosis of pediatric fractures.

ACCREDITATION

The Elsevier Office of Continuing Medical Education (EOCME) is accredited by the Accreditation Council for Continuing Medical Education (ACCME) to provide continuing medical education for physicians.

The EOCME designates this journal-based CME activity enduring material for a maximum of 12 *AMA PRA Category 1 Credit*(s)™. Physicians should claim only the credit commensurate with the extent of their participation in the activity.

All other healthcare professionals requesting continuing education credit for this enduring material will be issued a certificate of participation.

DISCLOSURE OF CONFLICTS OF INTEREST

The EOCME assesses conflict of interest with its instructors, faculty, planners, and other individuals who are in a position to control the content of CME activities. All relevant conflicts of interest that are identified are thoroughly vetted by EOCME for fair balance, scientific objectivity, and patient care recommendations. EOCME is committed to providing its learners with CME activities that promote improvements or quality in healthcare and not a specific proprietary business or a commercial interest.

The planning committee, staff, authors and editors listed below have identified no financial relationships or relationships to products or devices they or their spouse/life partner have with commercial interest related to the content of this CME activity:

Erin F. Alaia, MD; Gina M. Allen, BM, MRCGP, MRCP, FRCR, MFSEM, MScSEM; Sooheib Andoulsi, MD; Sammy Badr, MD, MSc; Sarah D. Bixby, MD; Frederik Bosmans, MD; Nathalie Boutry, MD, PhD; Francesco Pio Cafarelli, MD; Étienne Cardinal, MD; Victor Cassar-Pullicino, LRCP, MRCS, DMRD, FRCR, MD; Anne Cotten, MD, PhD; Julien Dartus, MD; Ioan N. Gemescu, MD; Paola Cecy Kuenzer Goes, MD; Giuseppe Guglielmi, MD; Thibaut Jacques, MD, MSc; Jérémy Jeantroux, MD; Rowena Johnson, MB ChB, FRCR; Alison Kemp; Pradeep Kuttysankaran; Guillaume Lefebvre, MD; Antonello Leone, MD; Héloïse Lerisson, MD; Dana J. Lin, MD; Jacques Malghem, MD; Adriana P. Martinez, MD, MSc, FRCSC; Paul Michelin, MD, MSc; Thomas P. Moser, MD, MSc; Charbel Mourad, MD; Suresh K. Mukherji, MD, MBA, FACR; Patrick Omoumi, MD, PhD; Mini N. Pathria, MD; Christoph Rehnitz, MD; Monique Reijnierse, MD, PhD; Zehava Sadka Rosenberg, MD; Ignacio Martín Rossi, MD; Lynne S. Steinbach, MD, FACR; Kolja M. Thierfelder, MD, Msc; Céline Tillaux, MD; Prudencia N.M. Tyrrell, MBBCh, BAO, FRCR; Bruno C. Vande Berg, MD, PhD; Filip M. Vanhoenacker, MD, PhD; John Vassallo; Timothy Woo, MBChB, MA, FRCR; Jonathan Zember, MD.

The planning committee, staff, authors and editors listed below have identified financial relationships or relationships to products or devices they or their spouse/life partner have with commercial interest related to the content of this CME activity:

Marc-André Weber, MD, MSc: participates in speakers bureau for and receives research support from Bayer Vital GmbH.

UNAPPROVED/OFF-LABEL USE DISCLOSURE

The EOCME requires CME faculty to disclose to the participants:
1. When products or procedures being discussed are off-label, unlabelled, experimental, and/or investigational (not US Food and Drug Administration [FDA] approved); and
2. Any limitations on the information presented, such as data that are preliminary or that represent ongoing research, interim analyses, and/or unsupported opinions. Faculty may discuss information about pharmaceutical agents that is outside of FDA-approved labelling. This information is intended solely for CME and is not intended to promote off-label use of these medications. If you have any questions, contact the medical affairs department of the manufacturer for the most recent prescribing information.

TO ENROLL

To enroll in the *Magnetic Resonance Imaging Clinics of North America* Continuing Medical Education program, call customer service at 1-800-654-2452 or sign up online at http://www.theclinics.com/home/cme. The CME program is available to subscribers for an additional annual fee of USD 260.

METHOD OF PARTICIPATION

In order to claim credit, participants must complete the following:

1. Complete enrolment as indicated above.
2. Read the activity.
3. Complete the CME Test and Evaluation. Participants must achieve a score of 70% on the test. All CME Tests and Evaluations must be completed online.

CME INQUIRIES/SPECIAL NEEDS

For all CME inquiries or special needs, please contact elsevierCME@elsevier.com.

Foreword

Musculoskeletal Imaging: Radiographic/MR Imaging Correlation

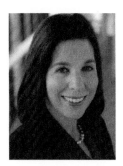

Lynne S. Steinbach, MD, FACR
Consulting Editor

Until the 1990s, Radiologists relied on radiographs and computed tomographic scans for imaging evaluation of osseous and soft tissue abnormalities of the musculoskeletal system. Many of us who trained in that era were taught about the subtle abnormalities on radiographs that could be quite meaningful for diagnosis of pathologic conditions. Osseous fracture might signify other soft tissue injury associated with trauma, including anterior cruciate ligament tears with Segond fractures of the knee, and labral tears with Hill-Sachs impaction injury of the humeral head. Periosteal reaction, cortical thinning, bowing, joint space narrowing, erosions, and effusion would also be important to recognize to indicate underlying infection, tumor, trauma, osteopenia, metabolic disease, or arthritis. Over the last 3 decades, we have learned a lot more about the bones and soft tissues of the musculoskeletal system through our correlation of these findings with MR imaging. Bone marrow changes related to infiltration by tumor and infection, internal derangement of the soft tissue structures of the joints, and occult fractures and the like are best seen with MR imaging. However, as radiologists have become more dependent on MR imaging, those who are well trained in both radiographs and MR imaging can find that they are both complementary modalities and can also finesse a diagnosis with that added knowledge. That is what this issue is all about. The reader will find a cornucopia of pearls in each article

that will reinforce the value of looking close at radiographs to make some important diagnoses even before MR imaging is obtained, if it does end up being indicated. MR imaging provides added value in some of these cases, allowing one to recognize patterns and subtle, but important, signs on imaging.

I am grateful to Professor Dr Anne Cotten for undertaking this important topic. Anne is a leading musculoskeletal radiologist who has also served as President of several European musculoskeletal imaging societies and will soon be the President of the Sociètè Française de Radiologie. Throughout her career, Anne has spearheaded important research in musculoskeletal imaging, especially in the field of musculoskeletal MR imaging. In this issue, she demonstrates the importance of the radiograph and its correlation with MR imaging, along with her chosen authors of each subtopic, who are also luminaries in the field. I want to thank all of them for their excellent contributions.

Lynne S. Steinbach, MD, FACR
Department of Radiology and
Biomedical Imaging
University of California, San Francisco
505 Parnassus
San Francisco, CA 94143, USA

E-mail address:
lynne.steinbach@ucsf.edu

Magn Reson Imaging Clin N Am 27 (2019) xiii
https://doi.org/10.1016/j.mric.2019.07.011
1064-9689/19/© 2019 Published by Elsevier Inc.

mri.theclinics.com

Preface

Musculoskeletal Imaging: Radiographic/MR Imaging Correlation

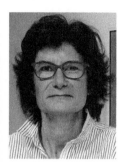

Anne Cotten, MD, PhD
Editor

Considering that advanced imaging techniques, such as MR imaging, computed tomography, and ultrasound, are now widely used in clinical practice, describing radiographic features in 2019 may seem somewhat obsolete. However, conventional radiograph prevails as the initial imaging modality in many musculoskeletal disorders as it provides excellent analysis of bone outlines. Moreover, it remains the simplest, most cost-effective, and most readily accessible imaging technique available.

Unfortunately, radiographic features are being taught less and less to radiologists, particularly to the younger generations, with a resulting decrease in skill level for this imaging modality. Rare nowadays are the meetings or scientific papers focusing on the description and significance of radiographic findings. Yet, a great deal of information can be obtained when systematic analysis of the different views is performed. The lack of recognition or understanding of radiographic features may lead to delayed diagnosis and persistent morbidity (prolonged suffering) for the patient. Moreover, some tiny radiographic features may be missed on MR imaging.

This issue of *Magnetic Resonance Imaging Clinics of North America* discusses typical radiographic findings in various disorders and joints, with correlative MR images used to explain and illustrate their significance. It begins with several articles involving the main anatomic regions. Kuenzer Goes and Pathria provide

an outstanding article on the common radiographic lesions associated with glenohumeral instability, rotator cuff pathology, and acromioclavicular joint injury. This is followed by an article written by Allen and Johnson on the main disorders of the elbow, focusing on the limitations of radiographs in this area. Then, Moser and colleagues describe a topographic approach of wrist pathologic conditions and explain how the radiographic findings correlate with MR imaging.

This is followed by 2 articles focusing on the spine, both of which are particularly useful in daily practice. The first one, written by Woo and colleagues, is based on the typical imaging changes that may affect the vertebral body, the end plates, the posterior arch, or the vertebral alignment. A systematic analysis of the main features affecting these structures is presented. Reijnierse then describes in detail the various paravertebral ossifications that are of practical interest in the diagnosis of specific diseases.

Three articles are devoted to the inferior limb. Mourad and colleagues provide a structured approach of the changes in radiological bone density and contours of the femoral head and on alterations of the joint space observed in common hip disorders. Jacques and colleagues then present a systematic analysis of the different types of joint effusion and of the bone outlines of the knee, highlighting several key points that are useful in daily

Magn Reson Imaging Clin N Am 27 (2019) xv–xvi
https://doi.org/10.1016/j.mric.2019.07.010
1064-9689/19/© 2019 Published by Elsevier Inc.

practice. Finally, Lin and colleagues provide the necessary tools needed to carefully examine the radiographs of the ankle so as to detect various disease entities that may otherwise remain undetected.

Subsequently, 2 articles are dedicated to the most common sources of pitfalls in the pediatric population. Bixby thoroughly describes the various imaging clues that allow for distinguishing fractures from mimics on plain radiographs, whereas Lerisson and colleagues discuss the normal aspects and main variants of endochondral ossification at the knee.

The article by Gemescu and colleagues focuses on bone tumors by highlighting their appearance on both radiographs and MR imaging, and accordingly, points out each technique's advantages and disadvantages. Finally, the last article, written by Vanhoenacker and colleagues, calls to mind the most valuable signs that may suggest the presence of soft tissue pathology on radiographs and discusses their diagnostic strength compared with MR imaging findings.

As guest editor of this issue, I would like to thank all the authors for spending the time to prepare excellent articles and for sharing their knowledge and expertise. I sincerely hope that the readers will enjoy this issue and improve their skills in depiction and understanding of findings on conventional radiography, as the latter can be very useful to guide further imaging and management. Enjoy!

Anne Cotten, MD, PhD
Service de Radiologie et
Imagerie Musculosquelettique
Centre de Consultations et
d'Imagerie de l'Appareil Locomoteur
Rue du Pr Emile Laine
59037 Lille Cedex, France

E-mail address:
anne.cotten@chru-lille.fr

Radiographic/MR Imaging Correlation of the Shoulder

Paola Cecy Kuenzer Goes, MD[a],*, Mini N. Pathria, MD[b]

KEYWORDS

- Shoulder • Radiography • MR imaging • Instability • Rotator cuff • Acromioclavicular joint

KEY POINTS

- Conventional radiograph is the first modality of imaging used in the evaluation of shoulder pain, allowing diagnosis of acute traumatic injuries and suggesting soft tissue pathology, especially in the setting of advanced disease.
- MR imaging plays an important role in the assessment of the shoulder, with high accuracy for both the osseous and soft tissue structures but can only be obtained in selected cases related to availability and cost considerations.
- Correlation with MR imaging allows the radiologist to improve his/her understanding of findings on conventional radiography and recognize signs indicating significant pathology, helping to guide further imaging and management.

INTRODUCTION

Shoulder pain is a common cause of pain and disability and can be due to a range of pathologies, most commonly related to trauma or degeneration.[1] The initial evaluation of the symptomatic shoulder consists of clinical examination, followed by conventional radiography. Conventional radiography, although limited in its visualization of the soft tissues about the shoulder, affords excellent spatial resolution and accurate assessment of osseous abnormalities. Advanced imaging, including ultrasound, computed tomography (CT), and MR imaging, is used for more accurate delineation of anatomy and pathology in selected cases. Increasing use of these modalities has resulted in less emphasis on teaching and understanding how lesions appear on conventional radiographs. In this article, the authors use MR imaging to illustrate the basis of the typical appearances on radiography of common lesions associated with glenohumeral instability, rotator cuff pathology, and acromioclavicular (AC) joint injury.

GLENOHUMERAL INSTABILITY

The glenohumeral joint (GHJ) is the most mobile joint in the human body, and the relatively small contact area between its glenoid and humeral articular surfaces and mismatch in their arcs of curvature results in inherent instability. At the midrange of shoulder motion, the concave articular surface of the glenoid and the labrum function as static stabilizers maintaining articular congruity. As movement progresses, the capsulolabral structures become the primary restraints, with the rotator cuff musculature contributing as a dynamic stabilizer of shoulder stability.[2] Instability of the GHJ occurs as a result from failure of these

Disclosure: Nothing to disclosure.
a Division of Musculoskeletal Radiology, Laboratorio Delboni Auriemo, DASA, Rua Dr. Diogo de Faria, 1379, São Paulo, SP 04037-005, Brazil; b Department of Radiology, University of California San Diego Health System, 200 West Arbor Drive, San Diego, CA 92103-8756, USA
* Corresponding author.
E-mail address: paolakuenzer@gmail.com

Magn Reson Imaging Clin N Am 27 (2019) 575–585
https://doi.org/10.1016/j.mric.2019.07.005
1064-9689/19/© 2019 Elsevier Inc. All rights reserved.

coordinated stabilizers, leading to displacement and abnormal contact between its articular surfaces.

Anterior Instability

The most common direction of GHJ dislocation is anterior, in which the humerus displaces anteroinferiorly to lie below the coracoid process or glenoid rim. Anterior dislocation is frequently associated with an impaction fracture at the posterosuperior humeral head (Hill-Sachs lesion) and/or a shearing fracture of the anteroinferior glenoid (Bankart lesion). Radiography is the initial modality used to detect, localize, and quantify displacement and these characteristic fractures. The standard anteroposterior (AP) view obtained in external rotation readily detects humeral displacement but is not tangential to the posterior humerus or GHJ, leading to suboptimal evaluation of fractures.

The Hill-Sachs lesion seems as a region of articular surface flattening at the posterior superior humeral head. An AP view in internal rotation is necessary to profile this region[3] (**Fig. 1**). The defect varies in size, location, and orientation depending on the position of the arm and force applied during dislocation. Variations in its appearance range from deep angular defects to a paradoxic "osteophyte-like" protuberance when the radiograph is tangent to the raised edge of the lesion relative to the affected segment.[4] The Hill-Sachs lesion should be distinguished from normal physiologic flattening at the posterior head-neck junction of the humerus. The Hill-Sachs lesion is located at the uppermost portion of the humeral head, whereas the physiologic depression lies further distally, typically 20 mm or more below the top of the humeral head. In the axial plane, the Hill-Sachs lesion is generally located farther laterally than the anatomic indentation.[5] Pseudocysts at the bare area of the humeral head, marginal erosions in inflammatory arthropathies, and

irregularity secondary to enthesopathy can also simulate a Hill-Sachs lesion.[4]

The Bankart lesion is less common and can be challenging to visualize on radiography, particularly when small. It appears as a disruption of the inferior half of the anterior glenoid rim, with an elongated bone fragment typically displaced medially and inferiorly. The Grashey view (AP view obtained obliquely along the plane of glenoid anteversion) is more sensitive (**Fig. 2**). The standard axillary projection is not sensitive, as the fracture is typically limited to the inferior glenoid below the profiled articular surface. The apical oblique projection (AP with 45° caudal angulation in internal rotation) is sensitive, although it and other specialized projections such as the West Point, Velpeau, and Bernageau views are less commonly used with the advent of cross-sectional imaging.[3,4,6] Soft tissue injuries associated with anterior dislocation such as tearing of the glenoid labrum and disruption of the glenohumeral capsule and supporting ligaments are best assessed with MR imaging (**Fig. 3**).

Posterior Instability

The primary restraints to posterior instability are the posterior capsule, posterior band of the inferior glenohumeral ligament, posterior labrum, and subscapularis.[7] Posterior glenohumeral instability is less common than the anterior form, accounting for only 2% to 4% of all shoulder dislocations; it may be bilateral when related to seizure or electric shock.[8] The humeral head is displaced posteriorly in internal rotation, producing impaction fractures at the contact zones at the anterior humeral head (reverse Hill-Sachs lesion) and posterior glenoid rim (reverse Bankart fracture). Avulsion fracture of the lesser humeral tuberosity and other fractures at the shoulder girdle may also be present.

Posterior shoulder dislocation can be challenging to identify on AP radiographs, with greater

A   **B**

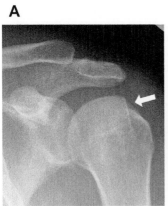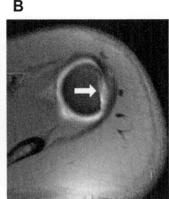

Fig. 1. Hill-Sachs lesion. (*A*) AP view in internal rotation shows a Hill-Sachs impaction fracture (*arrow*) at the posterosuperior humeral head. The size of the defect (*arrow*) is well shown on the (*B*) axial T1 fatsat MR arthrogram. Note that the flattening extends well above the greater tuberosity, helping to distinguish this injury from physiologic flattening.

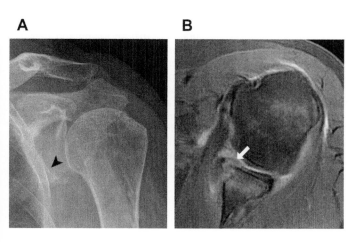

Fig. 2. Bankart fracture. (*A*) AP Grashey view shows loss of the normal cortical margin of the anteroinferior glenoid rim. The Bankart fracture fragment (*arrowhead*) is displacement medially. (*B*) Axial proton density fatsat MR shows glenoid edema and displacement of the bone fragment, as well as anterior labral irregularity and chondral injury (*arrow*). There is humeral edema related to a Hill-Sachs lesion (not included in this image, which is centered lower and shows the normal broad area of physiologic flattening).

than 50% missed at initial examination. Findings on AP radiographs include the "lightbulb sign" (fixed internal rotation of the humerus), "rim sign" (widening of the GHJ), absence of normal overlap of the humeral head and glenoid, and the "trough sign" (double contour of the medial humeral head, representing the normal cortex and the long axis of a reverse Hill-Sachs fracture).[8] When a posterior dislocation is suspected, a lateral scapula ("Y view") or axillary view should be obtained. The injury is most evident on the axillary

projection, which also profiles the trough and reverse Bankart fractures better (**Fig. 4**).

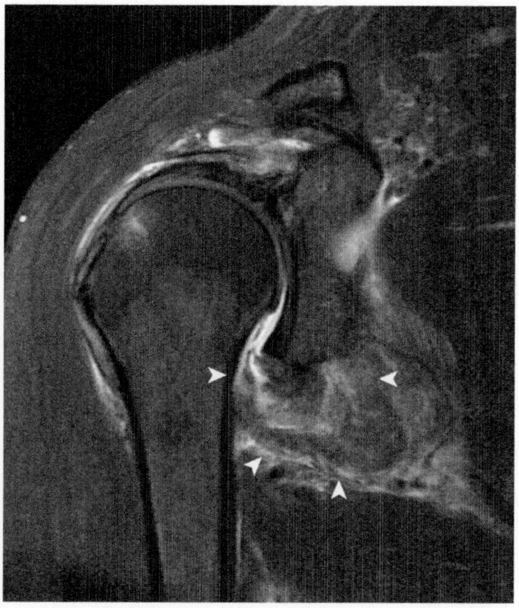

Frank posterior dislocation is less common than recurrent posterior subluxation. Chronic posterior instability may be related to repetitive trauma in competitive athletes or related to atraumatic factors such as soft tissue laxity and glenoid retroversion, hypoplasia, and dysplasia.[7] In repetitive trauma, as seen in overhead throwing sports, a Bennett lesion ("thrower's exostosis") may be seen as an extraarticular curvilinear bony spur along the posteroinferior glenoid rim related to traction at the posterior band of the glenohumeral ligament. The Bennett lesion itself is asymptomatic but is commonly associated with posterior labral and posterior undersurface rotator cuff tear.[9]

Advanced Imaging

Advanced imaging techniques play a critical role in the assessment of shoulder instability. CT is most useful for identifying and characterizing bone injuries, whereas MR imaging excels at identifying labral and soft tissue injury. Evaluation of the orientation of the fractures and the extent of humeral, glenoid, and combined (bipolar) bone loss is important for planning surgical repair to avoid recurrent shoulder instability (**Fig. 5**). Hill-Sachs fractures parallel to the anterior glenoid rim in abduction allow the humerus to engage the glenoid lip and redislocate.[2,10] Larger Hill-Sachs and Bankart defects require soft tissue augmentation or bone grafting to reestablish stability. The ontrack off-track method uses 3-dimensional CT scanning to assess fracture size and orientation. It applies the glenoid track definition, defined as the contact area between the humeral head and glenoid during shoulder abduction and external rotation.[11,12] It postulates that the risk of instability and engagement between the humeral defect and

Fig. 3. Capsular injury following shoulder dislocation. Coronal T2 fatsat MR following reduction of anteroinferior glenohumeral dislocation illustrates extensive injury of the axillary pouch (*arrowheads*) and inferior glenohumeral ligament with leakage of joint fluid and extensive surrounding edema.

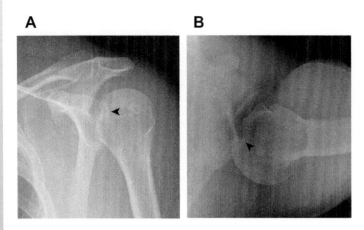

Fig. 4. Posterior glenohumeral dislocation. (*A*) The AP radiograph demonstrates internal rotation of the humeral head. Note the vertical sclerosis parallel to the glenoid, indicating a trough fracture (*arrowhead*). The dislocation and fracture are more evident on the (*B*) axillary view, showing posterior displacement and a trough fracture (*arrowhead*) of the anteromedial humeral head.

glenoid rim and redislocation is increased when the Hill-Sachs lesion approaches the medial margin of the residual glenoid. Inadequate reconstruction in such cases leads to persistent instability and a high incidence of redislocation.

ROTATOR CUFF

Rotator cuff pathology, a common cause of shoulder pain and dysfunction, may present acutely, typically caused by trauma or crystal-induced inflammation, or more commonly, resulting in chronic symptoms related to degeneration of the rotator cuff tissues causing loss of rotator cuff structure and function. Several radiographic findings can be used to diagnose rotator cuff pathology, supported by advanced imaging to confirm the diagnosis, delineate cuff morphology, identify associated abnormalities, and plan appropriate treatment.[13]

Acute Pathology

Trauma resulting in an acute tear of the rotator cuff is uncommon, representing a small minority of tears encountered in routine clinical practice.

Standard shoulder radiographs are typically normal in such patients unless there is an associated fracture. In the setting on an acute massive tear of the supraspinatus tendon, the active abduction view of the shoulder obtained with the shoulder at 90° from the horizontal plane may demonstrate decreased acromiohumeral distance ($\leq$ 2 mm), but only if there is significant medial retraction of the torn tendon.[14] Unfortunately, most of the acute tears do not immediately retract, so initial radiographs are insensitive.

Acute rotator cuff symptomatology is more commonly related to hydroxyapatite deposition disease (HADD), with symptoms related to crystal extrusion from the tendon into the peritendinous tissues, subacromial bursa, or less frequently, into the bone or muscle, producing acute inflammation. The shoulder is well recognized as the most common site of symptomatic HADD.[15] The imaging appearance depends on the phase of the disease, which varies from a dense ovoid homogeneous sharply marginated intratendinous calcification in the inactive phase to an irregular ill-defined amorphous calcification extending beyond the tendon footprint when active. AP

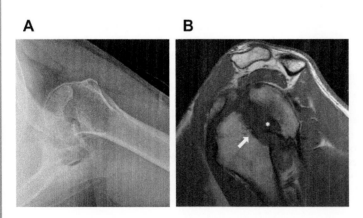

Fig. 5. Irreducible dislocation. (*A*) Axillary radiograph and (*B*) sagittal T1 MR in a patient with chronic shoulder instability demonstrate a chronic irreducible anterior glenohumeral dislocation. Note the large deep Hill-Sachs lesion (*white arrow*) and the compression deformity and bone loss of the anterior glenoid (*asterisk*). Such large deformities produce engaging lesions and make surgical reconstruction challenging.

radiographs with the shoulder in internal and external rotation allow identification and localization of calcific deposits.[15] Supraspinatus tendon calcifications are seen adjacent to the greater tuberosity in external rotation, whereas infraspinatus and teres minor calcifications are seen adjacent to the lateral edge of the greater tuberosity in internal rotation.[16] On MR imaging, calcific deposits appear as rounded areas of low signal intensity on all imaging sequences. Findings in the inflammatory phase include surrounding inflammation, bursal fluid and bone edema, mimicking infection, trauma, or neoplasm[17] (**Fig. 6**).

Degenerative Pathology

Degenerative rotator cuff disease is more common and its incidence increases with age, resulting in tendinosis and ultimately tearing.[18] The cause of cuff degeneration is multifactorial, caused by factors that include aging, repetitive microtrauma, hypovascularity, laxity, and impingement.[13] Clinical examination shows high sensitivity (90%) and specificity (54%) for full-thickness tears but has low accuracy for partial tears.[1] Similarly, radiographs show higher accuracy in large chronic complete tears than in early degeneration, when changes dominate at the entheseal attachment of the tendons at the tuberosities. Entheseal changes at the tendon insertion include osteopenia, bony sclerosis, surface irregularity, and cyst formation.[19,20]

The significance of cystic changes at the tuberosities depends on their precise position. These form as the tendon tearing at the footprint disrupts the normal barrier to synovial fluid intrusion, followed by further ingrowth of synovial and granulation tissue. In partial-thickness tears, such cysts are more common with those that are articular-sided rather than bursal-sided.[21] Cysts occur in 2 distinct locations that differ in their pathogenesis

and clinical significance. Cysts located anteriorly at the supraspinatus and subscapularis insertions are closely related to rotator cuff disorders, with a 94% positive predictive value[21] (**Fig. 7**). Conversely, posterior humeral cysts at the infraspinatus insertion and in the bare area of the anatomic neck have little correlation with cuff disease and are typically related to vascular intrusions and asymptomatic.[21,22] Cystic changes in the greater and lesser tuberosity appear as focal round lucencies with sharply defined margins, usually isolated on each location; these are typically 3 to 4 mm in diameter and uncommonly exceed 1 cm. Supraspinatus cysts are located at the upper anterior greater tuberosity and best seen in external rotation, whereas the less significant infraspinatus cysts are situated lower at the posterior tuberosity and anatomic neck and are profiled in internal rotation.[21] CT and MR imaging are more accurate in identifying and localizing these and other entheseal changes at the tendon attachment sites.

Subacromial impingement, caused by compression of the rotator cuff by the structures that form the coracoacromial arch, has been emphasized as a cause of rotator cuff tendinopathy. It is a clinical diagnosis, characterized by a painful arc of motion of the shoulder during abduction.[23] Radiographic findings that support the clinical diagnosis of impingement are related to alterations of the acromion, which can also be appreciated with CT and MR imaging. Findings associated with impingement and a secondary higher prevalence of rotator cuff tear include downward hooking of the anterior acromion, inferolateral acromial inclination, and prominent spur formation at the anterior acromial undersurface. The presence of an os acromiale, a nonunited acromial ossification center, is also a risk factor for impingement, as it can contribute to anterior acromial down-sloping. It may be unstable, leading to dynamic narrowing

A

B

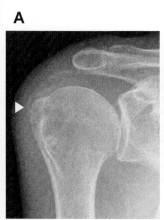
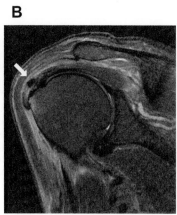

Fig. 6. Calcific tendinitis. (*A*) AP radiograph demonstrates linear calcifications along the supraspinatus tendon extending beyond the lateral edge of the tuberosity indicating extension into the subacromial bursa (*arrowhead*). (*B*) Coronal PD fatsat MR shows active calcific tendinitis with calcium extrusion (*arrow*) associated with inflammatory changes in the bursa and the adjacent soft tissue.

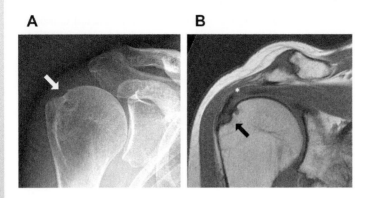

Fig. 7. Enthesopathic cysts. (*A*) The AP radiograph shows well-defined cysts (*white arrow*) at the junction of the humeral head articular surface and greater tuberosity. Corresponding cystic changes (*black arrow*) are seen on the (*B*) T1-w coronal MR, along with tendinosis of the supraspinatus tendon (*asterisk*).

of the subacromial space during deltoid contraction.[24,25] Acromion undersurface morphology is best assessed using the outlet-view radiograph (scapular Y-view with 15° caudal angulation) but can also be recognized on conventional projections[26,27] (**Fig. 8**).

Chronic Rotator Cuff Arthropathy

In the setting of a large rotator cuff, superior migration of the humeral head occurs due to loss of the normal depressing and centering effect of the rotator cuff tear against the upward pull of the deltoid.[28] Humeral head elevation correlates with tear size, extension to infraspinatus involvement of multiple tendons, and fatty atrophy of the rotator cuff muscles.[29,30] Superior migration of the humeral head causing narrowing of the subacromial space (<7 mm between the humeral head and acromion) is a poor prognostic factor for rotator cuff reconstruction.[29] Repetitive contact between the humeral head and the acromion leads to irregularity, sclerosis, and compression erosion of the humeral head, upper greater tuberosity, and the opposing acromial undersurface. These changes are usually seen during the late stages of rotator cuff dysfunction, in conjunction with the development of glenohumeral osteophytes in an attempt to maintain joint congruity. This final stage is known as cuff arthropathy[13,28] (**Fig. 9**).

With chronic acromial erosion, articular and bursal fluid can dissect superiorly into the AC joint through an eroded inferior AC capsule, producing the "geyser sign".[31] This finding is usually seen with chronic full-thickness tearing and suggests a difficult cuff repair.[31] Rarely, a soft tissue mass forms above the AC joint, appearing as focal swelling superior to a degenerative AC joint, usually accompanied with other findings of rotator cuff tear, such as humeral elevation and acromial erosion (**Fig. 10**). MR imaging is the optimal method for confirming the diagnosis of a cyst and excluding a neoplasm.[32]

Chronic rotator cuff tear results in profound muscle atrophy manifest as volume loss and fatty infiltration; severe atrophy correlates with worse function outcomes following surgical repair.[33] CT and MR imaging are used to identify and quantify the grade of fatty atrophy as it is challenging to identify atrophy on radiography, even in severe cases. A flattened ill-defined superior contour and heterogenous radiodensity of the supraspinatus on the AP view[34] and loss of infraspinatus bulk between the scapula and deep deltoid muscle on the scapular Y-view suggest atrophy, but the accuracy of radiography is too low to be reliable for treatment planning.

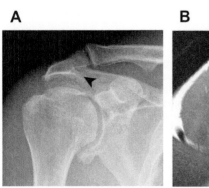
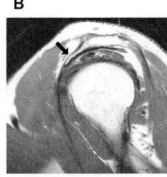

Fig. 8. Subacromial spur. (*A*) AP radiograph shows a subacromial spur (*arrowhead*) characterized as a large bony projection at the anterior end of the acromion at the site of the attachment of the coracoacromial ligament. (*B*) Sagittal T1 MR shows the spur (*arrow*) narrowing the subacromial space. A subacromial spur contributes to external impingement of the rotator cuff and bursa, located between the spur and humerus.

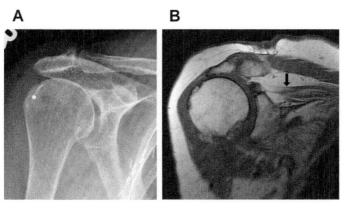

Fig. 9. Massive chronic cuff tear. (*A*) The radiograph demonstrates superior migration of the humeral head due to chronic rotator cuff arthropathy, with bone irregularity at the greater tuberosity (*asterisk*) and small osteophytes in the glenohumeral joint. On the (*B*) coronal T1 MR, the tendon is absent and humeral head contacts the acromion. There is atrophy and fatty infiltration in its muscle belly (*arrow*). Identifying the bony status at the tendon insertions, quality of the tendons, and muscle atrophy are important in the management of patients with rotator cuff tear, such as the long-term success of the surgical treatment that may depend on preoperative conditions of those.

ACROMIOCLAVICULAR JOINT INJURY

AC trauma represents 10% of all shoulder injuries and nearly 50% of shoulder injuries among athletes involved in contact sports, typically affecting young male adults.[35] The typical mechanism is a direct force applied to the superolateral acromion with the arm adducted, leading to sequential tensile failure beginning at the AC ligaments, progressing to the coracoclavicular (CC) ligaments, and ultimately involving the deltoid and trapezius muscle and fascia.[36]

Acromioclavicular Anatomy

The diarthrodial AC joint links the shoulder girdle to the axial skeleton and is stabilized by static capsuloligamentous (AC capsule, AC ligaments, CC ligaments) and dynamic muscle (deltoid, trapezius) restraints. Horizontal stability is provided by the AC capsule that is thickened and reinforced by the superior, inferior, anterior, and posterior AC ligaments. The superior ligament is most robust as it blends with fibers from the overlying deltoid and trapezial fasciae. The CC ligaments, consisting of the trapezoid and conoid, provide vertical stability and act as secondary restraints to AP translation when the AC capsule is torn.[37,38] The triangular trapezoid ligament runs from the anterior coracoid to the clavicular undersurface close to the AC joint. The quadrilateral-shaped conoid ligament arises farther posteriorly at the coracoid and inserts at the conoid tubercle of the clavicle, medial to the trapezoid.[39] In a small percentage of the population, the conoid ligament is replaced by an articulation between the coracoid and a flattened elongated facet on the inferior clavicle.[40–42] This facet should not be confused with the more irregular ossification seen in chronic CC ligament injury.

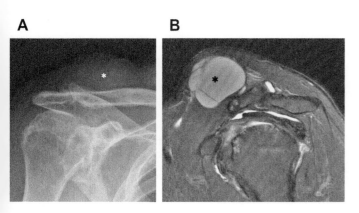

A   **B**

Fig. 10. Acromioclavicular cyst. (*A*) AP radiograph demonstrates swelling (*white asterisk*) superior to a degenerated AC joint associated with superior migration of the humeral head, cystic changes on the greater tuberosity, and erosion of the undersurface of the acromion. (*B*) Sagittal fluid sensitive MR demonstrates a cystic mass (*black asterisk*) corresponding to the swelling above the AC joint. The rotator cuff is degenerated and torn.

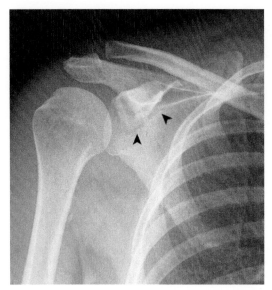

Fig. 11. Coracoid process fracture. AP radiograph demonstrating fracture at the base of the coracoid process (*arrowheads*) in the setting of acromioclavicular separation (type III variant). Note the elevation of the fractured coracoid fragment along with the clavicle, thereby maintaining the CC distance. The fracture can be difficult to appreciate on the AP projection and is best seen on scapular Y or axillary views.

Classification

The widely used Rockwood classification divides AC injuries into 6 types based on the direction and extent of clavicular displacement, which relate to the location and severity of the underlying soft tissue injury. Types I and II are treated conservatively, whereas types IV to VI injuries require surgery. The management of type III injuries is controversial although most are now managed conservatively.[43] Classification is based primarily on conventional radiography. The direction and degree of displacement is determined by AP and Zanca (10° cephalad angulated view centered on the AC joint) views of the clavicle. Bilateral views enhance detection of subtle degrees of joint widening and displacement. There is decreasing use of weight-bearing views, as upright radiographs with internal glenohumeral rotation demonstrate equivalent sensitivity.[44] Advanced imaging is not typically necessary but may be used to assess soft tissue damage in high-grade injury.

The type I injury is a sprain of the AC capsule, typically maximal at the superior capsule. There is no widening or malalignment, although swelling may be present. MR imaging shows soft tissue edema and partial AC capsule disruption, easily misinterpreted as degenerative disease in older adults.[36] In a type II injury, the AC capsule and ligaments are torn but the CC ligaments remain intact, although they may be sprained. The joint is typically widened (>6 mm) but there is little or no (<5 mm) superior displacement of the clavicle.[37] With further force, tearing of the CC ligaments produces a type III injury with greater than 5 mm superior displacement of the distal clavicle relative to the acromion, with the CC distance increased up to 100% greater than the contralateral side.

Some type III injuries do not exhibit much malalignment and are difficult to distinguish from type II injuries, even with weight-bearing. In one study, direct MR imaging assessment of the CC ligaments reclassified the radiographic grade into a less severe type in 36.4% and more severe type in 11.4%.[45] Discrepancies may be caused by intermediate CC injury patterns such as trapezial tearing without conoid injury, a variant not recognized in the Rockwood classification.[46] Another variant occurs when the CC ligaments remain intact but cause an avulsion fracture at the coracoid base, resulting in elevation of the fractured coracoid fragment along with the clavicle (**Fig. 11**).

The type IV injury is an uncommon pattern of posterior displacement of the clavicle into or through the trapezius, caused by the scapula being driven anteroinferiorly by a force applied to the posterior rather than superior acromion. On AP views, the AC and CC distances can appear

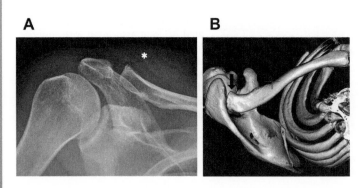

A   **B**

Fig. 12. Type IV acromioclavicular injury. (*A*) AP radiograph demonstrating swelling (*asterisk*) around the AC joint with normal AC and CC distances, which may be misinterpreted as a low-grade AC injury. (*B*) Three-dimensional reformatted tomography reveals the posterior displacement of the clavicle (*arrow*) relative to the acromion (grade IV injury).

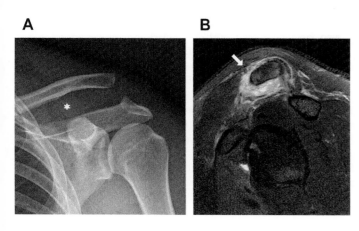

Fig. 13. Type V acromioclavicular injury. (*A*) AP external rotation radiograph demonstrating important superior displacement of the distal clavicle and widening of the AC joint and CC distance (*asterisk*). The apparent superior displacement of the clavicle is caused primarily by drooping of the acromion and shoulder girdle rather than true clavicular displacement. (*B*) Sagittal T2 fatsat MR shows tearing of coracoclavicular ligaments and the deltoid muscle attachment (*arrow*) to the clavicle (type V injury).

normal so the injury is easily overlooked. The axillary view, obtained supine with the arm abducted 90°, reveals posterior displacement of the clavicle relative to the acromion[35,47] (**Fig. 12**). The bipolar dislocation is a rare variant with simultaneous dislocation of both clavicular ends, with anterior dislocation at the sternoclavicular joint and posterior displacement at the AC joint.

In addition to complete rupture of the AC and CC ligaments, the type V injury shows tearing of the trapezius and deltoid muscles at their attachments to the clavicle and acromion. Disruption of the entire scapuloclavicular suspension mechanism leads to further inferior scapular drooping, accentuating AC displacement (>100% clavicle height elevation) and further widening the CC distance. The clavicle may assume a subcutaneous position or perforate the skin as it displaces through the deltotrapezial fascia. It can be challenging to distinguish it from type III injury on radiographs; the disruption of the trapezius and deltoid is best evaluated with MR imaging (**Fig. 13**). The rare type IV injury is caused by a direct force on the superior clavicle rather than the acromion, resulting in inferior clavicular displacement below the coracoid or acromion.

Posttraumatic Osteolysis of the Distal Clavicle

Posttraumatic osteolysis is a painful condition resulting from either a single trauma or chronic repetitive injury. Theories of pathogenesis include osteoclast activation, synovitis, ischemia, microfracture and autonomic dysfunction.[48] When caused by a single injury, osteolysis is unilateral and typically presents several months after direct trauma. Stress-induced osteolysis is most common in weightlifters and may be unilateral or bilateral. The imaging appearance of both forms is similar, although malalignment suggests discrete injury. Early radiographic findings are subtle; up to 50% of cases detectable on MR imaging are overlooked.[48] These include swelling, osteopenia, resorption of subchondral bone, and ultimately, erosions at the distal clavicle (**Fig. 14**). In advanced cases, osteolysis of the distal 0.5 to 3.0 cm clavicle results in AC widening.[49] On MR imaging, the most constant finding is intense marrow edema in the distal clavicle.[50] Swelling,

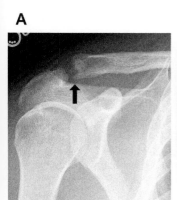
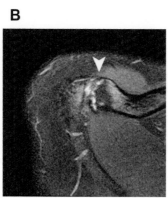

Fig. 14. Osteolysis of the distal clavicle. (*A*) AP radiograph demonstrating irregularity, osteopenia, and cortical undefinition in the distal clavicle (*arrow*), associated with widening of the AC joint. (*B*) Axial T2 fatsat MR demonstrating bone irregularity, cystic changes, and marrow edema in the distal clavicle (*arrowhead*).

effusion, subchondral cysts, cortical erosion, and subchondral stress fracture lines may also be present.[48]

SUMMARY

Conventional radiograph is the first modality of imaging used in the evaluation of shoulder pain, allowing diagnosis of acute traumatic injuries and suggesting soft tissue pathology, especially in the setting of advanced disease. MR imaging plays an important role in the assessment of the shoulder, with high accuracy for both the osseous and soft tissue structures but can only be obtained in selected cases related to availability and cost considerations. Correlation with MR imaging allows the radiologist to improve his/her understanding of findings on conventional radiography and recognize signs indicating significant pathology, helping to guide further imaging and management.

REFERENCES

1. Dinnes J, Loveman E, McIntyre L, et al. The effectiveness of diagnostic tests for the assessment of shoulder pain due to soft tissue disorders: a systematic review. Health Technol Assess 2003;7(29): 1–166.
2. Gyftopoulos S, Albert M, Recht MP. Osseous injuries associated with anterior shoulder instability: what the radiologist should know. AJR Am J Roentgenol 2014;202(6):W541–50.
3. Bianchi S, Prato N, Martinoli C, et al. Shoulder radiography. In: Davies AM, Hodler J, editors. Imaging of the shoulder: techniques and applications. Berlin: Springer; 2004. p. 3–13.
4. Vande Berg B, Omoumi P. Dislocation of the shoulder joint - radiographic analysis of osseous abnormalities. J Belg Soc Radiol 2016;100(1):89, 1–10.
5. Richards RD, Sartoris DJ, Pathria MN, et al. Hill-Sachs lesion and normal humeral groove: MR imaging features allowing their differentiation. Radiology 1994;190(3):665–8.
6. Gartth WP, Carter ES, Ochs CW. Roentgenographic demonstration of instability of the shoulder: the apical oblique projection. J Bone Joint Surg Am 1984; 66(9):1450–3.
7. Tannenbaum E, Sekiya JK. Evaluation and management of posterior shoulder instability. Sports Health 2011;3(3):253–63.
8. Cisternino SJ, Rogers LF, Stufflebam BC, et al. The trough line: a radiographic sign of posterior shoulder dislocation. AJR Am J Roentgenol 1978;130(5): 951–4.
9. Ferrari JD, Ferrari DA, Coumas J, et al. Posterior ossification of the shoulder: the bennett lesion: etiology, diagnosis, and treatment. Am J Sports Med 1994;22(2):171–6.
10. Burkhart SS, De Beer JF. Traumatic glenohumeral bone defects and their relationship to failure of arthroscopic Bankart repairs: significance of the inverted-pear glenoid and the humeral engaging Hill-Sachs lesion. Arthroscopy 2000;16(7):677–94.
11. Di Giacomo G, Itoi E, Burkhart SS. Evolving concept of bipolar bone loss and the Hill-sachs lesion: From "engaging/non-engaging" lesion to "on-track/off-track" lesion. Arthroscopy 2014; 30(1):90–8.
12. Yamamoto N, Itoi E, Abe H, et al. Contact between the glenoid and the humeral head in abduction, external rotation, and horizontal extension: a new concept of glenoid track. J Shoulder Elbow Surg 2007;16(5):649–56.
13. Moosikasuwan JB, Miller TT, Burke BJ. Rotator cuff tears: clinical, radiographic, and US findings. Radiographics 2005;25(6):1591–607.
14. Bloom RA. The active abduction view: a new maneuvre in the diagnosis of rotator cuff tears. Skeletal Radiol 1991;20(4):255–8.
15. Hayes CW, Conway WF. Calcium hydroxyapatite deposition disease. Radiographics 1990;10(6): 1031–48.
16. Steinbach LS. Calcium pyrophosphate dihydrate and calcium hydroxyapatite crystal deposition diseases: Imaging perspectives. Radiol Clin North Am 2004;42(1):185–205.
17. Chung CB, Gentili A, Chew FS. Calcific Tendinosis and Periarthritis: classic magnetic resonance imaging appearance and associated findings. J Comput Assist Tomogr 2004;28(3):390–6.
18. Yamaguchi K, Ditisos K, Middleton WD, et al. The demographic and morphological features of rotator cuff disease. A comparison of asymptomatic and symptomatic shoulder. J Bone Joint Surg Am 2006; 88(8):1699–704.
19. Jiang Y, Zhao J, van Holsbeeck MT, et al. Trabecular microstructure and surface changes in the greater tuberosity in rotator cuff tears. Skeletal Radiol 2002;31(9):522–8.
20. Caniggia M, Maniscalco P, Pagliantini L, et al. Titanium anchors for the repair of rotator cuff tears: preliminary report of a surgical technique. J Orthop Trauma 1995;9(4):312–7.
21. Fritz LB, Ouellette HA, O'Hanley TA, et al. Cystic changes at supraspinatus and infraspinatus tendon insertion sites: association with age and rotator cuff disorders in 238 patients. Radiology 2007;244(1): 239–48.
22. Pan Y-W, Mok D, Tsiouri C, et al. The association between radiographic greater tuberosity cystic change and rotator cuff tears: a study of 105 consecutive cases. Shoulder & Elbow 2011;3(4): 205–9.

23. Neer CS 2nd. Anterior acromioplasty for the chronic impingement syndrome in the shoulder: a preliminary report. J Bone Joint Surg Am 1972;54(1):41–50.

24. Sammarco VJ. Os acromiale : frequency, anatomy, and clinical implications. J Bone Joint Surg Am 2000;82(3):394–400.

25. Mellado JM, Calmet J, Domènech S, et al. Clinically significant skeletal variations of the shoulder and the wrist: role of MR imaging. Eur Radiol 2003;13(7): 1735–43.

26. Nicholson GP, Goodman DA, Flatow EL, et al. The acromion: morphologic condition and age-related changes. A study of 420 scapulas. J Shoulder Elbow Surg 1996;5(1):1–11.

27. Edelson JG, Taitz C. Anatomy of the coracoacromial arch. Relation to degeneration of the acromion. J Bone Joint Surg Br 1992;74(4):589–94.

28. Weiner DS, Macnab I. Superior migration of the humeral head. A radiological aid in the diagnosis of tears of the rotator cuff. J Bone Joint Surg Br 1970; 52(3):524–7.

29. Saupe N, Pfirrmann CWA, Schmid MR, et al. Association between rotator cuff abnormalities and reduced acromiohumeral distance. AJR Am J Roentgenol 2006;187(2):376–82.

30. Keener JD, Wei AS, Kim HM, et al. Proximal humeral migration in shoulders with symptomatic and asymptomatic rotator cuff tears. J Bone Joint Surg Am 2009;91(6):1405–13.

31. Craig EV. The geyser sign and torn rotator cuff: clinical significance and pathomechanics. Clin Orthop Relat Res 1984;191:213–5.

32. Coopper HJ, Milillo R, Klein DA, et al. The MRI geyser sign: acromioclavicular joint cysts in the setting of a chronic rotator cuff tear. Am J Orthop (Belle Mead NJ) 2011;40(6):E118–21.

33. Goutallier D, Postel J-M, Bernageau J, et al. Fatty muscle degeneration in cuff ruptures. Pre- and Postoperative evaluation by CT scan. Clin Orthop Relat Res 1994;304:78–83.

34. Stallenberg B, Rommens J, Legrand C, et al. Radiographic diagnosis of rotator cuff tear based on the supraspinatus muscle radiodensity. Skeletal Radiol 2001;30(1):31–8.

35. Alyas F, Curtis M, Speed C, et al. MR imaging appearances of acromioclavicular joint dislocation. Radiographics 2008;28:463–79.

36. Antonio GE, Cho JH, Chung CB, et al. Pictorial essay. MR imaging appearance and classification of acromioclavicular joint injury. AJR Am J Roentgenol 2003;180(4):1103–10.

37. Debski RE, Parsons IVIM, Woo SLY, et al. Effect of capsular injury on acromioclavicular joint mechanics. J Bone Joint Surg Am 2001;83–A(9): 1344–51.

38. Warth RJ, Martetschläger F, Gaskill TR, et al. Acromioclavicular joint separations. Curr Rev Musculoskelet Med 2013;6(1):71–8.

39. Rios CG, Arciero RA, Mazzocca AD. Anatomy of the clavicle and coracoid process for reconstruction of the coracoclavicular ligaments. Am J Sports Med 2007;35(5):811–7.

40. Cockshott WP. The coracoclavicular joint. Radiology 1979;131(2):313–6.

41. Nehme A, Tricoire JL, Giordano G, et al. Coracoclavicular joints. Reflections upon incidence, pathophysiology and etiology of the different forms. Surg Radiol Anat 2004;26(1):33–8.

42. Sener RN, Alper H, Sagtas E, et al. Bilateral synovial coracoclavicular joints: MRI demonstration. Eur Radiol 1996;6(2):196–8.

43. Fraser-Moodie JA, Shortt NL, Robinson CM. Injuries to the acromioclavicular joint. J Bone Joint Surg Br 2008;90(6):697–707.

44. Vanarthos WJ, Ekman EF, Bohrer SP. Radiographic diagnosis of acromioclavicular joint separation without weight bearing: Importance of internal rotation of the arm. AJR Am J Roentgenol 1994;162(1): 120–2.

45. Nemec U, Oberleitner G, Nemec SF, et al. MRI versus radiography of acromioclavicular joint dislocation. AJR Am J Roentgenol 2011;197(4):968–73.

46. Phadnis J, Bain GI, Bak K. Pathoanatomy of acromioclavicular joint instability. In: Bain GI, Itoi E, Di Giacomo G, et al, editors. Normal and pathological anatomy of the shoulder. Berlin, Heidelberg: Springer; 2015. p. 171–84.

47. Tauber M, Koller H, Hitzl W, et al. Dynamic radiologic evaluation of horizontal instability in acute acromioclavicular joint dislocations. Am J Sports Med 2010;38(6):1188–95.

48. Yu JS. Easily missed fractures in the lower extremity. Radiol Clin North Am 2015;53(4):737–55.

49. Kaplan PA, Resnick D. Stress-induced osteolysis of the clavicle. Radiology 1986;158(1):139–40.

50. Fiorella D, Helms CA, Speer KP. Increased T2 signal intensity in the distal clavicle: Incidence and clinical implications. Skeletal Radiol 2000;29(12):697–702.

Radiographic/MR Imaging Correlation of the Elbow

Gina M. Allen, BM, MRCGP, MRCP, FRCR, MFSEM, MScSEM[a],*, Rowena Johnson, MB ChB, FRCR[b]

KEYWORDS

• Elbow • Radiographs • MR imaging

KEY POINTS

• Radiographs are the mainstay of elbow imaging in trauma.
• Soft tissue disorders are common around the elbow, but radiographs are rarely helpful.
• MR imaging can be used to interrogate the soft tissues and bone.

INTRODUCTION

The emphasis of this article is on the use of radiographs and MR imaging for the diagnosis of elbow disorders. For completeness, the authors have included discussion relating to other imaging techniques, including computed tomography (CT), ultrasound, and nuclear medicine where they are of clinical importance.

Radiographs have been the mainstay of initial imaging of the elbow, particularly in the trauma setting. In the absence of traumatic injury, most of the disease processes encountered in the elbow relate to the soft tissues. Ultrasound examination will then be performed prior to radiographs when soft tissue disease is suspected. MR imaging has the advantage over radiographs and ultrasound in accurately examining both bone and soft tissue.

This article concentrates on the use of radiographs and MR imaging when the patient presents with particular symptoms. Fractures and children's abnormalities are covered in other articles.

GENERAL
Radiographs

Value

The value of conventional radiographs is that they typically clearly show fractures if at least 2 views of the affected area are undertaken. Furthermore, they are used in the initial assessment of bone pain as an examination to exclude bone tumors. They will demonstrate areas of lysis, calcification, and sclerosis within the bone. Bone textual changes may be observed including cortical scalloping and disturbance of the trabecular pattern of the medulla. Irregularity of the cortex may be seen in the enthesitis at the site of tendon insertion.

Displacement of fat pads in the soft tissues will identify larger joint effusions. Swollen soft tissues and calcification within the soft tissue may be observed. Fat-containing mass lesions may be seen as a radiolucent area within the soft tissue.

Limitations

A major limitation of conventional radiographs is that they are only a 2-dimensional image of a 3-dimensional object, and therefore abnormalities may be obscured by the overlying tissue. Microfracturing of bone will not be identified, and at least 80% of the bone must be destroyed before a radiograph will show a lucency when the destruction is centrally located. When there is cortical destruction, this will be identified sooner. This means that radiographs will not detect many cases of early cancer (**Figs. 1** and **2**).

Disclosure Statement: The authors have nothing to disclose.
[a] St Luke's Radiology Oxford Ltd, St Luke's Hospital, Latimer Road, Headington, Oxford OX3 7PF, UK;
[b] Nuffield Orthopaedic Centre, Oxford University Hospitals, Windmill Road, Oxford OX3 7HE, UK
* Corresponding author.
E-mail address: gina_m_allen@btinternet.com

Magn Reson Imaging Clin N Am 27 (2019) 587–599
https://doi.org/10.1016/j.mric.2019.07.006

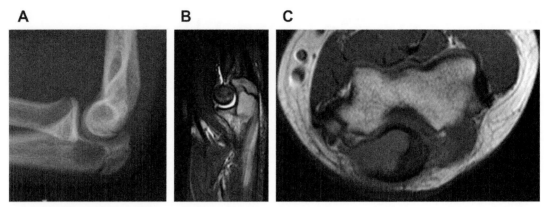

Fig. 1. (*A*) Radiograph of a giant cell tumor in the olecranon in a 12-year-old patient. (*B*) Sagittal STIR MR imaging of a giant cell tumor in the olecranon in a 12-year-old patient. (*C*) Axial T1 fast spin echo (FSE) MR imaging of a giant cell tumor in the olecranon in a 12-year-old patient.

In addition, the contrast between different soft tissue types is low, thus reducing the sensitivity of diagnosis, meaning many soft tissue abnormalities cannot be identified by radiographs.

MR Imaging

MR imaging will clearly show abnormality within the bone such as microfracturing, a bone tumor, or enthesitis. This of course depends on the correct sequences being performed-to optimize the conspicuity of bone lesions. T1 spin echo and short T1 inversion recovery (STIR) sequence should be performed. The use of T1 fast spin echo, proton density fat saturation, and T2 gradient echo sequences can obscure some bone lesions.

MR imaging will clearly identify abnormalities of the soft tissue when using the appropriate sequences. The tendons, ligaments, muscles, nerves, vessels, and subcutaneous soft tissue can be interrogated in detail.

The authors discuss the use of radiographs and MR imaging in the following clinical settings:

- Lateral elbow pain
- Medial elbow pain
- Anterior elbow pain
- Posterior elbow pain

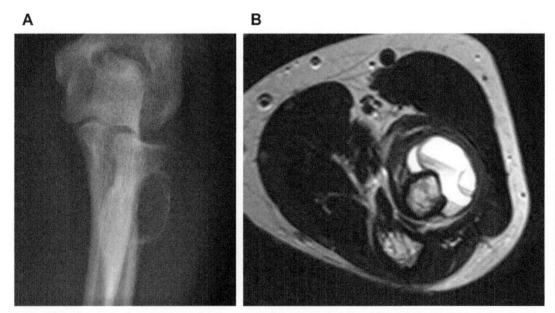

Fig. 2. (*A*) Radiograph of an Aneurysmal bone cyst in the proximal radius. (*B*) Axial T2 FSE MR imaging showing fluid levels in an aneurysmal bone cyst in the proximal radius.

- Generalised elbow pain
- A focal swelling
- Restriction of motion
- Locking
- Forearm and hand neurological symptoms

LATERAL ELBOW PAIN

The causes of lateral elbow pain are given in **Box 1**.

When a patient presents with pain on the radial side of the elbow, a radiograph is the initial investigation to exclude osteoarthritis of the radiocapitellar joint. This will be identified by the features including the presence of marginal osteophytes, irregular joint space narrowing, subchondral sclerosis, and subchondral cysts. In younger patients, there may be osteochondritis dissecans of the capitellum.

Calcification may be visible on the radiograph along the lateral epicondyle secondary to enthesitis. Please note that the presence of calcification is not limited to enthesitis; it can also be seen in soft tissue masses, including tumors and myositis ossificans and due to be calcification in an abnormal tendon (**Fig. 3**).

MR imaging may detect more subtle radiocapitellar osteoarthritis where there is cartilage loss and subchondral edema. The pseudodefect of the capitellum must be appreciated in the younger patient, and this can be misdiagnosed as an osteochondral fracture.[1]

The pain may arise from the lateral tendon insertions. The most commonly affected tendon group is the common extensor origin (CEO), commonly called tennis elbow or lateral epicondylitis.

On MR imaging, the extensor digitorum communis, extensor digiti minimi, and extensor carpi radialis brevis tendons have a common origin on the superior aspect of the lateral epicondyle. On the posterior inferior aspect of the lateral epicondyle is the insertion of the extensor carpi ulnaris, and this is separated from the insertion of the anconeus by fat.[2]

The common insertion of the radial collateral ligament and lateral ulnar collateral ligament on the superior aspect of the intertubercular sulcus and inferior aspect of the superior tubercle may also be identified.

Common extensor tendinosis occurs in patients who perform repeated extension of their wrists with gripping and supination. It is seen in novice tennis players because of poor backhand technique rather than in elite competitors (tennis elbow is never seen at Wimbledon). Interestingly, it is also more commonly seen in golfers than golfers' elbow and is reported in around 85% of golfers. In golfers, the left elbow is affected in right-handed players and vice versa. The disease commences at the origin of the extensor carpi radialis brevis and as the disease progresses, tearing of the undersurface of this tendon occurs.[3] This can sometimes lead to a more extensive tearing over time. This abnormality will be clearly seen by MR imaging but not on a radiograph. On an MR imaging fluid-sensitive sequence, the area of abnormality will be of high signal intensity because of mucoid degeneration of the tendon and/or tearing with fluid in the gap. If calcification is present, this will typically be of low signal on all sequences. There may be associated edema within the anconeus muscle.[4] The anconeus muscle is thought to be a lateral stabilizer of the elbow blending with the lateral joint capsule and lateral triceps muscle.[5] Avulsion injuries isolated to this muscle can therefore also be seen.[6] MR signal changes within the CEO can be seen following a recent injection and in the asymptomatic patient; hence clinical correlation is advised.[7]

The lateral collateral ligament is commonly thickened or torn when there is an extensive common extensor origin tendinosis, as it blends with the undersurface of the tendons.[8]

MEDIAL ELBOW PAIN

The causes of medial elbow pain are given in **Box 2**.

Established osteoarthritis of the medial humeroulnar joint will be detected on radiographs by the same features as described for lateral elbow pain.

MR imaging may detect more subtle medial osteoarthritis when there is cartilage loss and subchondral edema. The pseudodefect of the trochlear transverse ridge is a pitfall in MR imaging interpretation.[1]

Approximately 9.8% to 20% of epicondylitis relates to the common flexor origin. The pronator

---

Box 1
Causes of lateral elbow pain

Common

    Extensor tendinopathy (activity related)

    Referred pain (prolonged posture)

- Cervical spine
- Upper thoracic spine
- Neuromyofascial

Less common

    Radiocapitellar joint synovitis, osteoarthritis

    Posterior interosseous nerve entrapment

    Lateral collateral ligament injury

Not to be missed

    Osteochondritis dissecans

A
B

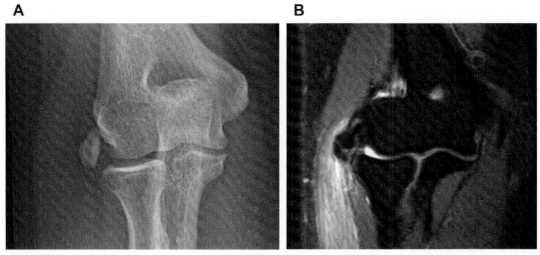

Fig. 3. (*A*) Radiograph of a common extensor origin calcific tendinosis. (*B*) Coronal STIR MR imaging showing the same common extensor origin calcific tendinosis. (*B*) Coronal STIR MRI showing the same common extensor origin calcific tendinosis. The oedema in the common extensor muscle is likely to be secondary to an acute absorption of the calcification.

teres and flexor carpi radialis tendons insert on the anterior aspect of the medial epicondyle and are the most commonly affected.[9] This is commonly known as golfers' elbow or medial epicondylitis. It can also occur in other daily activities with repeated wrist flexion and protonation such as bowling, pitching, carpentry, and in the playing of stringed instruments. Radiographs may show traction spurs around the humeral medial epicondyle.[10] It is best identified by MR imaging. The tendons do not commonly tear and if they do this usually occurs in combination with medial collateral ligament injury. Tendinosis will have similar appearances to common extensor origin tendinosis on MR imaging. Pronator teres muscle tears rarely occur when a bat or club hits the ground during a vigorous swing during cricket or golf, and flexor carpi ulnaris and digitorum superficialis muscle tears were observed at the London Olympic Games 2012[11,12]

The ulnar collateral ligament (UCL) of the elbow can be injured in throwing athletes. This will be a cause of medial-sided elbow pain. It can be injured at the same time as the medial tendons. In the United Kingdom, this is most commonly seen in javelin throwers, but in the United States, baseball pitchers are more frequently affected. If there is a complete tear, a radiograph can demonstrate widening of the medial joint line. Any associated avulsion fractures with this injury will often be identified on a radiograph. Calcification may also be seen within an injured UCL on a radiograph. The ligament will become thickened and edematous and will be seen on a fluid-sensitive MR sequence as

high signal intensity. The ligament can sometimes remain intact despite an avulsion fracture of the sublime tubercle of the coronoid process of the ulna and will be seen as a detached fragment of bone. For this, T1 spin echo sequences are useful.[13]

The ulnar nerve is in close proximity to these other structures and can be injured concomitantly or be a cause of pain in itself. Ulnar nerve abnormalities will be discussed in more detail in the section on neurologic symptoms.

Snapping triceps syndrome is caused by the medial head of the triceps muscle dislocating over the medial epicondyle in elbow flexion

---

Box 2
Causes of medial elbow pain

Common

    Flexor tendinopathy (activity related)

    Medial collateral ligament sprain

Less common

    Ulnar nerve compression

    Avulsion fracture of medial epicondyle (adolescents)

    Apophysitis (adolescents)

Not to be missed

    Referred pain (prolonged posture)

    • Cervical spine

    • Upper thoracic spine

    • Neuromyofascial

beyond 100°. It can be congenital or acquired. Congenital problems include an accessory triceps tendon or hypoplastic bone. Acquired hypertrophic musculature in weightlifters can lead to snapping. This can be a cause of pain in itself, but it can also cause ulnar neuritis.[14] There is no specific radiographic feature that relates to this diagnosis.

ANTERIOR ELBOW PAIN

Distal biceps tendon problems are the most common cause of anterior elbow pain. The distal biceps tendon is formed from both the short and long head of biceps muscles. An aponeurosis (lacertus fibrosis) is formed at the level of the musculotendinous junction. This lies superficial to the ulnar flexor muscles, radial flexor muscles, median nerve, and brachial artery. It then attaches to the proximal part of the ulna. The distal tendon has 2 attachments, with the long head being more proximally inserted into the radial tuberosity and the short head line more superficial and fanning out and attaching to the distal portion of the radial tuberosity.[15]

Distal biceps tendinosis can also be seen in patients who perform excessive lifting movements. Ruptures of the distal biceps tendon are more common than ruptures of the common extensor origin or flexor origin. This is because of the load exceeding the tendons' capacity and occurs in patients lifting unaccustomed weights. They are more common in males than females. Rupture is strongly associated with abuse of anabolic steroids.

A tear can occur within the biceps muscle. It is important to be able to identify the difference between a biceps muscle tear and a distal biceps tendon tear. This can be achieved by performing MR imaging, although others argue that dynamic ultrasound examination increases the precision of diagnosis. The distal biceps tendon can either be torn independently or along with the lacertus fibrosis. If the lacertus fibrosis is also torn, then the tendon will be retracted from the bicipital tuberosity. Clinically, an intact lacertus fibrosis can mimic an intact distal biceps tendon with preservation of the flexion power of the elbow. This is said to occur in approximately 15% of cases.

In order to optimize MR scanning to see the distal biceps tendon along the length of the tendon, the authors advise examination of the arm in a flexed, abducted, and supinated position.[16]

Another rare cause of anterior elbow pain is a brachialis muscle injury seen in weightlifters and those who practice judo.[17]

POSTERIOR ELBOW PAIN

The causes of posterior elbow pain are given in **Box 3**.

Olecranon bursitis can cause posterior elbow pain and swelling. This will be discussed further under focal swellings.

The triceps tendon can be affected by tendinosis and tears. Tearing often occurs in patients who put excess weight on this tendon (eg, weightlifters or patients who are wheelchair-bound and put the full weight on their elbow while transferring from wheelchair to chair or bed). This often leads to partial tears of 1 element of the triceps tendon. Tendon tears can be secondary to infection and steroid use (eg, injected steroid for the treatment of olecranon bursitis or ingesting anabolic steroids).[18,19]

If the elbow is in extension, the tendon may appear lax; therefore, a degree of flexion of the elbow is recommended when performing MR imaging to reduce artifact.[20] The appearance of tendinosis or tearing on MR imaging is the same as that seen for the other tendons.

GENERALIZED ELBOW PAIN

A plain radiograph is the initial investigation for generalized elbow pain. Generalized elbow pain is usually caused by an arthropathy. Osteoarthritis will be identified by a plain radiograph. Erosions may also be seen on a radiograph if there is an inflammatory arthropathy, gout, or rarely hemophilia (**Fig. 4**).

The patient with an inflammatory arthropathy such as rheumatoid arthritis will often present with an effusion and synovitis and potentially an olecranon bursitis. Clinically there will usually be swelling of the elbow and sometimes an increase of temperature. MR imaging will identify synovitis, erosions, marrow edema, and olecranon bursitis. If there is difficulty in differentiating between an

---

Box 3
Causes of posterior elbow pain

Olecranon bursitis - repeated trauma on hard surfaces or infection or arthropathy including gout

Triceps tendinopathy or tear

Posterior impingement – fixed flexion deformity

- Young age – hyperextension valgus overload – posterolateral impingement
- Older age – radio-capitellar joint osteophytes

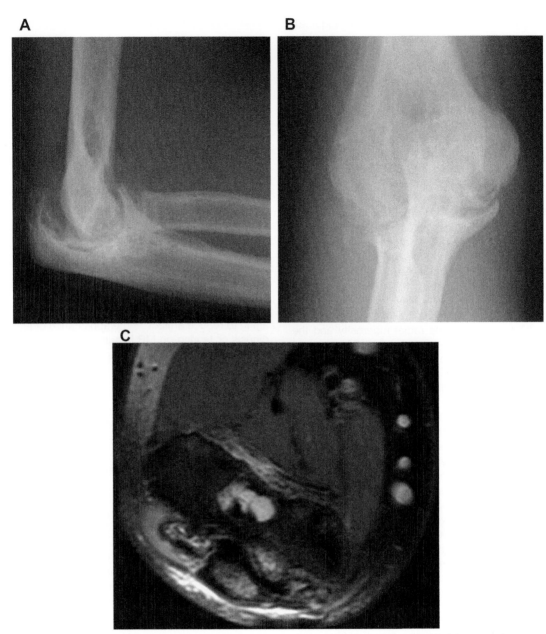

Fig. 4. (*A*, *B*) Lateral and AP Radiograph of haemophiliac elbow joint in a 28 year old. (*C*) An axial STIR MR showing the haemophiliac joint in same patient.

effusion and synovitis, gadolinium enhancement can be undertaken to assess for active synovitis. In practice this is rarely needed and should only be performed if it will make a difference to the patient's treatment. This is particularly relevant in view of the recent warnings regarding gadolinium deposition in the brain.[21]

An alternative cause for pain could be enthesitis. MR imaging is useful in detecting the inflammatory element of enthesitis at the insertion of the common extensor tendon and common flexor tendon origins, as well as the triceps tendon in an inflammatory arthropathy (typically rheumatoid and psoriatic). This will be seen as bone edema and edema within the enthesis, as well as perientheseal soft tissue oedema.[22]

The presence of a bone tumor will be seen by MR imaging. It is still important to correlate the appearances with the plain radiograph, as the presence of calcification on the radiograph may refine the differential diagnosis of the bone tumor. The bone tumor site, size, and signal characteristics will help refine the differential diagnosis (**Fig. 5**). The tumor itself can often only be given a definitive diagnosis by histologic analysis of a biopsy. Gadolinium prior to MR imaging does not need to be routinely given for tumor analysis.

A septic arthritis can cause generalized elbow pain. There will also be erythema of the skin and increased temperature of the joint. This may be because of an inoculation or de novo, perhaps because the patient is immunocompromised. An effusion will be seen on a conventional radiograph, and there may be soft tissue swelling and osteopenia. There will be subsequent bone erosion and joint destruction if left untreated.

MR imaging will detect the effusion, synovitis, and bone edema as well as any focal areas of abscess formation. Bone edema may indicate the presence of osteomyelitis. To diagnose osteomyelitis, the authors would advocate interrogation of the T1 sequence to assess for low signal indicative of marrow replacement, as well as assessing for supporting features. Osteomyelitis has a range of radiographic and MR features including initial localized osteopenia, a periosteal reaction, bone lysis, and eventual sclerosis. Untreated or chronic cases can result in a sequestrum, involucrum, or cloaca. The type of infection will not be identified by MR imaging, and this can only be ascertained by an aspiration or biopsy. The most common organism involving the joint will be *Staphylococcus*

aureus. Gadolinium enhancement does not need to be given to make a diagnosis of infection. It does, however, offer better definition of intraosseous or soft tissue infections and can be of use in the assessment of potentially necrotic bone (**Fig. 6**).

FOCAL SWELLING

Clinically it may be difficult to determine from which structure the soft tissue swelling is arising.

If there is a posterior swelling, this can be secondary to an olecranon bursitis, which is the most frequent cause. There may, however, be an elbow effusion that is mimicking this.

Olecranon bursitis is septic in approximately one-third of cases. On aspiration and culture most of these are caused by *S aureus* (90%), and the remainder predominantly caused by beta hemolytic *Streptococcus*. Impaired immunity makes sepsis more likely. This can be caused by alcohol abuse, renal impairment, steroid use, and diabetes mellitus. Bursitis is more common in occupations resting on the elbow, an inflammatory arthropathy such as rheumatoid and gout, where it may contain tophi (**Fig. 7**).

The MR appearances of a septic and nonseptic olecranon bursitis show much overlap, and both can be associated with elbow effusions and triceps edema. If there is surrounding soft tissue

A **B**

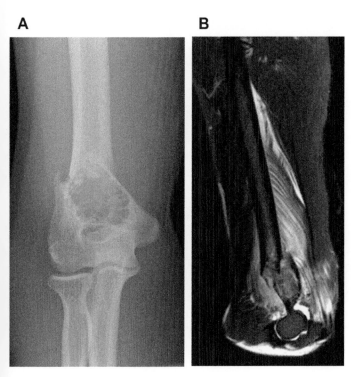

Fig. 5. (*A*) Radiograph of a sarcoma in the distal humerus that has fractured. (*B*) MR imaging sagittal STIR of the same elbow showing a sarcoma in the distal humerus that has fractured.

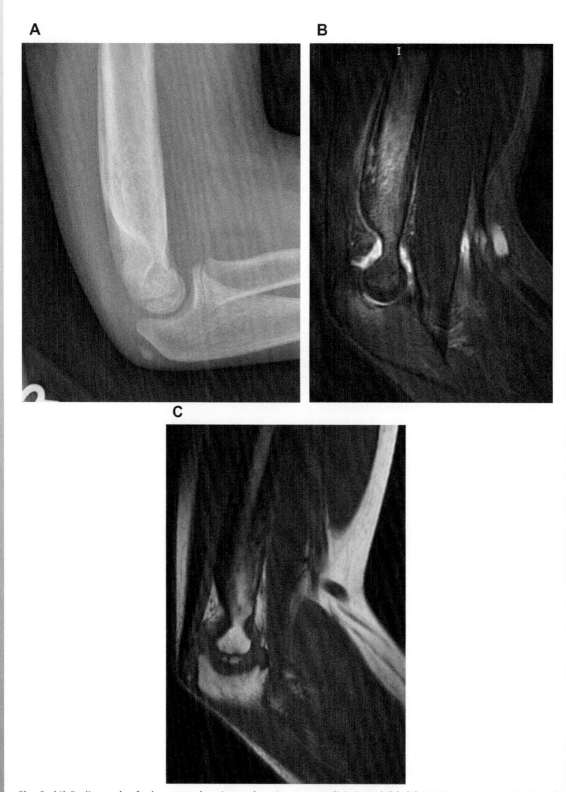

Fig. 6. (*A*) Radiograph of a humerus showing a chronic osteomyelitis in a child. (*B*) MR imaging sagittal STIR of the elbow showing a chronic osteomyelitis in a child. (*C*) MR imaging sagittal T1 FSE of the elbow showing a chronic osteomyelitis in a child.

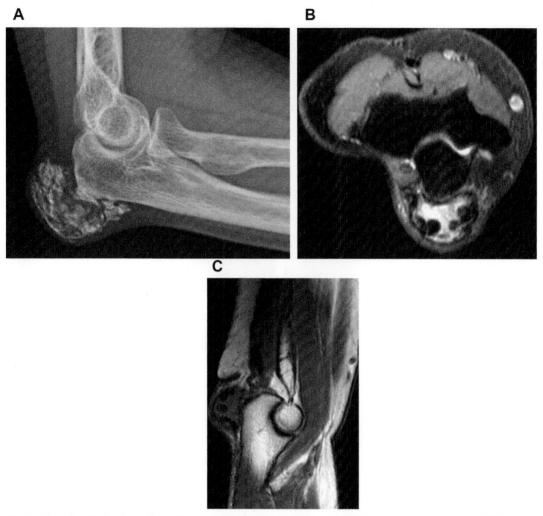

Fig. 7. (A) Radiograph of an elbow showing calcification in the region of the olecranon bursa. (B) MR imaging axial STIR of the elbow showing an olecranon bursitis with gouty tophi present. (C) MR imaging sagittal T1 FSE of the elbow showing an olecranon bursitis with gouty tophi present.

edema, complexity of the bursal fluid, triceps tendon thickening, and marked lobulation of the bursa walls, diagnosis leans more toward infection. Bone edema within the olecranon may be caused by osteomyelitis in the presence of a septic bursitis but can also be present with or without sepsis of the bursa and is therefore nonspecific.[23]

A focal swelling may also be a soft tissue tumor. The most common is a lipomatous tumor, and the most frequently encountered is a benign lipoma. This is most likely in the subcutaneous tissue that can occur in a muscle. If large and in the muscle, it may be identified on a radiograph as a radiolucent area. More commonly, MR imaging will identify this as a high-signal lesion on both T1 and T2. If it is a benign lesion, it will also be completely

far suppressed and of uniform low signal on a fat-suppressed sequence or STIR (Fig. 8).

Soft tissue tumors can involve the muscles, nerves, and subcutaneous soft tissue most frequently. MR imaging will be able to identify from which structure the soft tissue tumor is arising and its extent. It can also assess for bone involvement at the same time. By the use of a T1 and STIR sequence, a soft tissue lump can be determined to be benign or malignant. MR imaging can help refine the differential diagnosis, but histologic analysis from biopsy is the only way to give a complete diagnosis if the lesion has any appearances of possible malignancy.

Several infections may be encountered within soft tissues. These will cause a focal soft tissue

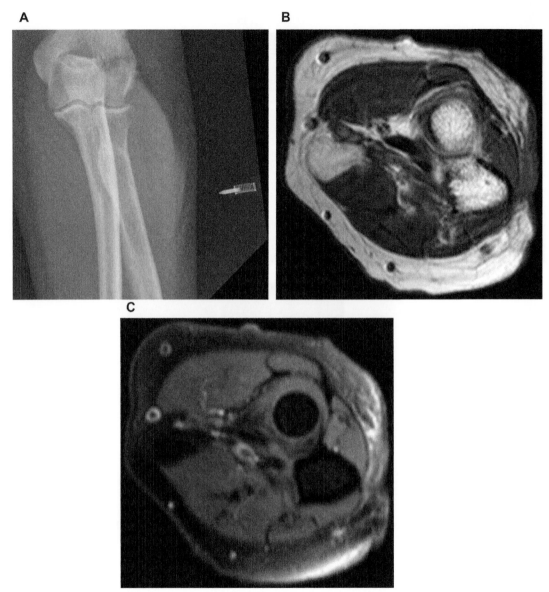

Fig. 8. (*A*) Radiograph of an elbow showing a subtle change in the extensor muscles. (*B*) MR imaging axial T1 FSE of the elbow showing an intramuscular lipoma. (*C*) MR imaging axial STIR of the elbow showing the same intramuscular lipoma.

swelling if there is an abscess or a generalized swelling of the muscle if involved globally. Infections of the muscle can occur, otherwise known as pyomyositis, and may be secondary to other systemic infections such as hepatitis A.

A painless swelling of the elbow may be seen in a neuropathic joint with destruction of the bone seen on the radiograph and MR imaging with synovitis. The cause for the Charcot joint should also be investigated, especially when both elbows are involved, suggesting a lesion in the cervical spine (**Fig. 9**).

RESTRICTION OF MOTION

A patient may not be able to bend his or her elbow because of a large effusion and synovitis. The way of assessing an elbow for reduced motion is the same as that for generalized elbow pain.

LOCKING

Locking of the elbow can occur in a certain position. It is usually caused by the presence of a loose body within the joint. A plain radiograph may show

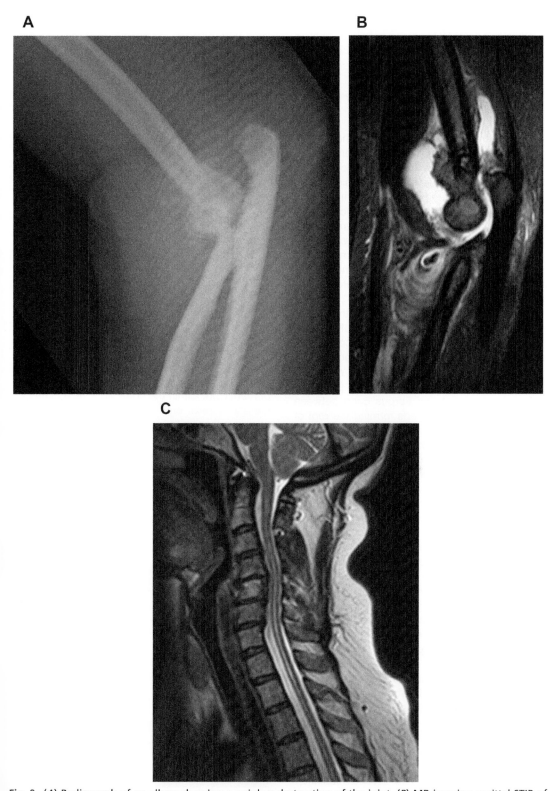

Fig. 9. (*A*) Radiograph of an elbow showing a painless destruction of the joint. (*B*) MR imaging sagittal STIR of the elbow showing destruction of the joint with an effusion. (*C*) MR imaging sagittal T2 FSE of the cervical spine showing a syrinx – the cause of bilateral Charcot elbow joints.

a loose body unless it is obscured by the surrounding bone. An MR imaging scan may show a loose body if it is large enough within a joint or effusion.

FOREARM AND HAND NEUROLOGIC SYMPTOMS

The most common nerve involved at the level of the elbow is the ulnar nerve as it progresses through the ulnar groove. The nerve shows proximal enlargement before the compression and a measurement of 11 mm² 1 cm proximal to the medial epicondyle is thought to be a good indicator of significant compressive ulnar neuropathy.[24] On water-sensitive MR sequences, it can be of increased signal intensity in 60% of asymptomatic individuals, so clinical correlation and increase in size are important in confirming compression at this site.[25]

Ulnar nerve entrapment can occur within the ulnar groove and may be exacerbated by ulnar nerve subluxation. Other entrapments can occur at the level of Struthers arcade (a tunnel produced by the aponeurosis of the medial triceps muscle)[26] cubital tunnel because of osteophytes, ganglions or Osborne ligament (the fibrous band between the flexor carpi ulnaris heads forming the roof of the tunnel), or unusually a snapping triceps.

Nerve entrapment may be caused by the presence of an anomalous muscle, the most common of which is the Anconeus Epitrochlearis. This arises from the posterior aspect of the medial epicondyle in up to 34% of individuals. Because its muscle lies within the cubital tunnel, on top of the ulnar nerve, it may protect the nerve from dislocation, but it also decreases the available space in the cubital tunnel.[1] The Osbourne ligament is absent in the presence of this muscle. These structures can all be identified by MR imaging.[27]

The median nerve can be compressed by Struther ligament, a thickened lacertus fibrosis, between the deep and superficial heads of the pronotor teres muscle (pronator syndrome) and by a thickened sublimis arch (the proximal edge of the flexor digitorum superficialis).[28]

The radial nerve is the least commonly involved at the elbow. Compression can occur at the level of the radial head from fibrous bands between the joint capsule and brachialis muscle, at the leash of Henry (the arcade of branches of the recurrent radial artery), the extensor radialis brevis tendon edge, the arcade of Frohse (supinator edge), and the distal supinator muscle.[14]

The posterior interosseous nerve (the terminal motor branch of the radial nerve) is also compressed at the level of the arcade of Frohse and can mimic lateral epicondylitis. This occurs in athletes who perform repetitive supination and pronotation such as kayakers, tennis players, and throwing athletes (**Fig. 10**).

OTHER IMAGING TECHNIQUES
Ultrasound

Ultrasound is used as a screening tool for soft tissue lumps around the elbow and the presence of tendinosis. Its advantages are that it can be directed to the site of the patient's pain, and the radiologist is able to obtain a history and undertake a clinical assessment. It can be used in a patient who is claustrophobic or cannot undergo MR imaging because of contraindications, such as MR-incompatible pacemakers. Its line pair resolution is superior to MR imaging; therefore the presence of small areas of abnormality within nerves can be detected. It is superior to unenhanced MR imaging in the assessment of active synovitis. Its greatest strength in elbow imaging is offering a dynamic assessment, such as in identifying the presence of ulnar nerve subluxation or in other problems like a snapping triceps. It can also be used to assess the soft tissues in the presence of metalwork within the bone, such as a plate single and screws crossing a fracture or an elbow prosthesis, when MR imaging is difficult to perform because of artifact.

Computed Tomography

CT will give more detail of bone trabeculae in the context of fracturing and identifies small loose bodies in the joints that may be missed by other techniques.

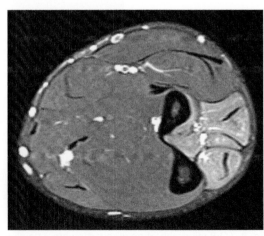

Fig. 10. MR imaging axial T2FSE showing the edema within extensor muscle of the forearm affected by a compression of the posterior interosseous nerve (PIN). The radiograph of the forearm was normal.

Nuclear Medicine

Nuclear medicine does not have any specific advantages over other techniques in the elbow.

SUMMARY

A radiograph is a good primary imaging technique when assessing a patient with pain. It can be useful in trauma, arthritis, and bone tumors.

MR imaging may be the only investigation needed in the presence of a soft tissue lump or when the diagnosis is thought to be caused by a soft tissue problem such as tendinosis.

REFERENCES

1. Rosenberg ZS, Bencardino J, Beltran J. MRI of normal variants and interpretation pitfalls of the elbow. Semin Musculoskelet Radiol 1998;2(2): 141–55.
2. Zoner CS, Buck FM, Cardoso FN, et al. Detailed MRI-anatomic study of the lateral epicondyle of the elbow and its tendinous and ligamentous attachments in cadavers. AJR Am J Roentgenol 2010; 195(3):629–36.
3. Sonin A. Tendon disorders. Semin Musculoskelet Radiol 1998;2(2):163–74.
4. Coel M, Yamada CY, Ko J. MR imaging of patients with lateral epicondylitis of the elbow (tennis elbow): importance of increased signal of the anconeus muscle. AJR Am J Roentgenol 1993;161(5):1019–21.
5. Ulnar compression neuropathy secondary to the anconeus epitrochlearis muscle. J Hand Surg Am 1989;14(5):917–9.
6. Al-Kashmiri A, Sun K, Delaney JS. Lateral humeral epicondyle fracture secondary to avulsion of the anconeus muscle. Clin J Sport Med 2007;17(5):408–9.
7. Tuite MJ, Kijowski R. Sports-related injuries of the elbow: an approach to MRI interpretation. Clin Sports Med 2006;25(3):387–408, v.
8. Bredella MA, Tirman PF, Fritz RC, et al. MR imaging findings of lateral ulnar collateral ligament abnormalities in patients with lateral epicondylitis. AJR Am J Roentgenol 1999;173(5):1379–82.
9. Walz DM, Newman JS, Konin GP, et al. Epicondylitis: pathogenesis, imaging, and treatment. Radiographics 2010;30(1):167–84.
10. Ciccotti MC, Schwartz MA, Ciccotti MG. Diagnosis and treatment of medial epicondylitis of the elbow. Clin Sports Med 2004;23(4):693–705, xi.
11. Niebulski HZ, Richardson ML. High-grade pronator teres tear in a cricket batsman. Radiol Case Rep 2011;6(3):540.
12. Bethapudi S, Robinson P, Engebretsen L, et al. Elbow injuries at the London 2012 Summer Olympic Games: demographics and pictorial imaging review. AJR Am J Roentgenol 2013;201(3):535–49.
13. Schwartz ML. Collateral ligaments. Semin Musculoskelet Radiol 1998;2(2):155–62.
14. Sutter R. MRI of the Elbow. ESSR Sports Imaging Subcommittee. Breitenseher Publisher; 2018.
15. Eames MH, Bain GI, Fogg QA, et al. Distal biceps tendon anatomy: a cadaveric study. J Bone Joint Surg Am 2007;89(5):1044–9.
16. Giuffre BM, Moss MJ. Optimal positioning for MRI of the distal biceps brachii tendon: flexed abducted supinated view. AJR Am J Roentgenol 2004; 182(4):944–6.
17. Sharma P, Mehta N, Narayan A. Isolated traumatic brachialis muscle tear: a case report and review of literature. Bull Emerg Trauma 2017;5(4):307–10.
18. Koplas MC, Schneider E, Sundaram M. Prevalence of triceps tendon tears on MRI of the elbow and clinical correlation. Skeletal Radiol 2011;40(5): 587–94.
19. Stannard JP, Bucknell AL. Rupture of the triceps tendon associated with steroid injections. Am J Sports Med 1993;21(3):482–5.
20. Fritz RC, Boutin RD. Musculotendinous disorders in the upper extremity: part 2. MRI of the elbow, forearm, wrist, and hand. Semin Musculoskelet Radiol 2017;21(4):376–91.
21. Gulani V, Calamante F, Shellock FG, et al. Gadolinium deposition in the brain: summary of evidence and recommendations. Lancet Neurol 2017;16(7): 564–70.
22. Groves C, Chandramohan M, Chew NS, et al. Clinical examination, ultrasound and MRI imaging of the painful elbow in psoriatic arthritis and rheumatoid arthritis: which is better, ultrasound or MR, for imaging enthesitis? Rheumatol Ther 2017;4(1): 71–84.
23. Floemer F, Morrison WB, Bongartz G, et al. MRI characteristics of olecranon bursitis. AJR Am J Roentgenol 2004;183(1):29–34.
24. Terayama Y, Uchiyama S, Ueda K, et al. Optimal measurement level and ulnar nerve cross-sectional area cutoff threshold for identifying ulnar neuropathy at the elbow by MRI and ultrasonography. J Hand Surg Am 2018;43(6):529–36.
25. Husarik DB, Saupe N, Pfirrmann CW, et al. Elbow nerves: MR findings in 60 asymptomatic subjects–normal anatomy, variants, and pitfalls. Radiology 2009;252(1):148–56.
26. Caetano EB, Sabongi Neto JJ, Vieira LA, et al. The arcade of Struthers: an anatomical study and clinical implications. Rev Bras Ortop 2017;52(3):331–6.
27. Granger A, Sardi JP, Iwanaga J, et al. Osborne's ligament: a review of its history, anatomy, and surgical importance. Cureus 2017;9(3):e1080.
28. Bilecenoglu B, Uz A, Karalezli N. Possible anatomic structures causing entrapment neuropathies of the median nerve: an anatomic study. Acta Orthop Belg 2005;71(2):169–76.

Radiographic/MR Imaging Correlation of the Wrist

Thomas P. Moser, MD, MSc[a],*, Adriana P. Martinez, MD, MSc, FRCSC[b], Sooheib Andoulsi, MD[a], Jérémy Jeantroux, MD[c], Étienne Cardinal, MD[d]

KEYWORDS

- Wrist • Carpal bones • Radiographs • MR imaging • Fractures • Arthritis • Avascular necrosis
- Tendinopathies

KEY POINTS

- The wrist can be divided into 3 functional columns (radial, central, and ulnar) as a practical way to discuss the different pathologic conditions.
- There is a synergy between radiographs and MR imaging that complements the diagnosis of these pathologic conditions; it is important to understand the advantages and limitations of each modality.
- Radiographically occult fractures of the wrist (eg, distal radius, scaphoid, hook of the hamate) are common, and the imaging strategy has evolved over the years thanks to a greater availability of MR imaging and multidetector computed tomography.
- Avascular necrosis of the carpal bones (eg, scaphoid and lunate) poses specific diagnostic and therapeutic difficulties.

INTRODUCTION

The wrist is one of the most complex articular structures in the human body owing to its multiple constitutive bones and intricate joints. This complexity makes it difficult to assess radiologically and stresses the importance of using an adequate imaging technique and a thorough systematic analysis of the images to reach the correct diagnosis.

In this article, the authors focus on the correlation between radiographs and MR imaging. Because MR imaging is now routinely obtained in the workup of wrist symptoms, the interpretation of subtle radiographic findings has been refined, and these will be emphasized here. There are also circumstances whereby MR images can be misleading when not analyzed together with the radiographs.

THE THREE COLUMNS OF THE WRIST

On a biomechanical point of view, the wrist is commonly divided into 3 functionally distinct columns (**Fig. 1**).[1] This approach is also valuable to narrow the differential diagnosis based on the location of the clinical symptoms and to ascertain that a specific anatomic area has been adequately investigated with the imaging protocol.

The lateral or radial column encompasses the scaphoid fossa and radial styloid: the scaphoid, the trapezium, the trapezoid, and the bases of the first and second metacarpals. In addition to the standard posteroanterior (PA) and lateral views, these bones are best demonstrated with dedicated radiographic views, including the semipronated oblique view, the scaphoid views, as well as the Kapandji views of the thumb.[2] The pathologic conditions of the lateral column of the wrist are summarized in **Table 1**.

The medial or ulnar column contains the distal ulna and ulnar styloid, the medial aspect of the lunate, the triquetrum, the pisiform, the hamate, and the bases of the fourth and

[a] Department of Radiology, Centre Hospitalier de l'Université de Montréal, 1000, rue Saint-Denis, Montréal, Québec H2X 0C1, Canada; [b] Department of Orthopedic Surgery, University of Ottawa, The Ottawa Hospital Civic Campus, 1053 Carling Avenue, Ottawa, Ontario K1Y 4E9, Canada; [c] Service d'Imagerie Médicale, Clinique St-François, 1-5, rue Colomé, Haguenau 67502, France; [d] Medvue, 5811 Côte-des-Neiges Road, Montreal, Québec H3S 1Z2, Canada
* Corresponding author.
E-mail address: thomas.moser@umontreal.ca

Magn Reson Imaging Clin N Am 27 (2019) 601–623
https://doi.org/10.1016/j.mric.2019.07.012

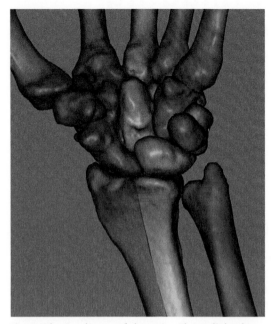

Fig. 1. The 3 columns of the wrist. The radial column (*pink*) includes the scaphoid fossa and radial styloid, the scaphoid, the trapezium, the trapezoid, and the first and second metacarpals. The central column (*white*) includes the ulnar side of the radius, the lunate, the capitate, and the third metacarpal. The ulnar column (*orange*) includes the ulna, the triquetrum, the pisiform, the hamate, and the fourth and fifth metacarpals.

fifth metacarpals. A thorough analysis of these bones may require additional specific radiographic views, such as the semisupinated view, and the carpal tunnel view for the hook of hamate.[3] The pathologic conditions of the medial column of the wrist are summarized in **Table 2.**

Table 1 Pathologic conditions responsible for radial-sided wrist pain and symptoms	
Bones	• Scaphoid fracture • Avascular necrosis of the scaphoid
Joints	• SLAC and SNAC patterns of osteoarthritis • Trapeziometacarpal osteoarthritis
Ligaments	• Scapholunate ligament tear
Tendons	• De Quervain tenosynovitis • Proximal and distal intersection syndromes • Flexor carpi radialis tenosynovitis
Nerves	• Wartenberg syndrome

Table 2 Pathologic conditions responsible for ulnar-sided wrist pain and symptoms	
Bones	• Hook of the hamate fracture
Joints	• Ulnocarpal impingement syndrome • Other impingement syndromes: distal radioulnar, styloidocarpal, hamatolunate • Pisotriquetral osteoarthritis
Ligaments	• Triangular fibrocartilage complex tears • Lunotriquetral ligament tear
Tendons	• Extensor carpi ulnaris tenosynovitis and instability • Flexor carpi ulnaris enthesopathy
Nerves	• Guyon canal syndrome

The central column of the wrist includes the rest of the bone structures, namely, the lunate fossa of the radius, the lunate, the capitate, and the base of the third metacarpal. Additional oblique semipronated and semisupinated views may be helpful; these bones are often difficult to assess on radiographs because of their central position with many overlapping structures. The pathologic conditions of the medial column of the wrist are summarized in **Table 3.**

Table 3 Pathologic conditions responsible for central wrist pain and symptoms	
Bones	• Kienböck disease • Carpal boss
Joints	• Inflammatory arthritis
Ligaments	• Perilunar instability • Ganglion cysts
Tendons	• Extensor and flexor tendons tenosynovitis and tears
Nerves	• Carpal tunnel syndrome

IMAGING PROTOCOLS
Wrist Radiographs

A recommended routine radiographic protocol for the wrist includes the PA, lateral, oblique semipronated, and oblique semisupinated views.[4,5]

In an appropriate clinical context, this protocol can be supplemented with the ligamentous instability series, including additional PA views in radial and ulnar deviations and a PA view with a clenched fist.[6] Selected views of the scaphoid and carpal tunnel can also be useful in specific circumstances.[7]

Wrist MR Imaging

A routine protocol typically includes a combination of T1-weighted and fat-suppressed T2- or intermediate-weighted sequences in the coronal, transverse, and sagittal planes. A dedicated wrist coil is required in order to obtain an optimal image quality with adequate signal-to-noise ratio and spatial resolution. The section's thickness is routinely set between 2 and 3 mm. Contiguous thinner sections or even isotropic submillimetric acquisition can be obtained with 3-dimensional gradient-echo or spin-echo sequences and may be useful for the evaluation of ligaments and cartilage.[8] In the authors' institutions, computed tomography (CT) arthrography and occasionally MR arthrography are still favored for the evaluation of wrist ligaments and cartilage abnormalities.[9–11]

RADIAL COLUMN OF THE WRIST
Helpful Radiographic Signs and Pitfalls

The scaphoid and pronator quadratus fat stripes
The normal scaphoid fat pad is located between the radial capsule and the abductor longus and the extensor brevis tendons (**Fig. 2**).

It appears as a thin linear or triangular lucency adjacent to the scaphoid on the PA view. Its obliteration may indicate a scaphoid fracture.[12]

The pronator quadratus fat pad is seen on the lateral view of the wrist as a thin lucent area superficial to the opacity of the pronator quadratus muscle. Its obliteration can be seen in the presence of distal radius fractures.[13]

In a recent study,[14] it was observed that these signs are not really reliable and had sensitivity and specificity values of only 50% and 50%, respectively, for the scaphoid fat stripe, and 26% and 70%, respectively, for the pronator fat stripe.

The scaphoid cortical ring sign
It corresponds to the end-on view of the scaphoid tubercle when the scaphoid is flexed (**Figs. 3** and **4**). Because a flexed scaphoid can be normal, the value of this sign depends on the position of the other carpal bones, mainly the lunate. The association of an abnormally extended lunate with a flexed scaphoid manifests as an increased scapholunate angle over 70° (normal values 30°–60°) and indicates scapholunate dissociation, usually associated with a complete scapholunate ligament tear.[15,16]

Fractures

Scaphoid fractures
Fractures of the scaphoid are the second most frequent fracture of the wrist after the

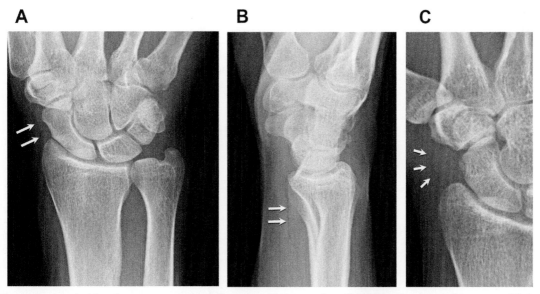

A   **B**   **C**

Fig. 2. The scaphoid and pronator quadratus fat stripes. The normal scaphoid fat stripe (*arrows*) is seen on (*A*) the PA view and the pronator quadratus fat stripe (*arrows*) is seen on (*B*) the lateral view. (*C*) A 23-year-old man with a fracture of the scaphoid tubercle; the scaphoid fat stripe (*arrows*) is displaced and deformed because of hematoma or effusion.

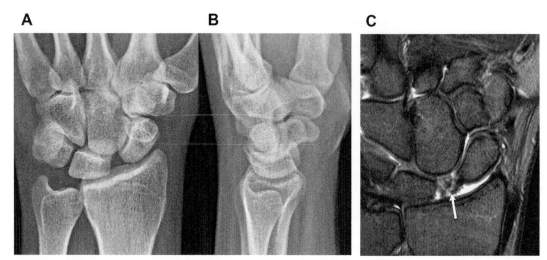

Fig. 3. (*A, B*) The scaphoid cortical ring sign corresponds to the end-on view of a flexed scaphoid. (*C*) For this 37-year-old man, there is a traumatic scapholunate dissociation (*arrow*) associated with a complete scapholunate ligament tear as evidenced on a coronal fat-suppressed T2-weighted MR image.

distal radius and represent 70% of carpal fractures. They involve, by decreasing order of frequency, the waist (70%), the proximal pole (20%), and the distal tubercle (10%) of the scaphoid.[17]

It is estimated that radiographs allow the diagnosis of only 40% to 60% of these fractures, leaving a large proportion undetected.[18,19] The strategy to demonstrate radiographically occult scaphoid fractures has evolved over the years from immobilization and follow-up radiographs to bone scintigraphy, and finally, early MR imaging or multidetector computed tomography (MDCT).[20–22] Both MR imaging and CT with submillimetric collimation have a sensitivity of nearly 100% for the detection of scaphoid fractures with cortical involvement.[23,24] The high sensitivity of MR imaging for recent fractures is due to the fact that the fracture line is highlighted by bone marrow edema (**Fig. 5**). However, there is a potential for false positives, corresponding to purely trabecular fractures or bone bruises.[25]

Other fractures

Fractures of the distal radius are the most frequent fractures of the wrist, and about 20% are radiographically occult (**Fig. 6**).[18] Fractures of the trapezium and base of the first metacarpal fractures are seen less frequently.

Ligament Injuries

Scapholunate ligament tear

The scapholunate ligament is the primary stabilizer of the scapholunate joint, and tears may occur

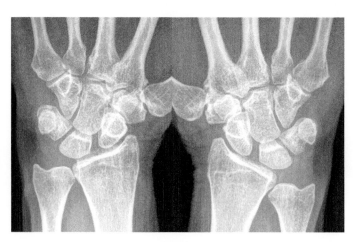

Fig. 4. A 67-year-old woman presenting with a bilateral scaphoid cortical ring sign and no history of trauma. There is a scapholunate diastasis and faint calcifications involving the scapholunate, lunotriquetral, and triangular fibrocartilage ligaments, suggesting calcium pyrophosphate dihydrate deposition disease.

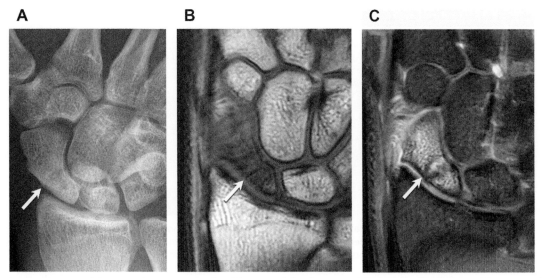

Fig. 5. A 28-year-old man with a recent scaphoid fracture. (*A*) A fracture of the proximal pole (*arrow*) is suspected on the scaphoid. (*B, C*) Coronal T1-weighted and fat-suppressed T2-weighted MR images confirm the fracture line surrounded by bone marrow edema (*arrow*).

following a fall on an outstretched hand. Disruption of this ligament and the secondary stabilizers (dorsal and palmar capsular ligaments) releases the natural tendency of palmar flexion for the scaphoid and dorsal flexion for the lunate, which results in a scapholunate dissociation.[26,27]

Scapholunate dissociation manifests on radiographs as a scapholunate diastasis on the PA view and an increased scapholunate angle over 70° (normal 30°–60°) on the lateral view (see **Fig. 3**). As a general rule, measuring carpal angles on CT and MR images should be avoided because of a different position of the wrist causing unreliable values. However, the scapholunate angle appears relatively independent of the wrist position

and demonstrates a low variability between different modalities.[28]

Scapholunate ligament tears are well demonstrated with MR imaging when they are complete (see **Fig. 3**). However, its sensitivity is insufficient for partial tears that are better demonstrated with MR arthrography or CT arthrography.[9,29]

Scapholunate ligament cyst
The dorsal aspect of the wrist is one the most common locations for ganglion cysts, where they can be seen in an area recently known as the dorsal capsuloscapholunate septum.[30] A nonspecific bulge of the dorsal soft tissues may be noted on

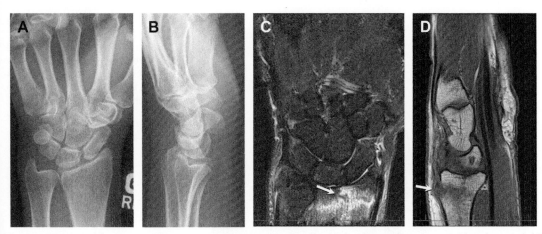

Fig. 6. A 58-year-old woman with posttraumatic wrist pain. (*A, B*) Initial radiographs were considered normal. (*C, D*) Coronal fat-suppressed T2-weighted and sagittal T1-weighted MR images demonstrate an occult nondisplaced fracture of the distal radius (*arrows*).

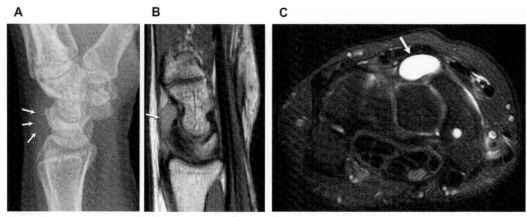

Fig. 7. A 42-year-old woman with dorsal wrist tenderness. (*A*) Lateral view shows subtle bulge of the dorsal soft tissues (*arrows*). (*B, C*) Sagittal intermediate-weighted and transverse fat-suppressed T2-weighted MR images demonstrate a ganglion cyst of the dorsal capsulo-scapholunate septum (*arrows*).

radiographs if the cyst is large. The diagnosis is more straightforward with ultrasound (US) or MR imaging (**Fig. 7**).[31,32]

Arthropathies

Trapeziometacarpal osteoarthritis

Osteoarthritis at the base of the thumb is common with aging and regularly associated with osteoarthritis of the hand. It is a frequent cause of pain and disability at the radial aspect of the wrist. It can be treated by arthroplasty or excision of the trapezium with good results (**Fig. 8**).[33,34]

Radioscaphoid osteoarthritis

Occurrence of degenerative changes between the radius and the scaphoid is the consequence of an altered kinematic of the intercalary segment and particularly the scaphoid. The scapholunate advanced collapse (SLAC-wrist) is a complication of scapholunate ligament tear and scapholunate dissociation, where rotatory subluxation of the scaphoid causes progressive cartilage damage.[35] Different stages of osteoarthritis starting between the distal radius and scaphoid, and extending to the capitolunate space, have been described (**Table 4**). In absence of traumatic history, calcium pyrophosphate dihydrate crystal deposition disease is another cause of SLAC-wrist (see **Fig. 4**).[36] Similarly, a pattern of scaphoid nonunion advanced collapse (SNAC-wrist) complicating scaphoid fractures has been described (**Fig. 9**, **Table 5**).[37] Treatment options include proximal row

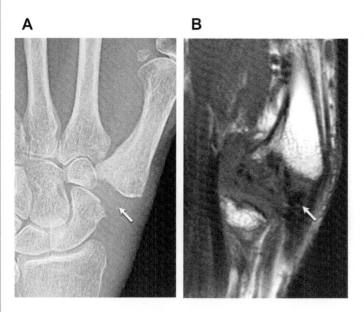

Fig. 8. A 58-year-old man followed up after surgery for trapeziometacarpal osteoarthritis. (*A*) PA view shows the resection of the trapezium (*arrow*). (*B*) Coronal T1-weighted MR image demonstrates the interposed flexor carpi radialis tendon (*arrow*), which is pleated in the cavity to stabilize the thumb (anchovy technique).

Table 4 Stages of scapholunate advanced collapse	
Stage 1	Osteoarthritic changes limited to the radial styloid
Stage 2	Osteoarthritic changes extending to the whole scaphoid fossa of the radius
Stage 3	Proximal migration of the capitate with osteoarthritic changes between the capitate and lunate

Data from Watson HK, Ballet FL. The SLAC wrist: scapholunate advanced collapse pattern of degenerative arthritis. J Hand Surg Am 1984;9(3):358-365.

Table 5 Stages of scaphoid nonunion advanced collapse	
Stage 1	Osteoarthritic changes limited to the radial styloid
Stage 2	Osteoarthritic extending between the distal scaphoid and capitate
Stage 3	Osteoarthritic changes between the capitate and lunate

Data from Moritomo H, Tada K, Yoshida T, et al. The relationship between the site of nonunion of the scaphoid and scaphoid nonunion advanced collapse (SNAC). J Bone Joint Surg Br 1999;81(5):871-876.

carpectomy, scaphoid excision with 4-corner arthrodesis, or total wrist arthrodesis depending on the stage and need for grip strength.[38]

Bone Abnormalities

Avascular necrosis of the scaphoid

Because the scaphoid is covered with cartilage over 75% of its surface, most of its vascularization derives from a branch of the radial artery entering the bone at the level of the waist and following a retrograde intraosseous path. Avascular necrosis complicates 13% to 50% of scaphoid fractures depending on their location (risk is high for the proximal third, moderate for the middle third, and low for the distal third) and displacement.[17,39] Coexistence with fracture nonunion is common, albeit occurrence of avascular necrosis after fracture consolidation has been described.[40] There is also an uncommon nontraumatic avascular necrosis of the scaphoid known as Preiser disease (Fig. 10).[41]

On radiographs, a denser appearance of the scaphoid proximal to the fracture line is frequently observed at follow-up, resulting from either the absence of physiologic carpal demineralization or true osteosclerosis. Its significance is uncertain, because it is not systematically associated with irreversible avascular necrosis.

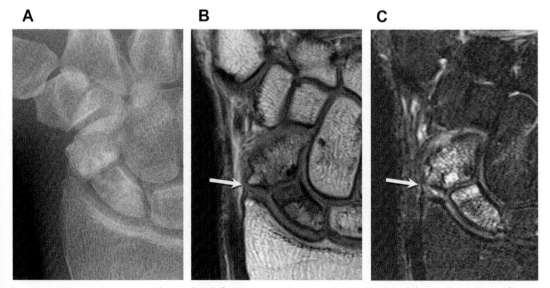

A   **B**   **C**

Fig. 9. A 24-year-old man with scaphoid fracture nonunion and SNAC-wrist. (*A*) PA view shows fracture nonunion. (*B, C*) Coronal T1-weighted and fat-suppressed T2-weighted MR images demonstrate signal abnormalities of the scaphoid (*arrow*) and early osteoarthritis (*arrow*) between the radial styloid and the distal portion of the scaphoid.

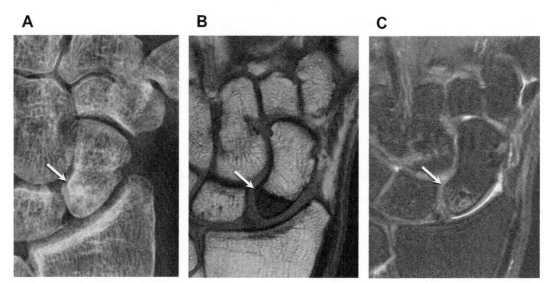

Fig. 10. A 57-year-old man with Preiser disease. (*A*) PA view shows a dense appearance of the proximal scaphoid (*arrow*) and no evidence of fracture. (*B, C*) Coronal T1-weighted and fat-suppressed T2-weighted MR images demonstrate the abnormal signal intensity of the proximal scaphoid (*arrows*).

MR imaging with administration of intravenous contrast media has been presented as a more reliable modality to assess for avascular necrosis of the scaphoid. The sensitivity and specificity vary greatly between studies, with divergent results regarding the usefulness of contrast administration and dynamic sequences as opposed to unenhanced sequences (**Fig. 11**).[42–46]

Tendinopathies

De Quervain tenosynovitis
Stenosing tenosynovitis of the first extensor compartment is the most frequent tenosynovitis of the wrist (**Fig. 12**). It is more frequent in women, noticeably in the postpartum period, where it is known as "baby wrist," but also affects people with different professional activities.

De Quervain tenosynovitis can be suspected on the radiographs in the presence of soft tissue swelling along the radial styloid and occasionally accompanying bone erosion.[47]

With MR imaging, there is a corresponding thickening and increased signal of the abductor longus and extensor brevis tendons and their retinaculum.[48] US is a valid alternative to MR imaging that offers superior spatial resolution and notably the capability to demonstrate an intracompartmental septum, which can have therapeutic implications.[49,50]

CENTRAL COLUMN OF THE WRIST
Helpful Radiographic Signs and Pitfalls

Gilula arcs
On a PA radiograph of the wrist, the proximal arc corresponds to the proximal aspect of the first carpal row; the second arc corresponds to the distal aspect of the first carpal row, and the distal arc corresponds to the proximal aspect of the capitate and hamate. These arcs are normally concentric and smooth, and any interruption, offset, or overlap should alert for a fracture or dislocation of the carpus.[16]

Sagittal alignment of the lunate
On a lateral view of the wrist, the lunate is normally aligned with the distal radius, capitate bone, and third metacarpal. Loss of this normal alignment should raise suspicion for wrist dislocation or perilunar instability.[16]

Fractures and Ligament Injuries

Perilunar dislocations and fractures
A pattern of traumatic perilunar instability implying the disruption of the ligamentous attachments (lesser-arc type) or fractures of the adjacent bones (greater-arc type) has been described, usually as a consequence of a high energy trauma. These lesions may remain clinically occult when other visceral or musculoskeletal injuries are at the forefront.[51,52]

These lesions should be recognized on radiographs, and a CT scan is usually performed secondarily for therapeutic planning. MR imaging is not required for the diagnosis, but may be performed for chronic pain and disability after a remote injury, and occasionally may reveal occult lesions (**Fig. 13**).

Bone Abnormalities

Kienböck disease
Avascular necrosis of the lunate is typically seen in young workers presenting with progressive pain, loss of grip strength, and mobility.

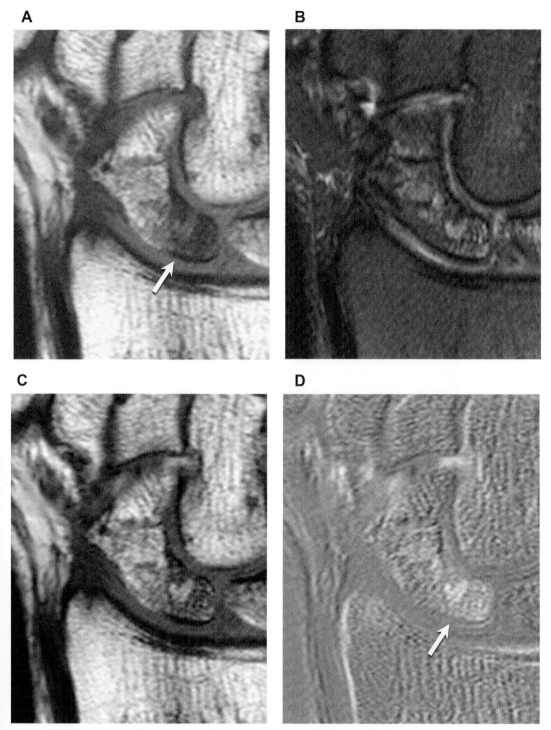

Fig. 11. A 45-year-old man followed up after bone graft for scaphoid fracture nonunion with concern for avascular necrosis. (*A–D*) Coronal T1-weighted, fat-suppressed T2-weighted, gadolinium-enhanced fat-suppressed T1-weighted and with subtraction MR images demonstrate hypointense T1 signal of the proximal pole (*arrows*) but persistent vascularization, which is better appreciated by subtracting the images (*A*) from (*C*).

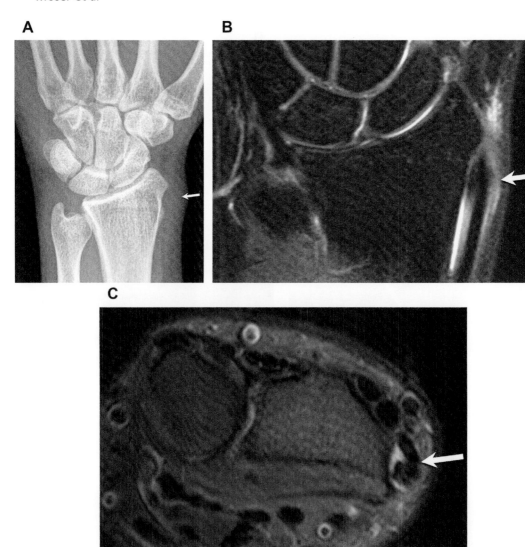

Fig. 12. A 41-year-old woman with radial-sided wrist pain. (*A*) PA view of the wrist demonstrates soft tissue swelling along the radial styloid and pressure erosion (*arrow*). (*B, C*) Coronal and transverse fat-saturated T2-weighted MR images confirm the presence of tenosynovitis of the first extensor compartment (*arrows*).

On radiographs, a negative ulnar variance is frequent as a contributory etiologic factor. The lunate appears normal at the earliest stage of the disease and demonstrates progressive osteosclerosis as well as fragmentation and collapse evolving toward radiocarpal and midcarpal osteoarthritis. These abnormalities are best described with the Lichtman classification (**Table 6**).[53]

With MR imaging, avascular necrosis can be demonstrated before radiographic abnormalities. Accompanying synovitis is frequent (**Fig. 14**).[54,55]

The carpal boss

The carpal boss manifests as a protuberance and occasional pain at the level of the carpometacarpal joint and is related to the presence of an accessory ossicle known as os styloideum, or sometimes osteophytes.

On radiographs, the abnormal bony protuberance articulating with the base of the third metacarpal can be recognized on the lateral and oblique views (**Fig. 15**).[56]

With MR imaging, associated abnormalities of the adjacent extensor carpi radialis brevis and longus tendons are infrequently seen.[57]

The carpal boss is the second cause of dorsal wrist lump after ganglion cysts (see **Fig. 7**). Other tumors can occasionally be revealed by a focal bulge of the soft tissues (**Fig. 16**).

Tendinopathies

Other tendinopathies of the extensor and flexor compartments owing to various causes (overuse,

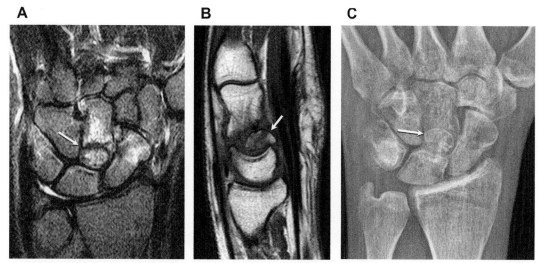

Fig. 13. A 22-year-old man presenting a few months after wrist trauma. (*A, B*) Coronal short-TI inversion recovery and sagittal T1-weighted MR images show bone marrow edema of the scaphoid and capitate (*arrows*). A transverse fracture of the capitate is associated with a rotation of its proximal pole. (*C*) PA view also demonstrates a subacute fracture of the scaphoid and the fracture of the capitate (*arrow*). This association is known as the scaphocapitate or Fenton syndrome.

inflammatory, sepsis, crystals) can present with symptoms along the central column. Radiographs are rarely contributive, and the diagnosis is usually made with MR imaging, or preferably US, which can also guide needle aspiration and therapeutic injections.

ULNAR COLUMN OF THE WRIST
Helpful Radiographic Signs and Pitfalls

The ulnar variance
The ulnar variance refers to the relative lengths of the distal radius and ulna. A normal neutral variance measures between +2 and −2 mm on a PA view with the wrist in neutral pronosupination (elbow flexed 90° and shoulder abducted 90°).[58] It is important to assess the ulnar variance in the presence of ulnar-sided wrist symptoms. A positive ulnar variance increases the load transmitted through the ulnocarpal joint and predisposes to ulnocarpal abutment syndrome (**Fig. 17**). A negative ulnar variance is associated with an increased radiolunate load, which has a role in the pathophysiology of Kienböck disease and is also seen with radioulnar impingement.[59] It is important to remember that ulnar variance changes with wrist position, being more positive in pronation and during a forceful grip, explaining the possibility of ulnocarpal abutment with an apparent neutral variance. This dynamic variation of the ulnar variance can be better evaluated with a pronated grip view of the wrist.[60]

As shown with carpal angles, there are discrepancies with the measurements of ulnar variance from MR images, and the radiographs remain the gold standard.[61]

The hook of hamate ring sign
The hook of the hamate is normally seen on the PA view of the wrist as an ovoid ring projecting over the hamate body (**Fig. 18**). An absent or poorly defined ring may indicate a fracture of the hook. An increased density of the ring may be seen with fracture nonunion and avascular necrosis.[62]

Table 6	
Lichtman classification of Kienböck disease	
Stage 1	Normal radiographs (abnormal MR imaging)
Stage 2	Lunate sclerosis without collapse
Stage 3	Lunate fragmentation and collapse A: With normal carpal height B: With decreased carpal height (flexed scaphoid)
Stage 4	Carpal osteoarthritis

From Lichtman DM, Degnan GG. Staging and its use in the determination of treatment modalities for Kienböck's disease. Hand Clin 1993;9(3):409-416; with permission.

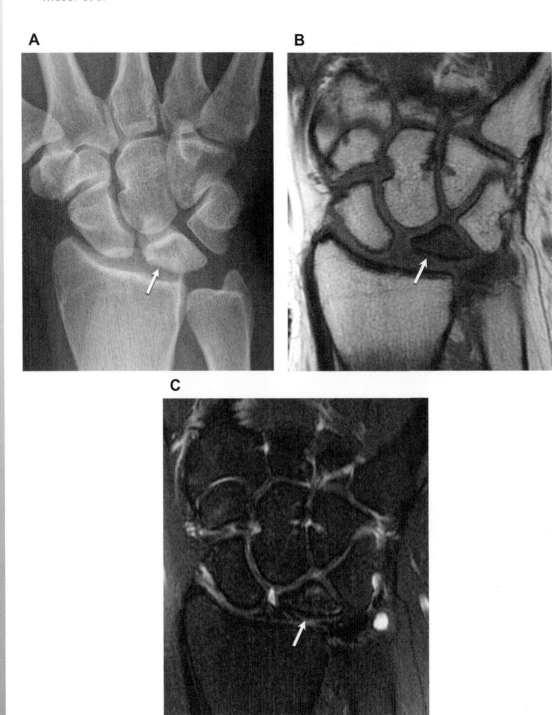

Fig. 14. A 21-year-old woman presenting with central wrist pain. (*A*) PA view shows moderate sclerosis of the lunate with a mild collapse of its proximal and radial aspect (*arrow*). (*B, C*) Coronal T1-weighted and fat-suppressed T2-weighted MR images demonstrate the abnormal signal intensity of the lunate and early collapse indicative of Kienböck disease stage 2 (*arrows*).

Fractures

Hook of the hamate fractures

Hook of the hamate fractures represent 2% of carpal fractures and are the most common type of hamate fractures. Different mechanisms, including direct trauma, avulsion, and stress, are responsible for these fractures, which are particularly frequent in sports involving a racket, club, stick, or bat. Based on their location, they are classified

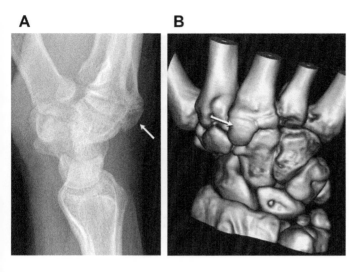

Fig. 15. A 49-year-old man with a dorsal tumefaction of the wrist. (*A*) Lateral view shows a bony prominence at the dorsal aspect of the carpometacarpal joint (*arrow*). (*B*) Volume-rendering CT better shows the supernumerary styloideum bone (*arrow*), articulating with the base of the third metacarpal, consistent with a carpal boss.

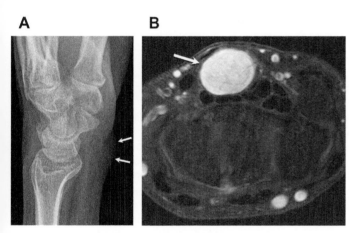

Fig. 16. A 42-year-old man with central wrist pain. (*A*) Lateral view shows a subtle bulge of the soft tissues at the anterior aspect of the wrist (*arrows*). (*B*) Transverse gadolinium-enhanced fat-suppressed T1-weighted MR image demonstrates a tumor of the median nerve (*arrow*) consistent with a schwannoma.

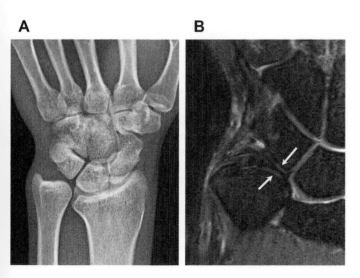

Fig. 17. A 25-year-old woman with chronic wrist pain. (*A*) PA view shows a markedly positive ulnar variance. (*B*) The corresponding coronal fat-suppressed T2-weighted MR image shows the stretching and thinning of the triangular fibrocartilage ligament (*arrows*) with no obvious tear or bone marrow edema.

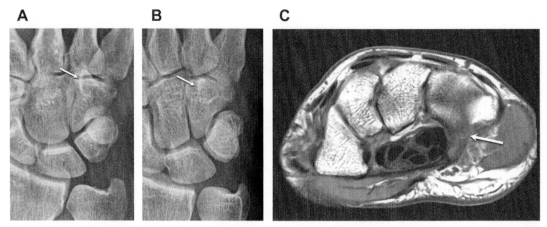

Fig. 18. The hook of hamate ring sign. (*A*) PA view shows a normal well-delineated hook of the hamate (ring sign) (*arrow*). (*B*) The margins of the ring (*arrow*) are less well defined in this 24-year-old man presenting after a fall. (*C*) The corresponding transverse proton density-weighted MR image shows a fracture of the hook of the hamate (*arrow*).

as type 1 (distal tip), type 2 (middle part), and type 3 (base of the hook). The type 3 accounts for 75% of these fractures.[63]

On radiographs, the diagnosis is difficult, especially if dedicated views (carpal tunnel, Papilion) are not obtained, with a reported sensitivity between 53% and 90%.[63]

CT is considered the standard reference with a sensitivity of nearly 100%. MR imaging performs equally well for acute fractures but could fail to detect chronic fractures or nonunion (**Fig. 19**).[63]

As a differential diagnosis, a bipartite hook of the hamate presents with round well-corticated margins on radiographs and CT and normal bone marrow signal with MR imaging.

Dorsal fractures of the triquetrum

The dorsal tubercle of the hamate gives insertion to the dorsal radiocarpal and intercarpal ligaments of the wrist.[64] Dorsal fracture of the triquetrum may result from an avulsion of these ligaments or from an impaction of the hamate or the ulnar styloid.[65,66]

With radiographs, a small displaced fragment can be seen at the dorsal aspect of the carpus on the lateral view. Nondisplaced fractures are easily overlooked.[39]

With MR imaging, bone marrow edema is inconsistent, and a small fragment can remain unnoticed; however, associated ligament tears are frequently depicted.[67]

Other fractures

Fractures involving the pisiform, the hamate body, the base of the fifth metacarpal may also be encountered in the setting of posttraumatic ulnar-sided wrist pain.

Ligament Injuries

Lesions of the triangular fibrocartilage ligament complex

The triangular fibrocartilage complex (TFCC) encompasses different structures providing stability to the distal radioulnar joint and ulnocarpal compartment.[68] Lesions of these structures can be traumatic or degenerative, and the classification of Palmer separates these into class I and class II, respectively (**Fig. 20, Table 7**).[69]

On radiographs, lesions of the TFCC can be suspected in the presence of a positive ulnar variance and signs of ulnocarpal impingement, a subluxation of the distal radioulnar joint, or a fracture nonunion of the ulnar styloid (**Fig. 21**).

With routine MR imaging, it is often difficult to assess adequately the different structures of the TFCC. The ulnar insertion of the triangular fibrocartilage is particularly challenging because of the ligamentum subcruentum, which can mimic a tear, with a sensitivity as low as 17% in one study.[70,71] For this reason, CT arthrography or MR arthrography should be preferred when these structures have to be evaluated.[9,11,72] With these imaging modalities, it is important to opacify the distal radioulnar compartment in order to demonstrate partial-thickness lesions at the proximal aspect of the TFCC.[73]

Lunotriquetral ligament injuries

Traumatic lunotriquetral injuries are much less frequent than their scapholunate counterpart.

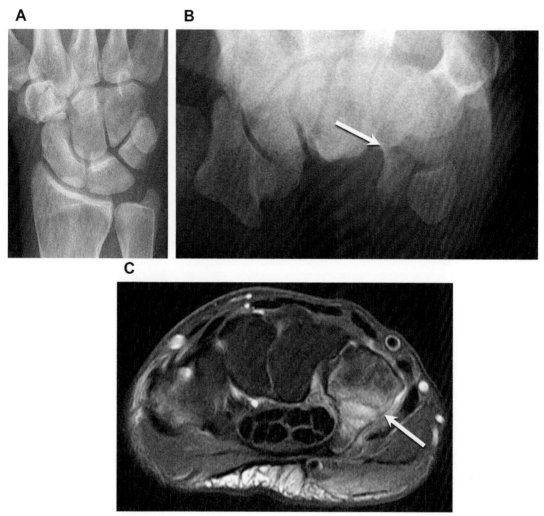

Fig. 19. A 66-year-old man presenting after a fall. (*A*) The PA view appears normal. (*B*) The carpal tunnel view reveals a fracture at the base of the hook of the hamate (*arrow*). (*C*) This fracture (*arrow*) is confirmed on the transverse fat-suppressed T2-weighted MR image.

Their diagnosis is mostly based on MR arthrography and CT arthrography.[9,72]

Arthropathies and Impingement Syndromes

Radioulnar impingement syndrome

Caused by a short ulna, which can be idiopathic, caused by skeletal growth disturbance (juvenile arthritis, hereditary multiple exostosis), or more frequently after surgical resection, radioulnar impingement syndrome is characterized by a radioulnar convergence with an abnormal distal radioulnar joint and progressive erosion of the radius (**Fig. 22**). The diagnosis is usually based on radiographs.[74]

Ulnocarpal impingement syndrome

Ulnocarpal impingement syndrome is the most common impingement syndrome of the

wrist and a frequent cause of ulnar-sided wrist pain (see **Fig. 21**). The positive ulnar variance can be constitutional or acquired, most frequently by posttraumatic shortening of the radius.

With radiographs, it is possible to observe a positive ulnar variance, subchondral cysts, and sclerosis involving the ulnar head, the medial aspect of the lunate, or the radial aspect of the triquetrum.[75]

With MR imaging, ulnocarpal impingement syndrome is well recognized in the presence of bone marrow edema in these same locations, by order of frequency the medial lunate (87%), the radial triquetrum (43%), and the ulnar head (10%).[74–76]

Styloidotriquetral impingement syndrome

In this an uncommon syndrome, a prominent ulnar styloid impinges on the medial aspect of the

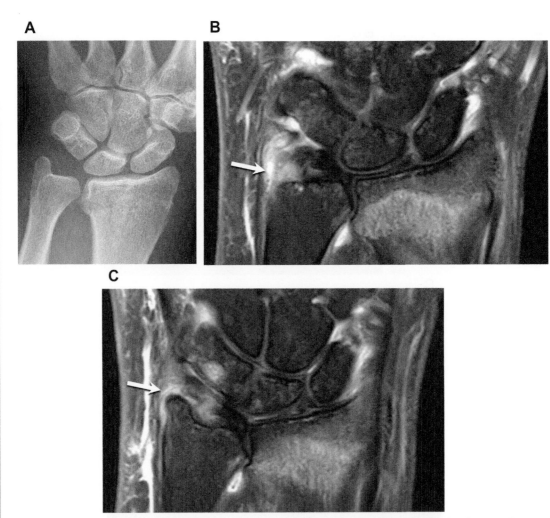

Fig. 20. A 49-year-old man complaining of ulnar-sided wrist pain 2 months after a distal radius fracture. (*A*) Initial PA view of the wrist shows a nondisplaced distal radius fracture. (*B, C*) Coronal fat-suppressed T2-weighted MR images show an ulnar avulsion of the triangular fibrocartilage ligament in addition to the distal radius fracture (*arrows*).

Table 7 Palmer classification of triangular fibrocartilage complex injuries	
Class I (traumatic)	A: Central tear B: Ulnar avulsion C: Distal avulsion D: Radial avulsion

Class II
(degenerative)
	A: Central wear
	B: Central wear + lunate
	  or triquetrum
	  chondromalacia
	C: Central perforation
	D: Additional lunotriquetral
	  ligament perforation
	E: ulnocarpal osteoarthritis

Adapted from Palmer AK. Triangular fibrocartilage complex lesions: a classification. J Hand Surg Am 1989;14(4):596; with permission.

carpus, mostly the triquetrum, during ulnar deviation (**Fig. 23**).

With radiographs, it is possible to recognize an unusually long or large ulnar styloid, and occasionally, intraarticular loose bodies. MR imaging can demonstrate bone marrow edema of the ulnar styloid and triquetrum.[75]

Hamatolunate impingement syndrome
Hamatolunate impingement corresponds to osteoarthritic changes between the hamate and the lunate, occurring in the presence of a type 2 lunate with an extra facet articulating with the hamate (**Fig. 24**). Imaging can demonstrate cartilage ulceration and subchondral changes at the proximal aspect of the hamate.[77,78]

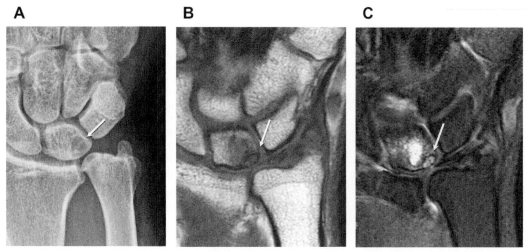

Fig. 21. A 51-year-old man with chronic ulnar-sided wrist pain. (*A*) The PA view of the wrist demonstrates a positive ulnar variance and subchondral cysts of the distal ulna and medial lunate (*arrow*). (*B, C*) Coronal T1 and fat-suppressed T2-weighted MR images from a 57-year-old woman show corresponding signal abnormalities of the lunate (*arrow*) and a central perforation of the triangular fibrocartilage (*arrow*).

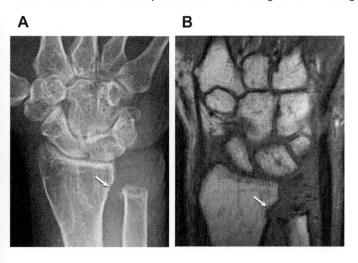

Fig. 22. A 53-year-old woman with ulnar-sided wrist pain after surgery. (*A*) PA view of the wrist indicates prior resection of the distal ulna (Darrach procedure) and shows a small erosion of the radius proximal to the sigmoid notch (*arrow*). (*B*) Coronal T1-weighted MR image better demonstrates the erosion (*arrow*), which is consistent with radioulnar impingement syndrome.

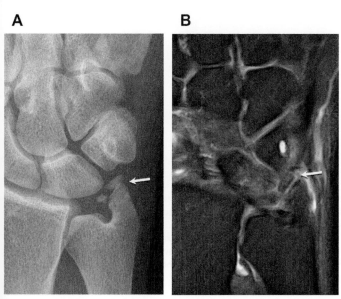

Fig. 23. A 26-year-old tennis player with ulnar-sided wrist pain. (*A*) PA view of the wrist shows bone fragments around the ulnar styloid (*arrow*). (*B*) Coronal fat-suppressed T2-weighted MR image shows additional bone marrow edema of the ulnar styloid and triquetrum and synovitis (*arrow*), consistent with styloidotriquetral impingement syndrome.

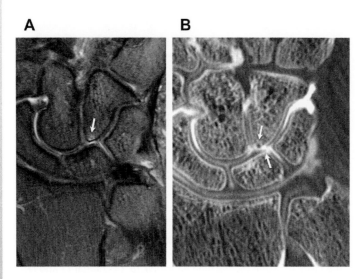

Fig. 24. A 52-year-old man with ulnar-sided wrist pain. (*A*) Coronal fat-suppressed T2-weighted MR image shows subtle subchondral edema of the proximal hamate (*arrow*). (*B*) Corresponding coronal CT arthrography image better demonstrates cartilage ulceration of the hamate and accessory lunate facet (*arrows*), indicative of hamatolunate impingement syndrome in the absence of other significant lesions.

Bone Abnormalities

Lunotriquetral coalition

Congenital fusion of the lunate and triquetrum is the most common synostosis of the wrist and is often bilateral (**Fig. 25**). It is usually an asymptomatic incidental imaging finding. Complete lunotriquetral coalition is frequently associated with a wider scapholunate space, which should not be mistaken for scapholunate ligament tear.[79] Incomplete fibrous or fibrocartilage coalitions are similar to a pseudoarthrosis and may be symptomatic.[80]

Tendinopathies

Extensor carpi ulnaris tendinopathy and instability

Because of its situation in the ulnar groove, the extensor carpi ulnaris tendon undergoes considerable stress during pronosupination and is prone to injuries such as tenosynovitis, tears, and instability (**Fig. 26**). It is also frequently involved in inflammatory arthropathies.

With radiographs, it is possible to observe soft tissue swelling and bone erosions at the

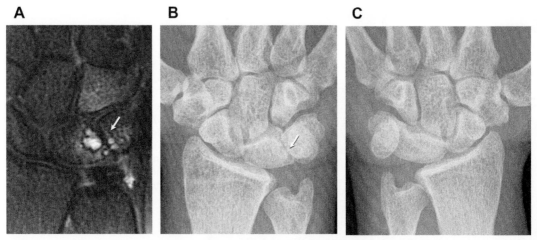

Fig. 25. A 38-year-old woman with ulnar-sided left wrist pain. (*A*) Coronal fat-suppressed T2-weighted MR image shows subchondral edema and cysts on both sides of the lunotriquetral joint and at the proximal hamate (*arrow*). An inflammatory arthropathy was considered based on MR imaging findings. (*B*) Corresponding PA view demonstrates narrowing and irregularities of the lunotriquetral joint space and proximal hamate erosion (*arrow*). No other abnormalities were evidenced at the rheumatological workup. (*C*) PA view of the right wrist demonstrates a complete lunotriquetral coalition. Therefore, the most likely diagnosis for the left wrist was incomplete lunotriquetral coalition and hamatolunate impingement.

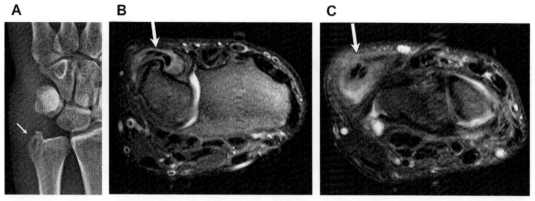

Fig. 26. A 39-year-old woman with ulnar-sided left wrist pain. (*A*) PA view of the wrist shows soft tissue swelling and erosion of the ulnar styloid (*arrow*). (*B, C*) Transverse fat-suppressed T2-weighted MR images show tenosynovitis, subluxation, and splitting of the extensor carpi ulnaris tendon (*arrows*).

ulnar styloid and the base of the fifth metacarpal. MR imaging better demonstrates the abnormalities of the tendon and its subsheath.[81]

Flexor carpi ulnaris tendinopathy

The flexor carpi ulnaris is another tendon frequently involved in ulnar-sided wrist pain (**Fig. 27**). It is usually an insertional tendinopathy because it has no synovial sheath and is frequently associated with hydroxyapatite deposition disease. The semisupinated oblique view is particularly useful to assess its insertion on the pisiform.[82]

COMMON PITFALLS
Calcium Apatite Deposition Disease

Inflammatory changes caused by the resorption of calcifications are frequently misleading with MR imaging and may be mistaken for infection or tumor (**Fig. 28**). Because calcifications are often unapparent on MR images, systematic correlation with radiographs is key.[83]

Undetermined Bone Marrow Edema

Demonstration of bone marrow edema with MR imaging is often helpful to pinpoint a lesion, and many of these have been discussed in the previous paragraphs. A few other causes can be challenging to diagnose and are worth mentioning: bone contusion, inflammatory arthropathies, osteomyelitis and septic joint, complex regional pain syndrome, and osteoid osteoma. Radiographic correlation remains essential and may be supplemented by CT in select cases.[84]

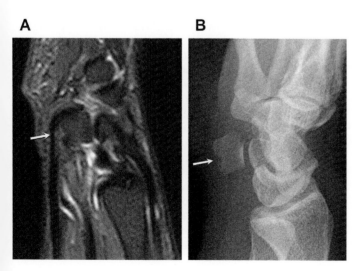

Fig. 27. A 44-year-old woman with ulnar-sided left wrist pain. (*A*) Sagittal fat-suppressed T2-weighted MR image shows a subtle signal abnormality of the pisiform at the insertion of the flexor carpi ulnaris tendon (*arrow*). (*B*) Semisupination oblique view better demonstrates bone erosion (*arrow*) indicative of insertional tendinopathy.

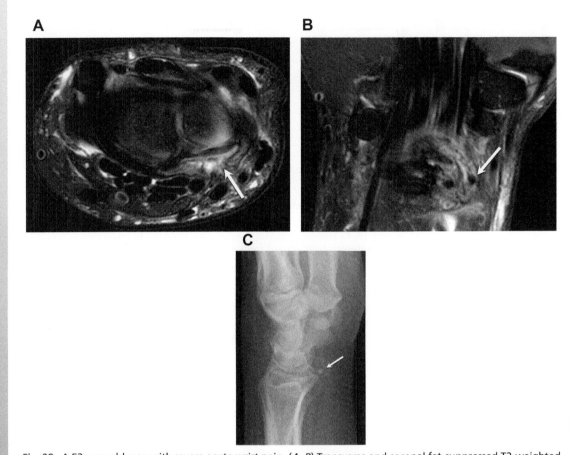

Fig. 28. A 53-year-old man with severe acute wrist pain. (*A, B*) Transverse and coronal fat-suppressed T2-weighted MR images show inflammatory changes involving the volar articular wrist capsule along the radiolunotriquetral and radioscaphocapitate ligaments (*arrows*). (*C*) Lateral view better demonstrates ill-defined calcifications (*arrow*) indicative of hydroxyapatite deposition disease at the resorption stage.

REFERENCES

1. Kauer JM. Functional anatomy of the wrist. Clin Orthop Relat Res 1980;(149):9–20.
2. Lee RK, Griffith JF, Ng AW, et al. Imaging of radial wrist pain. I. Imaging modalities and anatomy. Skeletal Radiol 2014;43(6):713–24.
3. Watanabe A, Souza F, Vezeridis PS, et al. Ulnar-sided wrist pain. II. Clinical imaging and treatment. Skeletal Radiol 2010;39(9):837–57.
4. Dalinka MK, Alazraki N, Berquist TH, et al. Chronic wrist pain. American College of Radiology. ACR Appropriateness Criteria. Radiology 2000; 215(Suppl):333–8.
5. Newberg A, Dalinka MK, Alazraki N, et al. Acute hand and wrist trauma. American College of Radiology. ACR Appropriateness Criteria. Radiology 2000;215(Suppl):375–8.
6. Gilula LA, Weeks PM. Post-traumatic ligamentous instabilities of the wrist. Radiology 1978;129(3): 641–51.
7. Demondion X, Boutry N, Khalil C, et al. Les radiographies simples du poignet et de la main. J Radiol 2008;89(5 Pt 2):640–51 [quiz: 652–3].
8. Stevens KJ, Wallace CG, Chen W, et al. Imaging of the wrist at 1.5 Tesla using isotropic three-dimensional fast spin echo cube. J Magn Reson Imaging 2011;33(4):908–15.
9. Moser T, Dosch JC, Moussaoui A, et al. Wrist ligament tears: evaluation of MRI and combined MDCT and MR arthrography. AJR Am J Roentgenol 2007;188(5):1278–86.
10. Moser T, Dosch JC, Moussaoui A, et al. Multidetector CT arthrography of the wrist joint: how to do it. Radiographics 2008;28(3):787–800 [quiz: 911].
11. Moser T, Khoury V, Harris PG, et al. MDCT arthrography or MR arthrography for imaging the wrist joint? Semin Musculoskelet Radiol 2009;13(1):39–54.
12. Terry DW Jr, Ramin JE. The navicular fat stripe: a useful roentgen feature for evaluating wrist trauma. Am J Roentgenol Radium Ther Nucl Med 1975; 124(1):25–8.

13. Macewan DW. Changes due to trauma in the fat plane overlying the pronator quadratus muscle: a radiologic sign. Radiology 1964;82:879–86.

14. Annamalai G, Raby N. Scaphoid and pronator fat stripes are unreliable soft tissue signs in the detection of radiographically occult fractures. Clin Radiol 2003;58(10):798–800.

15. Crittenden JJ, Jones DM, Santarelli AG. Bilateral rotational dislocation of the carpal navicular. Case report. Radiology 1970;94(3):629–30.

16. Gilula LA. Carpal injuries: analytic approach and case exercises. AJR Am J Roentgenol 1979; 133(3):503–17.

17. Taljanovic MS, Karantanas A, Griffith JF, et al. Imaging and treatment of scaphoid fractures and their complications. Semin Musculoskelet Radiol 2012; 16(2):159–73.

18. Balci A, Basara I, Cekdemir EY, et al. Wrist fractures: sensitivity of radiography, prevalence, and patterns in MDCT. Emerg Radiol 2015;22(3):251–6.

19. Edlund R, Skorpil M, Lapidus G, et al. Cone-beam CT in diagnosis of scaphoid fractures. Skeletal Radiol 2016;45(2):197–204.

20. Breitenseher MJ, Metz VM, Gilula LA, et al. Radiographically occult scaphoid fractures: value of MR imaging in detection. Radiology 1997;203(1): 245–50.

21. Hunter JC, Escobedo EM, Wilson AJ, et al. MR imaging of clinically suspected scaphoid fractures. AJR Am J Roentgenol 1997;168(5):1287–93.

22. Stevenson JD, Morley D, Srivastava S, et al. Early CT for suspected occult scaphoid fractures. J Hand Surg Eur Vol 2012;37(5):447–51.

23. Memarsadeghi M, Breitenseher MJ, Schaefer-Prokop C, et al. Occult scaphoid fractures: comparison of multidetector CT and MR imaging–initial experience. Radiology 2006;240(1):169–76.

24. Mallee W, Doornberg JN, Ring D, et al. Comparison of CT and MRI for diagnosis of suspected scaphoid fractures. J Bone Joint Surg Am 2011; 93(1):20–8.

25. De Zwart AD, Beeres FJ, Ring D, et al. MRI as a reference standard for suspected scaphoid fractures. Br J Radiol 2012;85(1016):1098–101.

26. Meade TD, Schneider LH, Cherry K. Radiographic analysis of selective ligament sectioning at the carpal scaphoid: a cadaver study. J Hand Surg Am 1990;15(6):855–62.

27. Short WH, Werner FW, Fortino MD, et al. A dynamic biomechanical study of scapholunate ligament sectioning. J Hand Surg 1995;20(6):986–99.

28. Tan S, Ghumman SS, Ladouceur M, et al. Carpal angles as measured on CT and MRI: can we simply translate radiographic measurements? Skeletal Radiol 2014;43(12):1721–8.

29. Schmid M, Schertler T, Pfirrmann C, et al. Interosseous ligament tears of the wrist: comparison of multi-detector row CT arthrography and MR imaging. Radiology 2005;237(3):1008–13.

30. Overstraeten LV, Camus EJ, Wahegaonkar A, et al. Anatomical description of the dorsal capsulo-scapholunate septum (DCSS)-arthroscopic staging of scapholunate instability after DCSS sectioning. J Wrist Surg 2013;2(2):149–54.

31. Cardinal E, Buckwalter KA, Braunstein EM, et al. Occult dorsal carpal ganglion: comparison of US and MR imaging. Radiology 1994;193(1):259–62.

32. Freire V, Guerini H, Campagna R, et al. Imaging of hand and wrist cysts: a clinical approach. AJR Am J Roentgenol 2012;199(5):W618–28.

33. Alnot JY, Muller GP. A retrospective review of 115 cases of surgically-treated trapeziometacarpal osteoarthritis. Rev Rhum Engl Ed 1998;65(2):95–108.

34. Eaton RG, Littler JW. Ligament reconstruction for the painful thumb carpometacarpal joint. J Bone Joint Surg Am 1973;55(8):1655–66.

35. Watson HK, Ballet FL. The SLAC wrist: scapholunate advanced collapse pattern of degenerative arthritis. J Hand Surg 1984;9(3):358–65.

36. Chen C, Chandnani VP, Kang HS, et al. Scapholunate advanced collapse: a common wrist abnormality in calcium pyrophosphate dihydrate crystal deposition disease. Radiology 1990;177(2):459–61.

37. Moritomo H, Tada K, Yoshida T, et al. The relationship between the site of nonunion of the scaphoid and scaphoid nonunion advanced collapse (SNAC). J Bone Joint Surg Br 1999;81(5):871–6.

38. Dacho AK, Baumeister S, Germann G, et al. Comparison of proximal row carpectomy and midcarpal arthrodesis for the treatment of scaphoid nonunion advanced collapse (SNAC-wrist) and scapholunate advanced collapse (SLAC-wrist) in stage II. J Plast Reconstr Aesthet Surg 2008;61(10):1210–8.

39. Kaewlai R, Avery LL, Asrani AV, et al. Multidetector CT of carpal injuries: anatomy, fractures, and fracture-dislocations. Radiographics 2008;28(6): 1771–84.

40. Filan SL, Herbert TJ. Avascular necrosis of the proximal scaphoid after fracture union. J Hand Surg 1995;20(4):551–6.

41. Allen PR. Idiopathic avascular necrosis of the scaphoid. A report of two cases. J Bone Joint Surg Br 1983;65(3):333–5.

42. Fox MG, Gaskin CM, Chhabra AB, et al. Assessment of scaphoid viability with MRI: a reassessment of findings on unenhanced MR images. AJR Am J Roentgenol 2010;195(4):W281–6.

43. Schmitt R, Christopoulos G, Wagner M, et al. Avascular necrosis (AVN) of the proximal fragment in scaphoid nonunion: is intravenous contrast agent necessary in MRI? Eur J Radiol 2011; 77(2):222–7.

44. Ng AW, Griffith JF, Taljanovic MS, et al. Is dynamic contrast-enhanced MRI useful for assessing

proximal fragment vascularity in scaphoid fracture delayed and non-union? Skeletal Radiol 2013; 42(7):983–92.

45. Larribe M, Gay A, Freire V, et al. Usefulness of dynamic contrast-enhanced MRI in the evaluation of the viability of acute scaphoid fracture. Skeletal Radiol 2014;43(12):1697–703.

46. Fox MG, Wang DT, Chhabra AB. Accuracy of enhanced and unenhanced MRI in diagnosing scaphoid proximal pole avascular necrosis and predicting surgical outcome. Skeletal Radiol 2015; 44(11):1671–8.

47. Chien AJ, Jacobson JA, Martel W, et al. Focal radial styloid abnormality as a manifestation of de Quervain tenosynovitis. AJR Am J Roentgenol 2001; 177(6):1383–6.

48. Meraj S, Gyftopoulos S, Nellans K, et al. MRI of the extensor tendons of the wrist. AJR Am J Roentgenol 2017;209(5):1093–102.

49. Rousset P, Vuillemin-Bodaghi V, Laredo JD, et al. Anatomic variations in the first extensor compartment of the wrist: accuracy of US. Radiology 2010; 257(2):427–33.

50. Choi SJ, Ahn JH, Lee YJ, et al. de Quervain disease: US identification of anatomic variations in the first extensor compartment with an emphasis on subcompartmentalization. Radiology 2011;260(2): 480–6.

51. Johnson RP. The acutely injured wrist and its residuals. Clin Orthop Relat Res 1980;Jun(149): 33–44.

52. Mayfield JK. Patterns of injury to carpal ligaments. A spectrum. Clin Orthop Relat Res 1984;(187): 36–42.

53. Lichtman DM, Degnan GG. Staging and its use in the determination of treatment modalities for Kienbock's disease. Hand Clin 1993;9(3):409–16.

54. Arnaiz J, Piedra T, Cerezal L, et al. Imaging of Kienbock disease. AJR Am J Roentgenol 2014;203(1): 131–9.

55. White C, Benhaim P, Plotkin B. Treatments for Kienbock disease: what the radiologist needs to know. Skeletal Radiol 2016;45(4):531–40.

56. Conway WF, Destouet JM, Gilula LA, et al. The carpal boss: an overview of radiographic evaluation. Radiology 1985;156(1):29–31.

57. Ghatan AC, Carlson EJ, Athanasian EA, et al. Attrition or rupture of digital extensor tendons due to carpal boss: report of 2 cases. J Hand Surg 2014;39(5): 919–22.

58. Palmer AK, Glisson RR, Werner FW. Ulnar variance determination. J Hand Surg Am 1982;7(4): 376–9.

59. Werner FW, Palmer AK, Fortino MD, et al. Force transmission through the distal ulna: effect of ulnar variance, lunate fossa angulation, and radial and palmar tilt of the distal radius. J Hand Surg 1992; 17(3):423–8.

60. Tomaino MM. The importance of the pronated grip x-ray view in evaluating ulnar variance. J Hand Surg 2000;25(2):352–7.

61. Kadzielski J, Qureshi AA, Han R, et al. Compared with magnetic resonance imaging, radiographs underestimate the magnitude of negative ulnar variance. Am J Orthop (Belle Mead NJ) 2014;43(3): 128–31.

62. Norman A, Nelson J, Green S. Fractures of the hook of hamate: radiographic signs. Radiology 1985; 154(1):49–53.

63. Davis DL. Hook of the Hamate: the spectrum of often missed pathologic findings. AJR Am J Roentgenol 2017;209(5):1110–8.

64. Viegas SF. The dorsal ligaments of the wrist. Hand Clin 2001;17(1):65–75.

65. Hocker K, Menschik A. Chip fractures of the triquetrum. Mechanism, classification and results. J Hand Surg 1994;19(5):584–8.

66. Levy M, Fischel RE, Stern GM, et al. Chip fractures of the os triquetrum: the mechanism of injury. J Bone Joint Surg Br 1979;61-B(3):355–7.

67. Becce F, Theumann N, Bollmann C, et al. Dorsal fractures of the triquetrum: MRI findings with an emphasis on dorsal carpal ligament injuries. AJR Am J Roentgenol 2013;200(3):608–17.

68. Palmer AK, Werner FW. The triangular fibrocartilage complex of the wrist–anatomy and function. J Hand Surg Am 1981;6(2):153–62.

69. Palmer AK. Triangular fibrocartilage complex lesions: a classification. J Hand Surg 1989;14(4): 594–606.

70. Haims AH, Schweitzer ME, Morrison WB, et al. Limitations of MR imaging in the diagnosis of peripheral tears of the triangular fibrocartilage of the wrist. AJR Am J Roentgenol 2002;178(2):419–22.

71. Burns JE, Tanaka T, Ueno T, et al. Pitfalls that may mimic injuries of the triangular fibrocartilage and proximal intrinsic wrist ligaments at MR imaging. Radiographics 2011;31(1):63–78.

72. Schmitt R, Christopoulos G, Meier R, et al. Direct MR arthrography of the wrist in comparison with arthroscopy: a prospective study on 125 patients. Rofo 2003;175(7):911–9.

73. Ruegger C, Schmid M, Pfirrmann C, et al. Peripheral tear of the triangular fibrocartilage: depiction with MR arthrography of the distal radioulnar joint. AJR Am J Roentgenol 2007;188(1):187–92.

74. Cerezal L, del Pinal F, Abascal F, et al. Imaging findings in ulnar-sided wrist impaction syndromes. Radiographics 2002;22(1):105–21.

75. Escobedo EM, Bergman AG, Hunter JC. MR imaging of ulnar impaction. Skeletal Radiol 1995;24(2): 85–90.

76. Imaeda T, Nakamura R, Shionoya K, et al. Ulnar impaction syndrome: MR imaging findings. Radiology 1996;201(2):495–500.

77. Malik AM, Schweitzer ME, Culp RW, et al. MR imaging of the type II lunate bone: frequency, extent, and associated findings. AJR Am J Roentgenol 1999;173(2):335–8.

78. Pfirrmann CW, Theumann NH, Chung CB, et al. The hamatolunate facet: characterization and association with cartilage lesions–magnetic resonance arthrography and anatomic correlation in cadaveric wrists. Skeletal Radiol 2002;31(8):451–6.

79. Metz VM, Schimmerl SM, Gilula LA, et al. Wide scapholunate joint space in lunotriquetral coalition: a normal variant? Radiology 1993;188(2):557–9.

80. Ritt MJ, Maas M, Bos KE. Minnaar type 1 symptomatic lunotriquetral coalition: a report of nine patients. J Hand Surg 2001;26(2):261–70.

81. Jeantroux J, Becce F, Guerini H, et al. Athletic injuries of the extensor carpi ulnaris subsheath: MRI findings and utility of gadolinium-enhanced fat-saturated T1-weighted sequences with wrist pronation and supination. Eur Radiol 2011;21(1):160–6.

82. Gandee RW, Harrison RB, Dee PM. Peritendinitis calcarea of flexor carpi ulnaris. AJR Am J Roentgenol 1979;133(6):1139–41.

83. Freire V, Moser TP, Lepage-Saucier M. Radiological identification and analysis of soft tissue musculoskeletal calcifications. Insights Imaging 2018;9(4):477–92.

84. Al Shaikhi A, Hebert-Davies J, Moser T, et al. Osteoid osteoma of the capitate: a case report and literature review. Eplasty 2009;9:e38.

Radiographic/MR Imaging Correlation of Spinal Bony Outlines

Timothy Woo, MBChB, MA, FRCR[a], Prudencia N.M. Tyrrell, MBBCh, BAO, FRCR[a],
Antonello Leone, MD[b], Francesco Pio Cafarelli, MD[c], Giuseppe Guglielmi, MD[c,d],
Victor Cassar-Pullicino, LRCP, MRCS, DMRD, FRCR, MD[a,*]

KEYWORDS

- Magnetic resonance imaging • Radiograph • Scoliosis • Spinal alignment • Spine

KEY POINTS

- Plain radiographs and MR images both have distinct strengths and weaknesses in the imaging of the spine.
- Disease processes predominantly affecting bone marrow or soft tissue can be difficult to detect on radiographs unless they affect the cortical outline, at which point changes on MR imaging are often extensive.
- Certain findings obvious on radiographs such as bony fusion and syndesmophyte formation can be difficult to discern on MR imaging.
- Radiographs have an advantage over MR imaging in assessing spinal alignment because they can be acquired erect and dynamic flexion examinations can also help in curve assessment. However, MR imaging is superior in assessing the neuraxis in these patients.

INTRODUCTION

The human spine is a highly specialized structure normally consisting of 33 bony elements and supporting soft tissues that support the body and protect the spinal cord and nerve roots while allowing remarkable flexibility and force distribution. The 24 mobile vertebrae with the exception of the atlas and axis consist of a roughly cylindrical body bounded at the cranial and caudal aspects by the "end plates," thin osseous and hyaline cartilage structures loosely connected to the underlying vertebra but closely associated with the fibrocartilaginous intervertebral discs,[1] which act to absorb and distribute axial load. Connected to the body by 2 pedicles, the posterior elements of the vertebrae serve as surfaces for articulation and ligamentous and muscular attachments.

The earliest documented imaging of the vertebral column dates to 1897, when a radiograph was used to locate a bullet lodged in the spine of a patient with Brown-Sequard syndrome by Harvey Cushing.[2] Imaging of the spine initially aimed to delineate the appearances and alignment of the bony structures of the spine, especially in blunt and penetrating trauma. However, the complex morphology of the vertebral bodies made accurate delineation of subtle abnormalities

Disclosure Statement: The authors report no conflicts of interest.
[a] Department of Radiology, Robert Jones and Agnes Hunt Orthopaedic Hospital NHS Foundation Trust, Oswestry SY10 7aG, UK; [b] Institute of Radiology, Catholic University, School of Medicine, Fondazione Policlinico Universitario A. Gemelli, IRCSS, 00168 Rome, Italy; [c] Department of Clinical and Experimental Medicine, Foggia University School of Medicine, Viale L. Pinto, 1, 71122 Foggia, Italy; [d] Department of Radiology, Scientific Institute Hospital "Casa Sollievo della Sofferenza", Viale Cappuccini, 1, 71014 San Giovanni Rotondo, Italy
* Corresponding author.
E-mail address: Victor.Pullicino@nhs.net

Magn Reson Imaging Clin N Am 27 (2019) 625–640
https://doi.org/10.1016/j.mric.2019.07.004

and injuries difficult to demonstrate on planar radiographs and soft tissue abnormalities were often completely occult.

It was not until MR imaging was realized in 1973 that the spinal soft tissues and neuraxis were directly visualized for the first time. Diagnostic images of the spine began to be documented in the early 1980s when the first clinical superconducting magnets were installed.[3] Since this time, MR imaging has completely revolutionized how the spine is investigated.

Today, imaging investigation of the spine consists of a multimodality approach of X-ray–based images and MR imaging. Plain radiographs afford a far greater resolution to detect structural change and can be acquired with the spine loaded to accurately delineate alignment, but MR imaging allows for the detection of subtle disturbances in soft tissues and bone marrow early on in disease and can demonstrate further lesions that may be occult on radiographs.

Radiography and MR imaging are therefore highly complementary with distinct strengths and weaknesses. In this review, we focus on nontraumatic conditions of the spine in which both plain radiographs and MR images play an important role and the correlation between modalities.

VERTEBRAL BODY

The vertebral body is the cylindrical anterior part of the C3 to L5 vertebrae and consists of a thin layer of compact bone enclosing cancellous bone occupied by highly hematopoietic red marrow. The anterior and posterior cortices are associated with the anterior and posterior longitudinal ligaments. The anterior longitudinal ligament is strongly associated with the anterior vertebral body periosteum, whereas the posterior longitudinal ligament is attached to the disc annulus and the superior and inferior vertebral corners corresponding to the location of the fused apophyseal growth centers.[4]

Radiographically, the vertebral body demonstrates slight concavity of the superior, inferior, and anterior aspects caused by the fusion of the ring apophyses to the centrum at skeletal maturity. There is normally a small cortical gap posteriorly corresponding with the foramen for the basivertebral vein(s). The cortical outline on radiographs is diagnostically most valuable and subtle cortical defects on radiographs can correspond to extensive MR imaging abnormalities within the cancellous bone occult radiographically. This finding is especially the case with sacral lesions.

On MR imaging, the vertebral body shows a low signal rim corresponding with compact bone and a variable signal marrow space depending on sequence and on the hematopoietic state of the marrow. However, the signal of the marrow on T1-weighted spin echo imaging is usually of higher signal than the corresponding disc or adjacent muscle.[5] A heterogenous marrow signal intensity is common in normal patients and can reflect hematopoietic foci in background yellow marrow, which sometimes can make interpretation difficult.[6]

Expanded or Eroded/Destroyed

An expanded or focally deficient contour implies a bone lesion or altered marrow process. Infection, which can also cause cortical erosion, is discussed in greater depth elsewhere in this article.

Vertebral body expansion can be due to benign processes or alternatively primary or metastatic malignancy. Plain radiographs can be helpful along with clinical and demographic information in narrowing the differential diagnosis. MR images may not add to the diagnosis of the primary lesion, but may reveal other radiologically occult lesions and delineate any soft tissue component or neuraxis impingement.

On plain radiographs, several features should be noted. The periphery of benign lesions is often sclerotic and narrow, whereas ill-defined destructive lesions are more likely to be aggressive. Some tumors such as giant cell tumors, hemangiomas, and myeloma favor the body over the posterior neural arch.[7] The presence of multiple levels of disease can also be helpful in narrowing the differential, with the most likely causes of multifocal or diffuse abnormality being metastases or hematological malignancy such as myeloma, whereas contiguous involvement generally tends to favor infection. In certain cases, plain radiography can be pathognomonic, such as in the picture frame appearance of Paget's disease (Fig. 1).

Compressed

Loss of height of a vertebral body on a radiograph implies a vertebral compression fracture, although normal variants such as cupid bow vertebrae and processes mimicking fractures should be excluded. For example, Scheuermann's disease, an osteochondritis characterized by anterior wedging of multiple adjacent vertebrae, end plate irregularity with Schmorl's nodes and hyperkyphosis is relatively common.

Once demonstrated, determining fracture acuity and distinguishing benign osteoporotic collapse from pathologic fracture caused by malignancy are the most important clinical questions. On the radiograph, acuity is very difficult to discern and

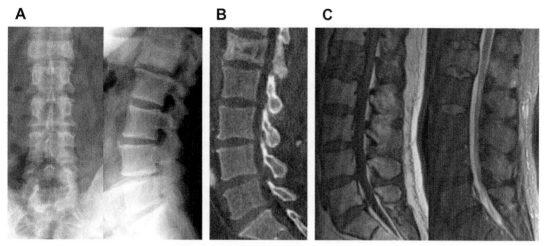

Fig. 1. Patient presented after a road traffic accident. Acute physicians querying pathologic fracture on plain radiograph. (*A*) Anteroposterior and lateral radiographs demonstrating a biconcave wedge of L1 with sclerotic appearances, lucent center and thickened cortices suggestive of Pagetic change. (*B*) Computed tomography sagittal reconstruction better demonstrating typical picture frame appearances. (*C*) T1 (*left*) and STIR (*right*) sagittal images are less specific for the bone pathology, but demonstrate retained marrow fat and acute edema changes further reassuring against a marrow infiltration pathology.

destructive bone lesions are often occult. Signs of malignancy such as pedicular destruction, an associated soft tissue mass, or a convex posterior bulge are helpful if present, although this finding is present in a minority of cases. Other characteristics may raise suspicion for malignant disease, such as multiple lytic lesions in the case of multiple myeloma or disseminated metastases (see **Fig. 9**).

By the time cortical destruction is visible on a radiograph or trabecular destruction is widespread enough to significantly affect bone density, disease is often extensive (**Fig. 2**). For this reason, the correlation of findings with MR imaging is critical to determine fracture etiology and neuraxis involvement.

MR imaging can evaluate bone marrow signal and in turn structural composition, being able to distinguish normal from pathologic patterns. In the case of a pathologic fracture owing to tumor, T1-weighted hypointensity represents malignant

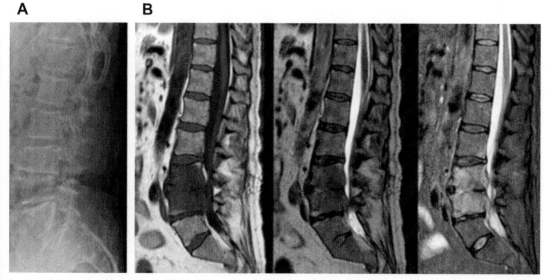

Fig. 2. (*A*) Lateral radiograph and (*B*) MR imaging of the spine (sagittal T1, *left*; sagittal T2, *middle*; and sagittal STIR, *right*). Patient presented with persistent low back pain. The radiograph does not show significant abnormality except for wedge deformation of L3. MR imaging demonstrates the extensive pathologic involvement of L3 and L4 owing to metastases.

substitution of normal marrow tissue and this abnormality may be seen asymmetrically involving the posterior elements. Although the T1 signal is reduced in an acute osteoporotic collapse, the foci of normal marrow fat can usually be observed using conventional sequences and these structures are seen to increase in extent on follow-up studies (**Fig. 3**). High signal in the posterior elements on fluid sensitive sequences is often seen as a stress phenomenon, but this is usually symmetric in distribution.[8]

Scalloped

The radiographic finding of vertebral body scalloping is most common posteriorly, but can less frequently affect anterior and even lateral aspects. The appearance implies a chronic pressure effect from a neighboring structure or tumor—in the posterior aspect, this finding is synonymous with canal pathology. The finding can be diffuse over many segments or localized, and there may be features on the radiograph such as congenital block vertebrae to hint at the cause. MR imaging is invaluable in assessment, because it will often reveal the etiology and can assess the effect on the neuraxis.

The most common cause of posterior scalloping is dural ectasia in which a deficient dura is thought to allow erosion of the vertebral body contour despite normal cerebrospinal fluid pressures.[9] However, longstanding high cerebrospinal fluid pressures in cases of chronic hydrocephalus and achondroplasia will also cause diffuse scalloping[10] (**Fig. 4**). Tumors of the spinal canal only rarely cause scalloping and the greatest effect is thought to occur with slow growing lesions such as ependymomas and lipomas that occur in the actively growing spine.[10]

Anterior and lateral scalloping are rarer and usually owing to pressure from pathologic local structures. Pulsations from an enlarged or pathologic aorta can erode posteriorly into the adjacent vertebral bodies (**Fig. 5**). Neurofibromata of the exiting nerve roots can cause lateral and anterior scalloping as well as exit foraminal enlargement on lateral radiographs. Down's syndrome is also a cause of anterior scalloping, although the cause is unknown.

Squaring and Shiny Corners

Loss of the normal anterior concavity of the vertebral body is most often observed in established axial spondyloarthropathy and most commonly in ankylosing spondylitis.[11] This loss only occurs after radiographic evidence of anterior longitudinal

A   **B**

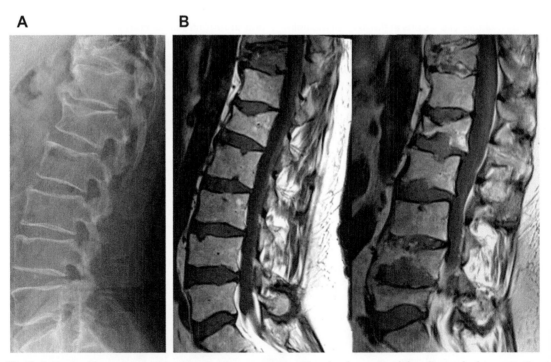

Fig. 3. Patient with acute onset low back pain presented with a lumbar spine (*A*) radiograph demonstrating several end plate fractures and collapse of T12 of indeterminate acuity. (*B*) MR imaging done at admission (*left*) and at 2 years (*right*): initial low T1 signal but retained marrow fat within the T12 body in keeping with an acute osteoporotic collapse. Normalization on the follow-up study is reassuring, but further osteoporotic collapses are noted in the adjacent vertebrae.

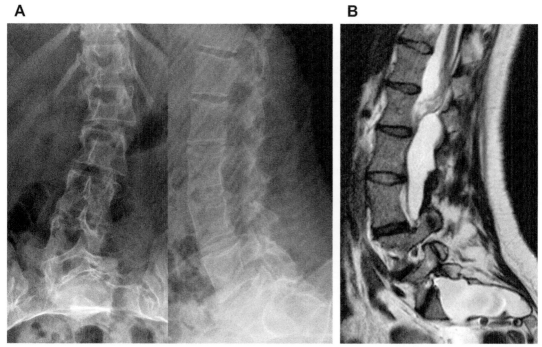

Fig. 4. (*A*) Anteroposterior and lateral radiographs of the lumbar spine demonstrating marked posterior vertebral scalloping with exit foraminal widening, wide spinal canal, and concave medial border to several pedicles. (*B*) Sagittal T2-weighted MR imaging demonstrating no intradural lesion, but typical appearances of dural ectasia. Patient had a background of neurofibromatosis type 1.

ligament enthesopathy becomes evident, and is due to an inflammatory osteitis and repair cycle centered on the enthesis, which "fills out" the anterior concavity. Although this finding may be subtle, other hallmarks such as syndesmophytes, Anderson lesions, and sacroiliac joint disease may also be present.

The first radiographically apparent abnormality is bony erosion at the entheses, but this process is difficult to detect because it is often transient

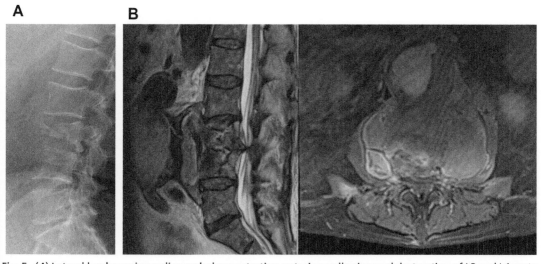

Fig. 5. (*A*) Lateral lumbar spine radiograph demonstrating anterior scalloping and destruction of L3 and L4 vertebral bodies with collapse of L3. (*B*) T2 sagittal (*left*) and postcontrast T1 axial (*right*) images demonstrating a large enhancing soft tissue mass continuous with the posterior wall of the aneurysmal aorta in keeping with a large mycotic aneurysm and abscess.

and the posterior body corner entheses are often obscured by other structures. However, on MR imaging, this early enthesopathic inflammation is easily visible as high signal "shiny corners" on fluid-sensitive sequences. Radiographic shiny corners correspond with healed entheseal lesions, which are seen as T1 low-signal quiescent areas on MR imaging. Other healed vertebral corner lesions can also demonstrate high T1 marrow signal reflecting fat content. Although early inflammatory changes are easily appreciable on MR imaging, subtle syndesmophytes are often difficult to appreciate and fusion between vertebral levels and of sacroiliac joints obvious on radiographs can sometimes be missed (**Fig. 6**).

Congenital Contour Abnormalities

The vertebral body develops from chondrification centers that arise within the sclerotome around the notochord. By the ninth gestational week, the notochord involutes and the ventral and dorsal ossification centers for the body arise within the cartilage; failure at any stage of this development results in a congenital contour abnormality such as a hemivertebra (chondrification center failure), wedge vertebra (ossification center failure), or butterfly vertebra (failure of notochord involution).[12]

On plain radiographs, vertebral body abnormalities are readily identified, usually situated at the apex of a scoliosis or kyphosis. MR imaging is used routinely now, especially if correction is being considered, because it can help to identify any levels of neuraxis compromise or associated

cord abnormalities (eg, diastomatomyelia, tethered cord, syrinx) to plan surgery (**Fig. 7**). Further discussion of the imaging and assessment of adult spinal deformity (ASD) is discussed in the section on vertebral malalignment.

END PLATES

The vertebral end plates are unique structures consisting of a thin, persistent layer of hyaline cartilage that, unlike in synovial joints, is not strongly attached by Sharpey's fibers to the underlying osseous end plate.[1] Instead, strong collagen fibrils attach the cartilaginous end plate to the adjacent disc,[13] which gives superior force distribution in axial loading, but is potentially weak in tension.[14] During development, a dense network of vessels perforate the end plate to supply the annulus, but these involute at skeletal maturity leaving areas of potential end plate weakness for disc herniation.[15] For all intents and purposes, reported end plate pathology usually refers to the osseous end plate because the cartilaginous end plate is not appreciable on radiographs and conventional MR imaging sequences.

Destruction and Erosion

Destruction of opposing end plates in most cases implies spondylodiscitis, an infectious process centered on the disc space. The subchondral end plate is thought to be the original site of infection owing to its supply by end arteries.[16] In pediatric patients, infection can also originate in the vascularized cartilaginous

A   **B**

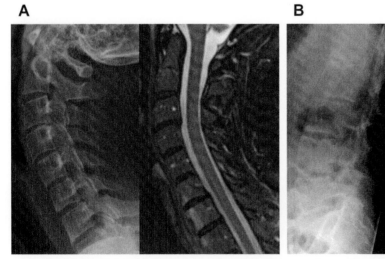

Fig. 6. Typical anterior vertebral body squaring with evidence of anterior corner enthesitis and spondylodiscitis changes evident both on lateral radiograph and sagittal STIR MR imaging in the (A) cervical and (B) lumbar spine of a patient with new presentation of inflammatory back pain in keeping with axial spondyloarthropathy. Note the syndesmophytes on the radiograph are difficult to appreciate on MR imaging.

A   B

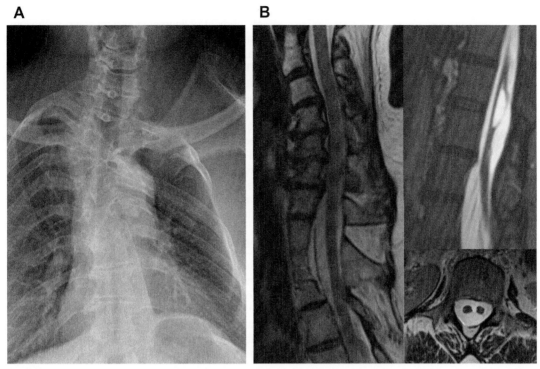

Fig. 7. (A) Anteroposterior radiograph demonstrating focal thoracic spine scoliosis, but the exact cause is difficult to determine. (B) Whole spine MR imaging demonstrated that this was caused by a T1 to T3 block vertebra (*left*), but also revealed diastomatomyelia in the lumbar spine (*right top* and *bottom*).

anlage and disc annulus. Multilevel contiguous involvement with large subligamentous and para-spinal abscesses are features thought to be suggestive of tuberculous rather than pyogenic spondylodiscitis.[17]

On conventional radiographs, the initial changes are often subtle with ill definition of the end plates. However, on MR imaging, these subtle changes often relate to marked bone marrow inflammation and bony destruction, and MR imaging changes can significantly precede discernible radiographic abnormality. Other involved levels occult on plain radiographs and associated paravertebral and epidural abscesses can be delineated on MR imaging allowing assessment of the full extent of disease (**Fig. 8**).

A   B

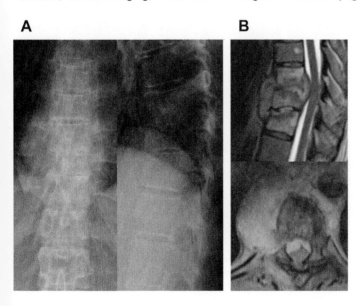

Fig. 8. (A) Anteroposterior and lateral radiographs of the thoracic spine demonstrate disc and vertebral height loss centered on T9 with a large fusiform soft tissue density. (B) T2-weighted sagittal (*top*) and post-contrast T1-weighted axial (*bottom*) MR images demonstrate typical subligamentous abscesses and contiguous involvement in tuberculous spondylodiscitis.

Schmorl's Nodes

Schmorl's nodes were first demonstrated in cadaveric specimens by Georg Schmorl in 1927 and usually occur in the thoracolumbar spine.[18] They relate to invagination of disc material through developmental weaknesses in the cartilaginous end plates.[15] A minority of end plate defects may also occur through pathologic processes such as infection, trauma, or malignancy—better termed cartilaginous nodes.[19] They are also associated with the idiopathic Scheuermann's disease in which end plate irregularities are associated with thoracolumbar kyphosis.

On plain radiographs, most (chronic) Schmorl's nodes are well-defined end plate defects with the region of disc material herniation into the vertebral body outlined by a sclerotic margin. Uncommonly, acute Schmorl's nodes can occur where there is a painful, acutely herniating intravertebral disc. In these cases, radiographs demonstrate ill-defined lucency, lacking a sclerotic margin and, on MR imaging, bone marrow edema can be seen, making these lesions more difficult to differentiate from early spondylodiscitis and tumor.

POSTERIOR ELEMENTS

The posterior neural arch or posterior elements (with the exception of C1) consist of 2 flat laminae that are attached to the body by 2 pedicles, forming the bony spinal canal. Projecting from this are 4 articular processes that form the zygoapophyseal (facet) joints and 3 apophyseal processes (1 spinous and 2 transverse) for the attachment of ligaments and muscles. In the lumbar spine, the pars interarticularis spans the articular processes.

The primary purpose of the posterior elements is not to bear weight (with the exception of L5, which does bear some weight on standing), but to serve to protect the neuraxis both directly and by allowing only limited directions and range of vertebral body movement.

Pathologies such as tumor and infection that affect the vertebral body and end plates also affect the posterior elements and can affect their radiographic contour, but certain pathologies favor the latter.

Pedicles

The pedicles are well-demonstrated on the anteroposterior spine radiograph and tumors and tumor-like processes affecting the vertebral body may involve the pedicles. Benign tumors such as osteoblastoma or processes such as Paget's disease can cause pedicle expansion. However, destruction of a pedicle, known radiographically as the "winking owl" sign, will more frequently be due to aggressive lesions such as metastases in adults or Ewing's sarcoma in children. It was previously thought that hematogenous metastases favored the pedicle, but with the increasing availability of cross-sectional imaging, it is likely that the clearly delineated cortical outline of the pedicle facilitates tumor identification on the radiograph rather than this being a true tropism[20] (**Fig. 9**).

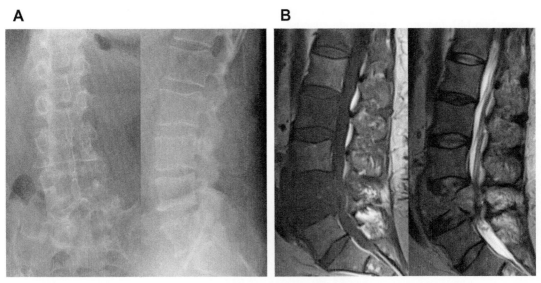

Fig. 9. (*A*) Anteroposterior and lateral lumbar spine radiographs show subtle loss of the left L4 pedicle. (*B*) T1-weighted (*left*) and T2-weighted (*right*) sagittal MR imaging images done 2 weeks later demonstrates a much wider extent of disease found to be secondary to metastases from lung adenocarcinoma.

The pedicles border both the spinal canal and neural exit foramen, and therefore causes of posterior scalloping such as slow-growing tumors of the canal or nerve sheath and dural ectasia can cause change in pedicle contour and in extreme cases widening of the exit foramen (**Fig. 10**). MR imaging is important for characterization, but can often demonstrate multilevel involvement, for example, in neurofibromatosis type 1.

Achondroplasia causes narrowing of the interpedicular distance in the lower lumbar spine and congenitally short pedicles and therefore a narrow spinal canal predisposing to stenosis and nerve root compromise (**Fig. 11**). MR imaging is often indicated to determine any levels of neuraxis impingement and plan if and which surgical interventions would be beneficial. Other congenital defects of pedicles are rarely reported, such as hypoplastic and hyperplastic pedicles and pediculate bars.[21] These entities can mimic pedicular destruction on radiographs and MR imaging is often required to demonstrate the abnormality.

Articular Processes and Facet Joints

The facet joints are synovial joints capable of limited range of movement and the lower lumbar facets are most commonly seen to be degenerate owing to their loadbearing role. However, other processes affecting synovial joints such as infectious and inflammatory arthritides should be considered.

It was previously thought that inflammatory arthritides such as rheumatoid arthritis favored the cervical spine and craniocervical junction, but more recent studies have found that thoracic and lumbar changes are also highly prevalent, even in asymptomatic patients.[22]

Septic arthritis of the facet joints is less common than spondylodiscitis (and the 2 entities can coexist) but is believed to share a similar hematogenous infective origin[23] and the predominant isolate is also *Staphylococcus aureus*.[24] Both of these etiologies are often occult on the radiograph, but joint widening and erosions are suggestive. On MR imaging, joint erosion and subluxation can be better appreciated and intense periarticular edema, effusions, and fluid collections help to distinguish it from other pathology (**Fig. 12**).

Pars defects are stress-related fractures through the pars interarticularis, a small span of bone between the articular processes in the lumbar spine. L5 is most commonly affected owing to its unique position exposing the pars to shearing between L4 and S1.[25] On oblique lateral radiographs, increased sclerosis of the pars is suggestive, but only late stages of pars fractures are reliably identified. MR imaging is usually required to identify early stress reactions that will require treatment to prevent development into a cortical break.

Transverse and Spinous Processes

The transverse and spinous processes serve as muscular attachments, and as such are most commonly involved by avulsion type injuries usually during major trauma.

Congenital spinal dysraphism is a common condition causing deficient closure of the posterior neural arch with or without an associated mass or neural tube defect. The mild occulta form is most commonly encountered incidentally in adults and is said to be present in up to 25% of births.[26] On radiographs, there is bony agenesis of the posterior neural arch (sparing the

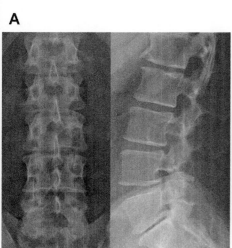

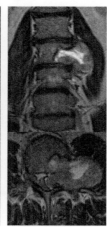

Fig. 10. (*A*) Anteroposterior and lateral lumbar spine radiographs demonstrate widening of the left L3 to L4 exit foramen and erosion of the inferior left pedicle and vertebral body suggestive of a long-standing lesion. (*B*) Coronal (*top*) and axial (*bottom*) T2-weighted MR imaging demonstrates a mass lesion in the exit foramen with mixed signal characteristics. Biopsy proved degenerated giant schwannoma.

A   **B**

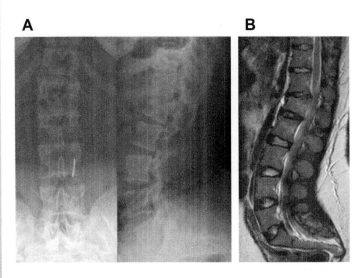

Fig. 11. (*A*) Anteroposterior and lateral lumbar spine radiographs demonstrating the typical narrowing interpedicular distance and horizontal sacrum in a patient with achondroplasia who sustained a fall. There is an acute fracture of the L1 vertebra. (*B*) Sagittal T2-weighted MR imaging demonstrates contusion to the conus owing to the considerably reduced canal dimensions secondary to short pedicles.

transverse processes and pedicles) most commonly seen at L5 to S2. Although in most cases it is neurologically benign, MR imaging is indicated in symptomatic patients as there is association with cord lipoma, dermoid cysts, and cord tethering[27] (**Fig. 13**).

VERTEBRAL MALALIGNMENT

In healthy individuals, the spine is straight in the coronal plane and exhibits an S-shape in the sagittal plane. This, together with a delicate balance between the spine and pelvis allow the standing posture to be maintained and the bipedal walk. A balanced posture is obtained when the spine and pelvis are aligned to minimize muscular energy expenditure. Orientation of the spine (sagittal spinal alignment, in particular) and resultant posture varies with the gender, weight, and age of the patient.

Spinal alignment disorders may malalign the spine in plane (eg, spondylolisthesis and

A   **B**

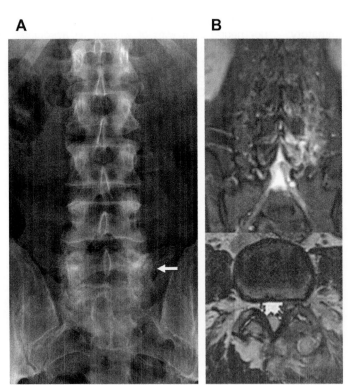

Fig. 12. (*A*) Anteroposterior radiograph of the lumbar spine demonstrates well-preserved facet joints but unilateral irregularity and erosion of the left L5 to S1 facet (*arrow*) can be seen in this patient with acute low back pain. (*B*) Coronal STIR (*top*) and axial T2 (*bottom*) images demonstrate intense soft tissue and bone edema centered on this joint with associated abscesses in keeping with septic arthritis.

A   B

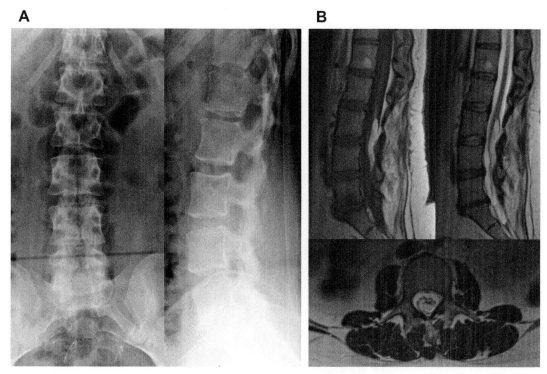

Fig. 13. (*A*) Anteroposterior and lateral radiographs on this patient with back pain incidentally demonstrating L2 to S1 spina bifida occulta. (*B*) Subsequent T1 (*top left*) and T2 (*top right*) sagittal and T2 axial (*bottom*) MR imaging demonstrate associated cord lipoma.

Scheuermann's kyphosis) or in all 3 planes, as in idiopathic scoliosis.[28]

ASD is an umbrella term covering various developmental, progressive, or degenerative entities that can involve deformity in any combination of planes.[29,30] ASD may occur as the result of poor bone quality and osteoporosis leading to vertebral body collapse, or a focal problem such as congenital or developmental osseous anomalies (eg, failure of segmentation), trauma, infection, and neoplastic disease. However, after skeletal maturity, the most prevalent spinal deformities are (1) iatrogenic deformities, (2) adult idiopathic scoliosis that commences before skeletal maturity and becomes symptomatic between the ages of 20 and 50 years owing to degenerative changes (**Fig. 14**), and (3) degenerative (de novo) scoliosis in adults more than 60 years of age and with no history of scoliosis. The latter develops as part of the aging process owing to cumulative asymmetrical degenerative changes focused on the intervertebral discs and facet joints producing sagittal and coronal imbalance, malalignment, and potentially neural element compression.[28–32] Some patients may be asymptomatic, whereas others experience pain and disability, which can be severe enough to impact daily activities.[30]

Imaging of a patient with suspected spinal deformity begins with static standing full-length 36-inch anteroposterior and lateral radiographs of the whole spine, iliac crests, and hip joints.[33] These views provide an assessment of global and regional spinopelvic alignment allowing the necessary measurements. Global coronal alignment is assessed by measuring the horizontal distance between a vertical line crossing the center of the sacrum and a plumb line dropped from the C7 centroid (C7PL). A C7PL passing to the left, through, or to the right of the vertical line crossing the center of the sacrum corresponds to negative, neutral, and positive coronal alignments, respectively.[30] The magnitude of the coronal deformity typically involves measurements of scoliotic curves using the Cobb angle method. The largest curve, as measured from the maximally angulated vertebra above and below the apex (the vertebra maximally displaced from midline and minimally angulated), is considered the major curve; adjacent curves are termed "minor."[30]

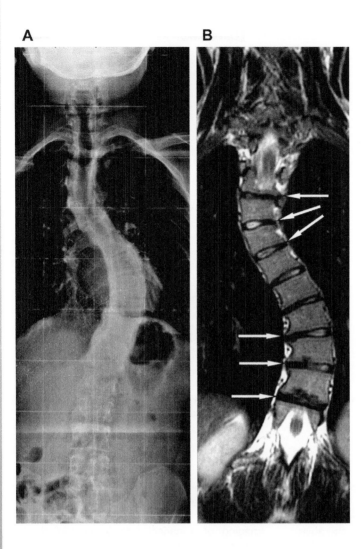

A

B

Fig. 14. A 29-year-old woman with adult idiopathic scoliosis. (*A*) Static standing full-length 36-inch Antero-posterior of the spinopelvic axis shows thoracic levoscoliosis with apex at T8 to T9 disc space. (*B*) Coronal T2-weighted MR image shows asymmetric degenerative changes in the intervertebral discs associated with 2 lumbar Schmorl's nodes (*arrows*).

Global and regional sagittal spinal alignment is assessed on lateral 36-inch radiographs by measuring the sagittal vertical axis (SVA) and the lumbar lordosis (LL) respectively. The SVA is the horizontal distance from the C7PL to the posterosuperior corner of the sacrum. By convention, a C7PL that passes anterior or posterior to the posterosuperior sacrum is designated as positive or negative, respectively. Thoracic kyphosis is measured between the cephalad end plate of T5 and the caudal end plate of T12, whereas LL is the angle between the inferior T12/superior L1 end plate to the inferior L5/superior S1 end plate.[34] Kyphosis and positive sagittal balance cause the body's center of gravity to move forward in space, which can cause severe pain and disability.

Sagittal spinal alignment is greatly influenced by 3 key pelvic parameters: pelvic incidence (PI), pelvic tilt (PT), and sacral slope (SS) (**Fig. 15**). The PI is the angle between the line perpendicular to the superior plate of the first sacral vertebra at its midpoint and the line connecting this point to the middle axis of the femoral heads. The PT is the angle between the vertical line and the line joining the middle of the sacral end plate to the middle axis of the femoral heads. The SS is the angle between the horizontal line and the cranial sacral end plate tangent. The PI is a fundamental anatomic parameter that is specific and constant for each individual and independent of the 3-dimensional orientation of the pelvis. Geometrically, the PI equals the sum of the SS and the PT. Therefore, as PI increases, the PT and/or SS will increase. Generally, the normal range of the PT is very narrow, from 10° to 15°. Thus, if the PI increases, the SS will increase more relative to PT and cause increasing LL.[35]

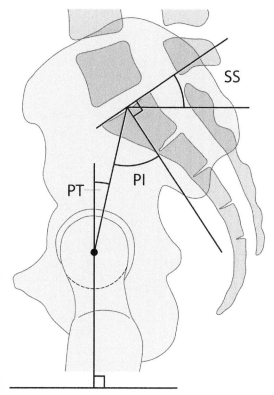

SS

PT

PI

Fig. 15. Diagram of a lateral radiograph of the lumbosacral spine showing PI, PT, and SS. PI is the angle formed by drawing a perpendicular line starting from the midpoint of the sacral end plate and a line connecting this point to the middle axis of the femoral heads. PT is the angle between the vertical line and the line connecting the midpoint of the sacral plate to the axis of the femoral heads. SS is the angle between the superior plate of S1 and the horizontal line. (*Modified from* Leone A, Cianfoni A, Cerase A, et al. Lumbar spondylolysis: a review. Skeletal Radiol 2011;40(6):686; with permission.)

Correlation between sagittal spinal malalignment and negative health-related quality-of-life has been demonstrated by various studies.[36,37] Although increased sagittal imbalance (SVA of >5 cm) highly relates to adverse patient-reported outcomes, SVA alone may underestimate the severity of sagittal spinal malalignment.[38] A multicenter, prospective study[37] demonstrated that PT and PI–LL mismatch (PI minus LL) combined with SVA predicts patient disability and provides a guide for patient assessment. Threshold values for severe disability (Oswestry Disability Index of $\geq$40) included a PT 22° or greater, an SVA of 46 mm or greater, and a PI–LL of 11° or greater. Furthermore, Merril and colleagues[38] demonstrated that with increasing SVA, an increase in the PI–LL mismatch (>10°) recruits compensatory mechanisms of increased pelvic retroversion, reduced thoracic kyphosis, increased knee flexion, and increased pelvic shift to balance the SVA, indicating that other sagittal parameters influence sagittal alignment. Additionally, cervical sagittal parameters, such as cervical lordosis (Cobb angle between C2 and C7) and C2 to C7 SVA (horizontal distance between plumb line from the C2 centroid and plumb line from the posterosuperior corner of C7), relate to health-related quality-of-life and disability, stressing the importance of considering the entire spine in sagittal deformity.[39,40]

Functional flexion and extension radiography in the sagittal plane, which should be obtained in lateral decubitus to maximize detection of abnormal translation, is important to identify spondylolisthesis.[41,42] Because of its simplicity and wide availability, it is also the most widely used method in the imaging diagnosis and study of lumbar intervertebral instability.[42]

Supine side-bending radiographs may help to assess the flexibility of the scoliotic curve distinguishing between the major and minor curves. Major curves will always be the largest and are always considered structural. Minor curves may be structural or nonstructural; curves are considered structural if they are 25° or greater on the anteroposterior radiograph and remain greater than 25° on side bending, whereas if they decrease to less than 25° they are considered nonstructural.[30] Curves less than 25° are nonstructural by definition.

In ASD, malalignment is associated with facet joint osteoarthritis and degenerative disc disease inducing canal stenosis and radicular impingement. MR imaging provides exceptional soft-tissue detail and should be used to determine the effect of deformity on the neuraxis (see **Fig. 14**; **Fig. 16**). Fu and colleagues[43] have reported a high prevalence of stenosis in degenerative scoliosis, with 86% of patients having central canal stenosis and 100% of patients showing foraminal stenosis. Furthermore, MR imaging may be useful in determining spinal flexibility for planning ASD surgery. Baker and colleagues[44] assessed spinal alignment on supine MR imaging in addition to standing radiographs and found that a change in the PI–LL mismatch on MR imaging can obviate the need for an invasive osteotomy. The drawback, however, is the routine supine and therefore unloaded patient position. However, recent advances in open MR imaging system design and upright MR imaging provides new opportunities to investigate spinal kinematics.[42]

A   **B**

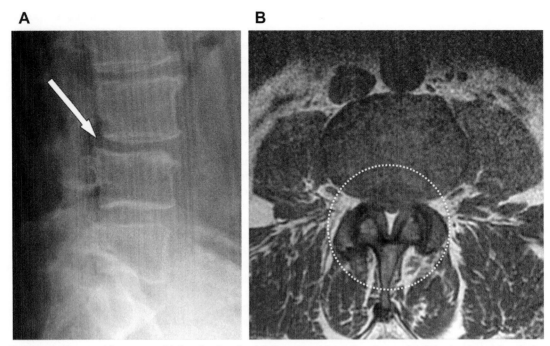

Fig. 16. A 48-year-old woman with low back pain. (*A*) Functional lateral radiograph of the lumbar spine during flexion shows grade I axial degenerative spondylolisthesis at L3 (*arrow*). (*B*) Axial T2-weighted MR image through the L3 to L4 intervertebral space demonstrates moderately severe central spinal stenosis owing to bulging disc with posterolateral protrusion associated with sagittal facet orientation, and hypertrophy of flaval ligaments (*circle*).

SUMMARY

With the advent of multidetector computed tomography and better and faster MR imaging scanners, radiologists find themselves being exposed to fewer plain radiographs in their daily reporting. However, plain radiographs are sufficient to recognize many disorders of the spine, and as we have explored in this article, can be highly complementary to MR imaging in characterizing lesions and planning and monitoring treatment. With the radiologist's ever-increasing workload, it will become increasingly more important to ensure that this skill does not disappear with time.

REFERENCES

1. Inoue H. Three-dimensional architecture of lumbar intervertebral discs. Spine (Phila Pa 1976) 1981; 6(2):139–46.
2. Cushing H. Haematomyelia from gunshot wounds of the spine: a report of a case, with recovering following symptoms of hemilesion of the cord. Am J Med Sci 1898;115:654.
3. Modic MT, Pavlicek W, Weinstein MA, et al. Magnetic resonance imaging of intervertebral disk disease. Clinical and pulse sequence considerations. Radiology 1984;152(1):103–11.
4. Bick EM, Copel JW. The ring apophysis of the human vertebra; contribution to human osteogeny. II. J Bone Joint Surg Am 1951;33-A(3):783–7.
5. Carroll KW, Feller JF, Tirman PF. Useful internal standards for distinguishing infiltrative marrow pathology from hematopoietic marrow at MRI. J Magn Reson Imaging 1997;7(2):394–8.
6. Shah LM, Hanrahan CJ. MRI of spinal bone marrow: part I, techniques and normal age-related appearances. AJR Am J Roentgenol 2011;197(6): 1298–308.
7. Korres DS, Zoubos AB, Kavadias K, et al. The "tear drop" (or avulsed) fracture of the anterior inferior angle of the axis. Eur Spine J 1994;3(3): 151–4.
8. Baker LL, Goodman SB, Perkash I, et al. Benign versus pathologic compression fractures of vertebral bodies: assessment with conventional spin-echo, chemical-shift, and STIR MR imaging. Radiology 1990;174(2):495–502.
9. Leeds NE, Jacobson HG. Spinal neurofibromatosis. AJR Am J Roentgenol 1976;126(3):617–23.
10. Mitchell GE, Lourie H, Berne AS. The various causes of scalloped vertebrae with notes on their pathogenesis. Radiology 1967;89(1):67–74.

11. Aufdermaur M. Pathogenesis of square bodies in ankylosing spondylitis. Ann Rheum Dis 1989;48(8): 628–31.

12. Cohen J, Currarino G, Neuhauser EB. A significant variant in the ossification centers of the vertebral bodies. Am J Roentgenol Radium Ther Nucl Med 1956;76(3):469–75.

13. Johnson EF, Chetty K, Moore IM, et al. The distribution and arrangement of elastic fibres in the intervertebral disc of the adult human. J Anat 1982;135(Pt 2):301–9.

14. Balkovec C, Adams MA, Dolan P, et al. Annulus fibrosus can strip hyaline cartilage end plate from subchondral bone: a study of the intervertebral disk in tension. Global Spine J 2015;5(5): 360–5.

15. Resnick D, Niwayama G. Intravertebral disk herniations: cartilaginous (Schmorl's) nodes. Radiology 1978;126(1):57–65.

16. Dagirmanjian A, Schils J, McHenry MC. MR imaging of spinal infections. Magn Reson Imaging Clin N Am 1999;7(3):525–38.

17. Moore SL, Rafii M. Imaging of musculoskeletal and spinal tuberculosis. Radiol Clin North Am 2001; 39(2):329–42.

18. Schmorl G. Uber die an den wirbelbandscheiben vorkommenden ausdehnungs—und zerreisungsvorgange die dadurch an ihnen und der wirbelspongiosa hervorgerufenen veranderungen. Verh Dtsch Ges Pathol 1927;22:250.

19. Pfirrmann CW, Resnick D. Schmorl nodes of the thoracic and lumbar spine: radiographic-pathologic study of prevalence, characterization, and correlation with degenerative changes of 1,650 spinal levels in 100 cadavers. Radiology 2001;219(2):368–74.

20. Algra PR, Heimans JJ, Valk J, et al. Do metastases in vertebrae begin in the body or the pedicles? Imaging study in 45 patients. AJR Am J Roentgenol 1992;158(6):1275–9.

21. Patel NP, Kumar R, Kinkhabwala M, et al. Radiology of lumbar vertebral pedicles: variants, anomalies and pathologic conditions. Radiographics 1987; 7(1):101–37.

22. Yamada K, Suzuki A, Takahashi S, et al. MRI evaluation of lumbar endplate and facet erosion in rheumatoid arthritis. J Spinal Disord Tech 2014;27(4): E128–35.

23. Muffoletto AJ, Ketonen LM, Mader JT, et al. Hematogenous pyogenic facet joint infection. Spine (Phila Pa 1976) 2001;26(14):1570–6.

24. Rombauts PA, Linden PM, Buyse AJ, et al. Septic arthritis of a lumbar facet joint caused by Staphylococcus aureus. Spine (Phila Pa 1976) 2000;25(13): 1736–8.

25. Capener N. Spondylolisthesis. Br J Surg 1932; 19(75):374–86.

26. Fidas A, MacDonald HL, Elton RA, et al. Prevalence and patterns of spina bifida occulta in 2707 normal adults. Clin Radiol 1987;38(5):537–42.

27. Burrows FG. Some aspects of occult spinal dysraphism: a study of 90 cases. Br J Radiol 1968; 41(487):496–507.

28. Cil A, Yazici M, Uzumcugil A, et al. The evolution of sagittal segmental alignment of the spine during childhood. Spine (Phila Pa 1976) 2005;30(1): 93–100.

29. Smith JS, Shaffrey CI, Fu KM, et al. Clinical and radiographic evaluation of the adult spinal deformity patient. Neurosurg Clin N Am 2013;24(2):143–56.

30. Ailon T, Smith JS, Shaffrey CI, et al. Degenerative spinal deformity. Neurosurgery 2015;77(Suppl 4): S75–91.

31. Cassar-Pullicino VN, Eisenstein SM. Imaging in scoliosis: what, why and how? Clin Radiol 2002; 57(7):543–62.

32. Kim H, Kim HS, Moon ES, et al. Scoliosis imaging: what radiologists should know. Radiographics 2010;30(7):1823–42.

33. Angevine PD, Kaiser MG. Radiographic measurement techniques. Neurosurgery 2008;63(3 Suppl): 40–5.

34. Polly DW, Kilkelly FX, McHale KA, et al. Measurement of lumbar lordosis. Evaluation of intraobserver, interobserver, and technique variability. Spine (Phila Pa 1976) 1996;21(13):1530–5 [discussion: 1535–6].

35. Leone A, Cianfoni A, Cerase A, et al. Lumbar spondylolysis: a review. Skeletal Radiol 2011;40(6): 683–700.

36. Schwab F, Ungar B, Blondel B, et al. Scoliosis Research Society-Schwab adult spinal deformity classification: a validation study. Spine (Phila Pa 1976) 2012;37(12):1077–82.

37. Schwab FJ, Blondel B, Bess S, et al. Radiographical spinopelvic parameters and disability in the setting of adult spinal deformity: a prospective multicenter analysis. Spine (Phila Pa 1976) 2013;38(13): E803–12.

38. Merrill RK, Kim JS, Leven DM, et al. Beyond pelvic incidence-lumbar lordosis mismatch: the importance of assessing the entire spine to achieve global sagittal alignment. Global Spine J 2017; 7(6):536–42.

39. Protopsaltis TS, Scheer JK, Terran JS, et al. How the neck affects the back: changes in regional cervical sagittal alignment correlate to HRQOL improvement in adult thoracolumbar deformity patients at 2-year follow-up. J Neurosurg Spine 2015;23(2):153–8.

40. Scheer JK, Passias PG, Sorocean AM, et al. Association between preoperative cervical sagittal deformity and inferior outcomes at 2-year follow-up in patients with adult thoracolumbar deformity:

analysis of 182 patients. J Neurosurg Spine 2016; 24(1):108–15.

41. Wood KB, Popp CA, Transfeldt EE, et al. Radiographic evaluation of instability in spondylolisthesis. Spine (Phila Pa 1976) 1994;19(15):1697–703.

42. Leone A, Guglielmi G, Cassar-Pullicino VN, et al. Lumbar intervertebral instability: a review. Radiology 2007;245(1):62–77.

43. Fu KM, Rhagavan P, Shaffrey CI, et al. Prevalence, severity, and impact of foraminal and canal stenosis among adults with degenerative scoliosis. Neurosurgery 2011;69(6):1181–7.

44. Baker J, Day L, Oren J, et al. Analysis of lumbar flexibility on supine MRI and CT may reduce the need for more invasive spinal osteotomy in adult spinal deformity surgery. Spine J 2016;16(10):S197.

Radiographic/MR Imaging Correlation of Paravertebral Ossifications in Ligaments and Bony Vertebral Outgrowths
Anatomy, Early Detection, and Clinical Impact

Monique Reijnierse, MD, PhD

KEYWORDS

- MR imaging • Radiograph • Spine • Paravertebral ossifications • Rheumatology
- Axial spondyloarthritis • DISH • Degeneration

KEY POINTS

- Calcifications and ossifications of paravertebral ligaments may cause clinical symptoms.
- Differentiation between hypertrophied ligaments and ligamentous calcifications is limited using MR imaging alone.
- A vertebral bony outgrowth can be characterized on radiographs based on its origin and growth direction.
- A suspected axial spondyloarthritis on radiograph or MR imaging of the spine can be followed by MR imaging of the sacroiliac joints for definite diagnosis.
- There is a high prevalence of degenerative changes in the spine, seen as early as the age of 16 years, without clinical significance.

INTRODUCTION

Radiographs have been the cornerstone in diagnostic imaging. In the case of back pain, a common complaint in the general population, conventional imaging of the spine is still one of the first imaging methods performed. However, there is a high prevalence of degenerative changes in the spine, described in up to 70% in a young population without clinical significance.[1] These findings will increase with age. Inflammatory back pain, on the other hand, is only present in a minority of patients, and specific imaging findings should raise the suspicion of spondyloarthritis. The availability of effective medication in rheumatology has shifted the attention toward early disease detection. MR imaging is the only imaging modality to detect bone marrow edema, and its role has become more important. Because MR imaging–detected sacroiliitis is part of the Assessment of SpondyloArthritis International Society (ASAS) criteria for the classification of patients at an early

Disclosure Statement: The author disclose any commercial or financial conflicts of interest and any funding sources.
Department of Radiology, Leiden University Medical Center, Albinusdreef 2, PO Box 9600, 2300RC Leiden, The Netherlands
E-mail address: m.reijnierse@lumc.nl

Magn Reson Imaging Clin N Am 27 (2019) 641–659
https://doi.org/10.1016/j.mric.2019.07.003
1064-9689/19/© 2019 Elsevier Inc. All rights reserved.

stage, MR imaging is increasingly used.[2] Here, attention is paid to radiographs and MR imaging of the spine, more specifically, to the variety of imaging features of paravertebral ossifications. Certain types of ossifications can be diagnostic for a disease, and others are merely correlated to aging. Therefore, correct interpretation is clinically important. These paravertebral ossifications can be primarily ligamentous or bony in origin. Differentiation between these two origins is not always possible and not always necessary if some general guidelines in interpretation are used. Because both radiographs and MR imaging of the spine are widely performed, knowledge of a correlation between these two imaging modalities might be useful in clinical practice.

Therefore, the purpose of this article is to review the anatomy of the spine, to describe paravertebral ligamentous ossifications, to understand the development of vertebral bony outgrowths and correlate these to specific diseases, and finally, to correlate radiographic and MR imaging findings in paravertebral ossifications.

ANATOMY

The vertebral column is built up from bony vertebra and fibrocartilaginous discs that are connected by strong ligaments and supported by a musculotendinous system.[3]

ANATOMY OF THE DISCOVERTEBRAL JUNCTION

The intervertebral disc consists of an outer layer, the annulus fibrosus, and a slightly posteriorly located central zone, the nucleus pulposus. In the superior and inferior endplates of the vertebral body is a central depression covered with cartilage, the fused epiphyseal rings form the periphery. The annulus fibrosus is attached to the vertebral endplate by strong fibers. The external fibers, Sharpey fibers, penetrate the outer bony ring. These fibers also extend beyond the confines of the disc and blend with the vertebral periosteum and anterior longitudinal ligament[3,4] (Fig. 1).

ANATOMY OF THE SPINAL LIGAMENTS

The anterior longitudinal ligament is a broad fibrous band located at the anterior part of the vertebral column, extending from skull to sacrum (see Fig. 1; Fig. 2). The posterior longitudinal ligament is a thinner band of fibers at the posterior vertebral column, located within the spinal canal anteriorly. It extends from the level of the axis and membrana tectoria to the sacrum. Both

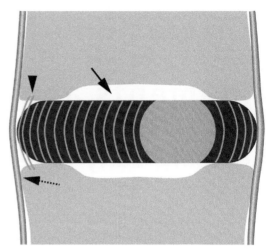

Fig. 1. Anatomy of the discovertebral junction (vertebral unit). Sagittal view. The intervertebral disc consists of concentric layers of fibrous tissue, the annulus fibrosus, and a slightly posterior central zone, the nucleus pulposus. A depression central in the endplate is covered by a cartilaginous endplate (arrow), and the fused epiphyseal rings form the periphery. The annulus fibrosus is attached to the vertebral endplate by strong fibers (Sharpey fibers) (arrowhead). The anterior longitudinal ligament is attached to anterior edge of the vertebral bodies (dotted arrow) and is less firm to the intervertebral disc. The posterior longitudinal ligament is firmly attached to the intervertebral disc and bows over the more concave formed posterior vertebra. (Adapted from Resnick D. Degenerative disease of the spine. In: Resnick D, editor. Diagnosis of bone and joint disorders, Vol 2, 4th edition. Philadelphia: Saunders; 2002; with permission.)

anterior and posterior longitudinal ligaments are attached to the margins of the vertebral bodies and loosely attached to the intervertebral discs. Whereas the anterior longitudinal ligament is adherent to the anterior surface of the vertebral body, the posterior longitudinal ligament forms a bow stretching over the concave posterior surface.[4] The ligamenta flava form the posterior ligamentous demarcation of the spinal canal. They are attached to the articular capsule of the apophyseal joints, connect the laminae, and meet in the midline. These ligaments increase in thickness from cranial to caudal. The interspinal ligaments interconnect the spinous process to each other, and the intertransverse ligaments extend between the transverse processes of the vertebrae. The ligamentum nuchae extends from the external occipital protuberance to C7. Below C7 extending to the sacrum, the supraspinal ligament connects the tips of the spinous processes.[3,4]

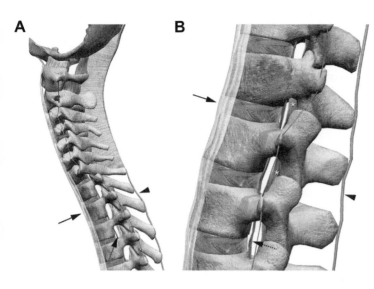

Fig. 2. Anatomy of the spinal ligaments. Sagittal view from (*A*) occiput-Th4 and (*B*) a detail of Th1-Th3. It shows the anterior longitudinal ligament (*arrows*), posterior longitudinal ligament (*dotted arrows*), ligamentum flavum (*asterisk*), and supraspinal ligament (*arrowheads*). The ligamentum nuchae extends from the external occipital protuberance to C7. The interspinal ligaments and intertransverse ligaments are not shown.

NORMAL AGING

The pediatric spine changes in appearances with aging, and ossification centers and synchondroses may be multiple and variable.[5] The normal appearance and fusion of the superior and inferior ring apophysis for different pediatric age groups have recently been reported.[6] An ununited secondary ossification center (limbus vertebra) is a normal variation, which is suggested to be the result of intervertebral disc herniation.[7]

When we age, the nucleus pulposus decreases its water content; the mucoid matrix is replaced by fibrocartilage, and it will resemble the annulus fibrosus.[3] The discs will lose their height. Calcifications or ossifications of spinal ligaments are part of normal aging and a physiologic process.[8]

PART 1
Paravertebral Ligamentous Ossifications

Ligamentous ossifications may become more prominent in time, and these are most frequently seen in the anterior longitudinal ligament as part of diffuse idiopathic skeletal hyperostosis (DISH). These ossifications are often asymptomatic and diagnosed on radiographs; however, specific criteria do exist and need to be met (see later discussion). Posterior spinal ligaments may ossify as well, and their close proximity to the spinal canal may cause neurologic symptoms. Diagnosing posterior ossifications on radiographs might be challenging because of overlying osseous structures, and computed tomography (CT) is used to confirm ossification. MR imaging is of additional value in the case of neurologic symptoms to evaluate spinal cord compression.[9] A limitation of MR imaging is that differentiation between hypertrophy of ligaments and calcifications is difficult.[10,11] Ligaments and calcifications are both low of signal intensity on T1-weighted and T2-weighted fat-saturated images. Ossifications can be confirmed in the presence of fatty marrow, which are of high signal intensity on T1-weighted images and suppressed on T2-weighted fat-saturated images. Because of the small size of ligamentous ossifications and their potential impact, CT can be used for further investigation.[9] Exceptions with extensive paraspinal ligament ossifications occur.

Anterior Longitudinal Ligament and Soft Tissues

Diffuse idiopathic skeletal hyperostosis
DISH is a skeletal disorder, with typical changes in the spine as well as extraspinal involvement. Because this disease is characterized in part by calcification and ossification of the anterior longitudinal ligament, this is discussed here. The extraspinal locations include hyperostosis at ligament insertions, usually the pelvis, calcaneus, tarsal bones, ulnar olecranon, and patella.[12,13] It has often been referred to as Forestier disease. DISH is a common entity, affecting middle-aged and elderly patients, predominantly men. Its origin is unknown. It may be asymptomatic or associated with mild to moderate restriction of motion.[14] It is suggested that certain symptoms and signs, including stiffness, range of motion, and tendinosis, are part of the disease spectrum, consistent with radiographic and radionuclide findings.[12,13]

Radiographic criteria The 3 following radiographic diagnostic criteria are defined for the definite diagnosis of DISH:

1. Flowing calcification and ossification along the anterolateral aspects of at least 4 contiguous vertebra.
2. A relative normal intervertebral disc space at these levels, without characteristics of degenerative disc disease, including vacuum phenomena and vertebral body marginal sclerosis.
3. Absence of apophyseal joint bony ankylosis and sacroiliac joint erosion, sclerosis, or bony fusion[12,13] (**Figs. 3** and **4**).

These criteria help to differentiate from the following:

1. Spondylosis deformans,
2. Intervertebral osteochondrosis, degenerative disc disease, and
3. Ankylosing spondylitis.[12,13]

A recent systematic review article shows that different classification criteria for DISH are available, and that there is a lack of consensus on the (early) diagnosis.[15] Hyperostosis is gradually formed at the anterior vertebral body, appearing at the anterior margin and extending downwards (see **Figs. 3** and **4**). The flowing ossification may show a radiolucent disc extension at the intervertebral level, with a small ossicle anterior tot the disc space.[16] Such an appearance is less frequently seen in the cervical spine than in the thoracic spine. CT might help to exclude a fracture (**Fig. 5**). DISH at the cervical spine may cause dysphagia owing to large ossifications, which are diagnosed on conventional imaging. It should be noted that in the cervical spine concomitant posterior vertebral abnormalities are not infrequent, including ossification of the posterior longitudinal ligament (OPLL) as well as hyperostosis of the posterior vertebral body and osteophytes.[17] A patient with DISH may show activity on a radionuclide study (**Fig. 6**). Involvement of the atlantoaxial level may show a crowned dens and can be extensive in some cases (**Fig. 7**).[18,19] In DISH, the role of MR imaging is limited, unless additional posterior spine involvement is causing neurologic complaints. Because in early stages disease activity on MR imaging might be visualized at the enthesis, looking at early radiographic changes may lead to the correct diagnosis.

Acute calcific tendinitis of the longus colli muscle

On normal conventional imaging of the lateral cervical spine, the anterior prevertebral soft tissues are closely approximated to the anterior vertebral bodies from C1-4. The anterior longitudinal ligament and the longus colli muscle form this 3- to 4-mm soft tissue shadow.[20] A widened prevertebral space C1-4 is abnormal and reason for further clinical and radiological investigation. In a clinical presentation of progressive severe pain in the cervical spine and subfebrile temperature, a retropharyngeal abscess is in the differential diagnosis. However, (subtle) prevertebral calcifications should raise the diagnosis of acute calcific tendinitis of the longus colli muscle (**Figs. 8** and **9**), an aseptic inflammatory response to deposition of calcium hydroxyapatite in the longus colli muscle tendons[20] (**Fig. 10**). On MR imaging, inhomogeneous enhancing prevertebral soft tissues are visualized. The calcific deposition is of low signal intensity on all sequences and not enhancing and should not be misinterpreted as an abscess. Calcifications either on conventional radiograph or on additional CT are diagnostic for acute calcific tendinitis of the longus colli muscle/retropharyngeal tendinitis.[21] Typically, the superior oblique fibers of the longus colli muscle are involved, extending from the anterior atlas to

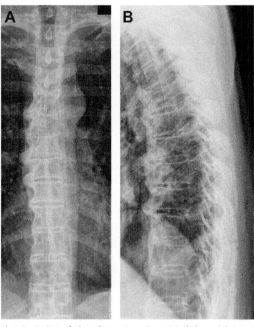

Fig. 3. DISH of the thoracic spine, PA (*A*) and lateral (*B*), in a 62-year-old man. Excessive flowing ossifications at the anterolateral spine on more than 4 levels. The left site is thought to be less involved secondary to aortic pulsations.

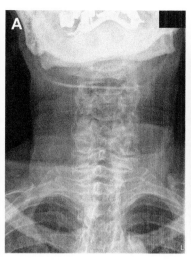
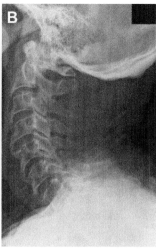

Fig. 4. Cervical spine radiograph (A) anteroposterior (AP) and (B) lateral view of a 63-year-old man. Bony outgrowths at the anterior margin of the vertebra, predominantly extending from the anterior endplate distally, characteristic of DISH. The intervertebral disc spaces are preserved.

anterior tubercles of the transverse processes C3-5[20,21] (see **Fig. 10**).

Conservative treatment includes the use of nonsteroidal anti-inflammatory drugs (NSAIDs). The specific location and clinical information differentiate this from enthesitis in spondylarthropathy (see later discussion).

Posterior Ligaments and Soft Tissues

Ossification of ligaments in the periphery of the spinal canal may decrease the subarachnoid space, leading to acquired spinal stenosis and neurologic symptoms and signs.

Calcification or ossification of the posterior longitudinal ligament

OPLL and the association with progressive cervical myelopathy in a Japanese patient were first published in 1960.[22] Its prevalence has been investigated in Japan, and among patients with cervical spine disorders on conventional radiographs, it varies between 1% and 1.7%. Among asymptomatic Japanese patients older than 30 years of age, it is reported to be 1.9% to 4.3%.[23,24] In non-Japanese patients, a much lower prevalence of 0.1% to 1.7% is described.[25,26] An explanation for the probably

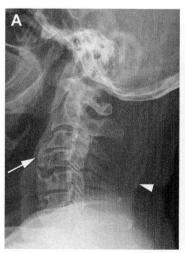
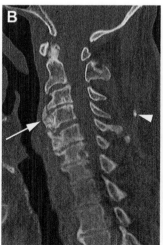
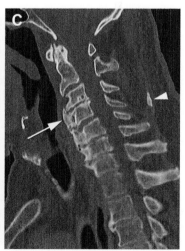

Fig. 5. (A) Lateral cervical spine radiograph performed to rule out a fracture after adequate trauma. The prevertebral soft tissues are normal, and flowing ossifications are consistent with DISH; an incidental ossification in the ligamentum nuchae is visualized (arrowhead). The arrow points to C3-4, where no fracture is visualized. Sagittally reconstructed CT at (B) baseline and (C) after 6 weeks. A radiolucent line is seen at C3-4; a definite differentiation between an incomplete ossification anteriorly at C-4 or a fracture line could not be made. (C) After 6 weeks of immobilization, the CT was repeated, and the radiolucent line was not recognized anymore.

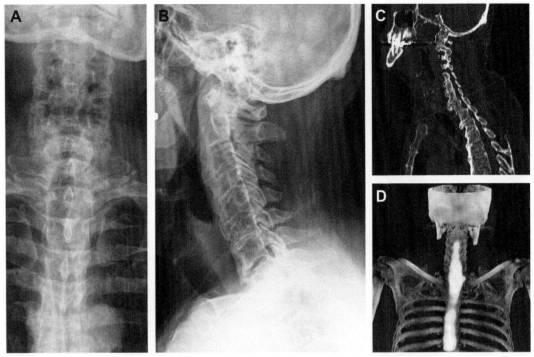

Fig. 6. Active DISH. Patient with progressive complaints of the cervical spine. Conventional radiograph (*A*) AP and (*B*) lateral view. (*B*) Flowing ossifications at the anterior spine, but also (*A*) intervertebral laterally. Ossifications at the facet joint C2-3, posterior in the spinal canal (ligatum flavum) C3, and (*B*) the ligamentum nuchae. (*C*) The sagittal reconstructed image of the single-photon emission computed tomography (SPECT) also shows ossification posterior to the upper thoracic supraspinal ligament. (*D*) Prominent radionuclide uptake is seen in the cervicothoracic spine.

of higher incidence of symptomatic patients in Japan may be the associated narrowing of the spinal canal.[9] Its cause is uncertain.[23] It has been reported in patients with DISH and ankylosing spondylitis.[19] It is most commonly seen in the midcervical region. The thoracic and lumbar spine is involved in about 20% of cases; of these, the fourth to seventh thoracic level is most frequently affected[26] (**Figs. 11–14**). OPLL is more frequent in men than in women and may be asymptomatic (**Fig. 15**). Neurologic symptoms and signs can be initiated by trauma.[9,27]

Imaging On lateral spine radiographs, a linear ossification of variable thickness can be seen posterior to the vertebral bodies and discs (see **Fig. 11**). Based on the anatomy of the posterior longitudinal ligament, the ossification is not always adherent to the vertebral body but separated by a thin radiolucent zone (see **Fig. 2**). The intervertebral disc space is unremarkable. OPLL can be localized or extended along several vertebrae.[28] On cervical spine radiographs, OPLL can be more easily detected than on

thoracic spine radiographs. CT can be used for diagnosis and (preoperative) evaluation.[26] MR imaging is the imaging method of choice to evaluate the spinal canal and cord compression (see **Figs. 11–14**).

Calcification or ossification of the ligamentum flavum

Enthesopathy of the ligamentum flavum at the insertion sites of the laminae is frequently present, predominantly at the lower thoracic level. These ligamentous ossifications are in general without clinical consequences.[9] On conventional radiographs, ossification of the ligamentum flavum (OLF) is not well appreciated, and it can be incidentally found on CT scans or MR imaging (see **Fig. 15**). OLF appears to be unrelated to the presence of OPLL or DISH. A combination of OPLL and OLF can cause myelopathy or radiculopathy, especially in combination with a congenital narrow spinal canal.[29,30]

A focal nodular radiodensity at the posterior part of the spinal canal on a conventional cervical spine radiograph is a typical finding (**Fig. 16**). This is calcium hydroxyapatite crystal deposition in the

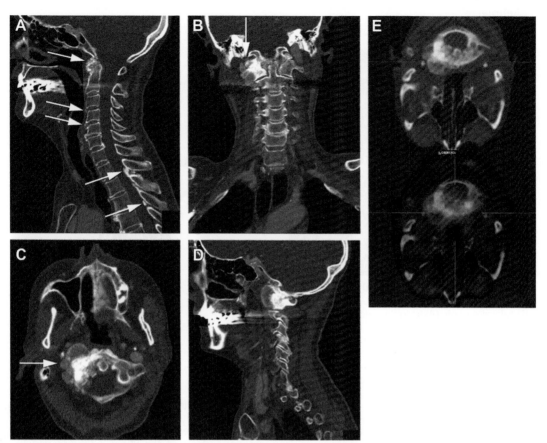

Fig. 7. Crowned dens in a patient with DISH. SPECT with multiplanar reconstructions. Multiple calcifications/ossifications at the atlantoaxial joint, forming a "crowned" dens. (*A*) On the sagittal reconstructed image, arrows point to the ossifications around the dens, the anterior longitudinal ligament, and ligamentum flavum. Sclerosis of the lateral mass C1 is appreciated on the (*B*) coronal (*arrow*) and (*C*) axial image (*arrow*). The (*D*) sagittal image shows hyperostosis at the base of the occiput and the lateral mass of C1 on the right. (*E*) The SPECT shows radionuclide uptake at the C0-C1 joint, consistent with disease activity.

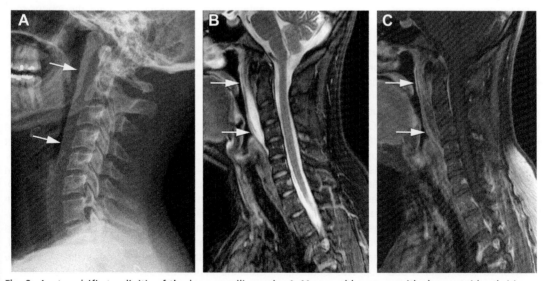

Fig. 8. Acute calcific tendinitis of the longus colli muscle. A 41-year-old woman with rheumatoid arthritis presents with neck pain and subfebrile temperature. (*A*) Conventional lateral radiograph of the cervical spine shows a prevertebral soft tissue swelling from C1-C4 (*arrows*). (*B*) Sagittal T2 turbo spin echo (TSE) and (*C*) sagittal T1 TSE FS with gadolinium. The high-signal intensity on T2 (*B*) (*arrows*) shows inhomogeneous enhancement (*C*) (*arrows*). No demarcated fluid collection with rim enhancement; thus no abscess or spondylodiscitis.

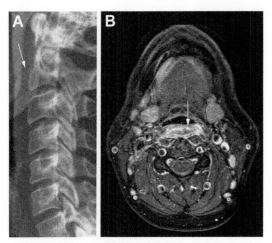

Fig. 9. Acute calcific tendinitis of the longus colli muscle (same patient as in **Fig. 8**). (*A, B*) On the conventional radiograph, (*A*) irregular calcifications anterior to C2 can be appreciated (*arrow*). (*B*) The axial T1 TSE FS with gadolinium shows enhancement in the periphery of the longus colli muscle and irregularly prevertebral (*arrow*). On flexible fiber-optic laryngoscopy, no abscess was found. Symptoms were relieved with NSAIDs.

ligamentum flavum, and only few exceptions, such as fibrocartilaginous or osseous tissue, occur. With additional CT scans or MR imaging, this can be differentiated. A rare case with spinal cord compression owing to an osteochondroma at the lamina C5 is shown in **Fig. 17**. The preferred site for OLF is the midcervical level, often seen in elderly women. No association with other spinal calcifications or ossifications is known. The cause might be degenerative in origin.[10]

Enthesitis in spondyloarthritis

One of the hallmarks of spondyloarthritis is enthesitis, which includes the inflammation of the insertion of muscles and ligaments.[31] Inflammatory back pain in spondyloarthritis is predominantly located in the lower spine and buttocks, but all the entheses in the spine can be involved.[32] On MR imaging, high-signal intensity on fluid-sensitive sequences can be observed at these insertion sites and surrounding connective tissue, consistent with active inflammation. In a patient with psoriasis and progressive cervical spine pain (no trauma), MR imaging shows both anterior and posterior enthesitis (**Fig. 18**). Anteriorly, the vertical fibers of the longus colli muscle from C4-7 are involved, and posteriorly, the intervertebral and supraspinal ligaments are involved (see **Figs. 2** and **10**). The location, absence of calcifications on the conventional radiograph, and concomitant anterior and posterior ligamentous involvement differentiate this from acute calcific tendinitis (see **Figs. 8** and **9**).

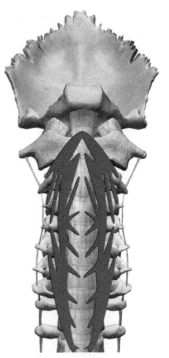

Fig. 10. Anatomic drawing of the longus colli muscles, anterior view. The longus colli muscle is the principal flexor of the cervical spine. It originates from the anterior surfaces of the upper 3 thoracic vertebral bodies and the lower 3 cervical vertebrae. It is divided into superior oblique, vertical, and inferior oblique fibers. The superior oblique fibers insert on the anterior tubercle of the atlas and the second, third, and fourth cervical vertebrae (transverse processes). These superior oblique fibers are the most vulnerable to calcific deposits. On a lateral view of the cervical spine, the anterior longitudinal ligament and the longus colli form a 3- to 4-mm soft tissue shadow anterior to the vertebral bodies of the cervical spine. (*Adapted from* Zibis AH, Giannis D, Malizoset KN, et al. Acute calcific tendinitis of the longus colli muscle: case report and review of the literature. Eur Spine J 2013;22(Suppl 3): S437; with permission.)

PART 2
Paravertebral Ossifications: Vertebral Bony Outgrowths

A variety of ossifications can develop secondary to degeneration or inflammatory disease involving the spine. The pattern and distribution of bony outgrowths are favorable for a certain diagnosis, and additional features of the vertebra can be of help. For instance, the findings of discovertebral erosions in the thoracolumbar spine and signs of osteitis favor the diagnosis of ankylosing spondylitis.

Appreciation of the type of vertebral bony outgrowth may be of important diagnostic value.

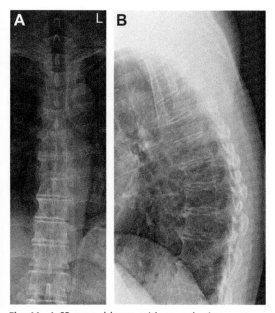

Fig. 11. A 62-year-old man with neurologic symptoms secondary to OPLL and cord compression. (*A, B*) Conventional imaging of the thoracic spine with ossifications on the anterolateral aspect of the spine, consistent with DISH. Calcifications/ossifications posterior to vertebra Th5-7 might be detected.

Type of Vertebral Bony Outgrowth

Routine radiographs form the basis for accurate diagnosis; the lateral view is especially important to analyze carefully.[33] The origin and the growth direction of the phyte as well as height of the adjacent intervertebral disc space may be of diagnostic help.

The commonest change is degenerative disease of the spine with osteophyte formation of the vertebra, combined with intervertebral disc space narrowing. These outgrowing osteophytes may form a bony bridge over the discs, which used to be called senile ankylosing hyperostosis.[14] In ankylosing spondylitis, ossification takes place in the outer layers of the annulus fibrosus itself, resulting in bridging of the intervertebral spaces, and in psoriatic arthritis, new paraspinal ossifications can progress rapidly, separate from the vertebral bodies and discs.[4,34,35] In the schematic drawing in **Fig. 19**, the morphology of different bony outgrowths of the vertebra in early and late stage of disease is shown. The vertical directed bony outgrowths are called syndesmophytes, a hallmark of spondyloarthritis. The horizontal directed extensions from the endplates, osteophytes, are seen in spondylosis and degenerative disc disease. A cutoff point of 45° might be used to differentiate syndesmophytes from osteophytes.[36] The intervertebral disc space may be normal in spondyloarthritis, DISH, and in spondylosis deformans; however, in the latter, this may decrease with aging, consistent with degenerative disc disease. Differentiation between primary ossified ligaments and bony outgrowths of the vertebral endplate might be challenging. However, the anatomy, the site attachment of the ligaments, and knowledge of inflammatory and degenerative processes involved can be of help (see **Fig. 1**). An example

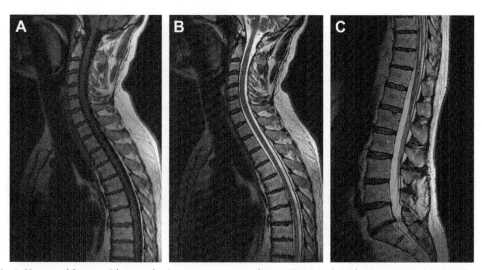

Fig. 12. A 62-year-old man with neurologic symptoms secondary to OPLL and cord compression. MR imaging of the spine: (*A*) sagittal T1-weighted turbo spin echo (T1 TSE), (*B, C*) sagittal T2 TSE. Directly posterior to Th6-7, a linear irregular demarcated area is seen, with high signal intensity on T1 and low on T2 TSE, in contact with the spinal cord. (*B, C*) A linear high-signal intensity central in the spinal cord extends from Th5-10, consistent with myelomalacia.

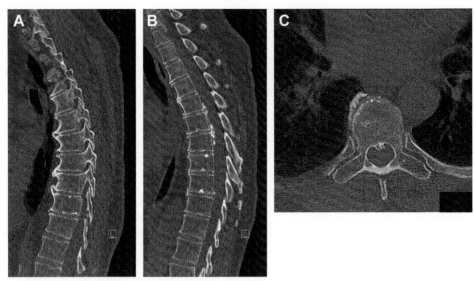

Fig. 13. A 62-year-old man with neurologic symptoms secondary to OPLL and cord compression. Sagittal reconstructed CT images show (*A*) flowing ossifications at the anterior longitudinal ligament (DISH) and (*B*) calcifications/ossifications at the area of the posterior longitudinal ligament extending from Th5 to Th7. (*C*) On the axial CT slice, anterior and posterior calcifications/ossification are appreciated.

is the exuberant hyperostosis at the ligament insertion, separate from the vertebral body in DISH, as is previously discussed (see **Fig. 4**). In **Table 1**, the different types of vertebral phytes, the matching disease, and origin are given. On lateral lumbar spine radiographs, typical examples of bony outgrowths in patients with ankylosing spondylitis, DISH, and degenerative disc disease, respectively, are shown (**Fig. 20**).

Spondyloarthritis

Background

Spondyloarthritis comprises a group of clinically and genetically interrelated rheumatic diseases, including ankylosing spondylitis, psoriatic arthritis, Reiter syndrome, and arthritis-associated inflammatory bowel disease.[37,38] In order to treat patients effectively, spondyloarthritis is nowadays divided into two groups: axial spondyloarthritis (axSpA) and peripheral spondyloarthritis. The predominant inflammatory involvement of the spine and sacroiliac joints requires different treatment. Early detection of AxSpA is of increasing interest, and the role of early imaging, especially MR imaging, has become more important. MR imaging is the only imaging method that shows bone marrow edema. In patients with axSpA, the presence of subchondral bone marrow edema on MR imaging of the sacroiliac joints is part of the new ASAS criteria for classification of disease.[2] Although axSpA primarily affects the sacroiliac joints, MR

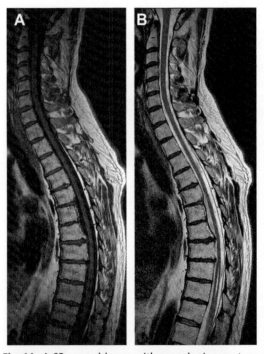

Fig. 14. A 62-year-old man with neurologic symptoms secondary to OPLL and cord compression. Postoperative MR after decompression Th5-7. Sagittal (*A*) T1 TSE and (*B*) T2 TSE. (*B*) Atrophy of the spinal cord with a normal signal at the postoperative level, persisting high signal on T2 TSE at Th9-10. (*A, B*) Bulging discs and osteophytes at Th7-9 with decrease of the subarchnoid space.

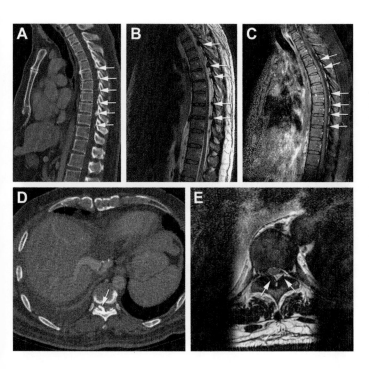

Fig. 15. Incidental ossifications of the ligamentum flavum (OLF). A 60-year-old woman with incidental multiple ligamentum flavum ossifications (*arrows*). (*A*) Sagittal CT reconstruction shows multiple OLF in the thoracic spine. In addition, ossifications of the anterior longitudinal ligament are present, and a midthoracic disc calcification. Sagittal (*B*) T2 TSE and (*C*) T1 TSE fat-saturated after intravenous (IV) contrast administration show bony prominences with a decrease of the subarachnoid space without myelum compression. (*D*) The corresponding axial CT and (*E*) T2 TSE images confirm the location of ossification in the ligamentum flavum. CT and MR are performed in an oncology setting; ascites and pleural fluid are present.

imaging of the spine can play a role.[39,40] In reporting MR imaging of the spine, knowledge of the early and late signs of inflammatory disease and their differential diagnosis is essential. Correlation with conventional radiographs might be useful. The goal is to be sensitive but also specific.

Developing Bony Outgrowths in Axial Spondyloarthritis: Radiograph and MR Imaging Correlation

Enthesitis is a prominent feature of spondyloarthritis[31] (see **Fig. 18**). At the site of ligament insertion,

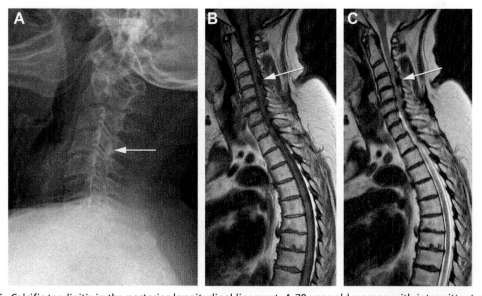

Fig. 16. Calcific tendinitis in the posterior longitudinal ligament. A 79-year-old woman with intermittent neurologic signs. (*A*) The lateral cervical spine radiograph shows a demarcated sclerotic area projecting at the posterior side of the spinal canal at level C4. Sagittal MR images (*B*) T1 TSE and (*C*) T2 TSE show a focal area of low signal intensity on both sequences. There is a congenital narrow spinal canal and cord compression C4-5; no myelomalacia. Arrows point to the calcium hydroxyapatite crystal deposition in the ligamentum flavum at level C4.

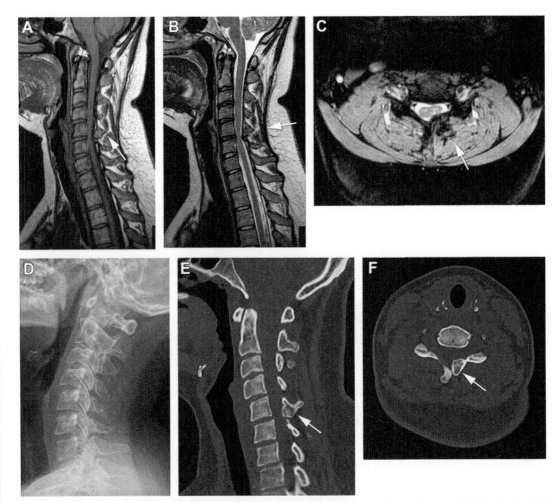

Fig. 17. Osteochondroma of lamina C5 in a young man with multiple osteochondroma. Sagittal (*A*) T1 TSE, (*B*) T2 TSE and axial, (*C*) 3DFFE show spinal cord compression at C5-6 without myelomalacia. There is a prominent mass at the left lamina C5 (*arrow*). On T1, the signal intensity is intermediate, similar to the vertebral bodies. (*D*) The lateral cervical spine radiograph shows an ossification caudal from the facet joints C5-6 (*arrow*). (*E*) The sagittal reconstructed CT and (*F*) axial CT images show a demarcated expanding osseous lesion continuous with the lamina C5 (*arrow*).

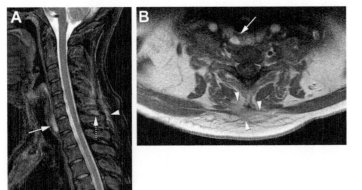

Fig. 18. A 64-year-old woman with psoriasis presents with progressive neck pain. (*A*) Sagittal T2 Dixon and (*B*) axial T1 TSE after IV Gadolinium without fat saturation. Prevertebral linear high-signal intensity on (*A*) T2 Dixon extending from C4 to C7 enhances (*B*) after IV contrast administration (*arrow*) and is located in the vertical part of the right longus colli muscle. There is no abscess, no bone marrow edema, and no spondylodiscitis. The interspinous ligaments (*dotted arrow*) and supraspinal ligament (*arrowheads*) show edema. This is consistent with anterior and posterior enthesitis of the cervical spine in psoriasis. The conventional radiograph (not shown) was unremarkable; especially no calcifications in the soft tissues were present.

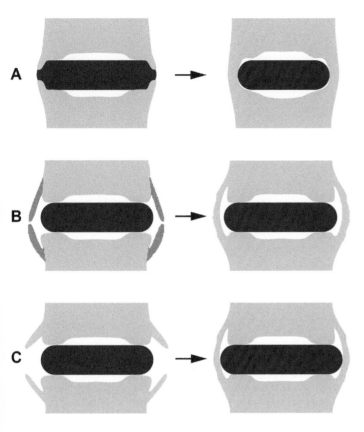

Fig. 19. Different bony outgrowths of the vertebral bodies: (A) ankylosing spondylitis, (B) spondyloarthritis (psoriasis, Reiter syndrome), and (C) spondylosis deformans. The early stage is on the left; the late stage is on the right. In (A) ankylosing spondylitis, the annulus fibrosus ossification forms a syndesmophyte, bridging the intervertebral disc space, forming a bamboo spine. The outgrowth is in the vertical direction. In (B) psoriasis, ossification is formed in the connective tissues; the bony outgrowth develops from irregular to well-defined and eventually bridges; it is vertically directed. In (C) spondylosis deformans, the bony outgrowth is triangular in shape a few millimeters from the corner of the vertebral body; bridging may occur. This horizontal direction is typical for a degenerative origin. A tear in the annular fibrosus insertion to the vertebral endplate facilitates protrusion of disc material. Stress on the ligament insertion site leads to osteophyte formation. (Adapted from Resnick D. Degenerative disease of the spine. In: Resnick D, editor. Diagnosis of bone and joint disorders, Vol 2, 4th edition. Philadelphia: Saunders; 2002; with permission.)

osteitis results in erosion of bone with surrounding sclerosis: a Romanus lesion (see Figs. 1, 2, and 19). As the lesion heals, squaring of the anterior surface of the vertebral body can be observed, and reactive sclerosis produces a shiny corner. A well-defined vertically directed bony outgrowth appears, a syndesmophyte, originating from ossification in the annulus fibrosus[34] (Fig. 21). Enlargement of the syndesmophyte includes ossification of the anterior longitudinal ligament and paravertebral connective tissue, and the end stage is a bridging syndesmophyte. On conventional radiographs of the spine, initial findings may be subtle or absent; MR imaging, however, is more sensitive and detects bone marrow edema.[41] Vertebral corner edema is mentioned as a precursor to syndesmophyte development (see Fig. 21; Fig. 22). Initial unremarkable conventional radiographs of the lumbar spine may detect anterior vertebral corner edema on MR of the lumbar spine and raise suspicion of spondyloarthritis. Additional MR imaging of the sacroiliac joints might help to diagnose AxSpA with certainty (see Figs. 21 and 22; Fig. 23).

Chronic AxSpA changes on MR imaging are detectable as fatty marrow replacement. On MR

Table 1
Bony paravertebral ossification

Type of Vertebral Phytes	Disease	Origin
Syndesmophytes	Ankylosing spondylitis	Annulus fibrosus outer margin
Focal paravertebral ossifications	Psoriasis/Reiter syndrome	Paravertebral soft tissues
Osteophytes/spondylophytes	Degenerative disc disease Spondylosis deformans	Vertebral endplate
Diffuse flowing paravertebral ossifications	DISH	Ligament insertion

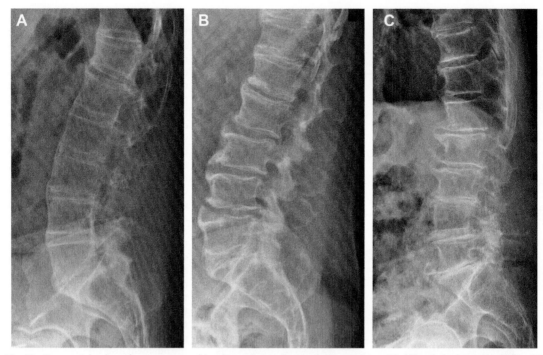

Fig. 20. Paravertebral ossification. Lateral lumbar spine radiograph in patients with (*A*) ankylosing spondylitis, (*B*) DISH, and (*C*) degenerative disc disease (DDD). In (*A*) ankylosing spondylitis, ossification takes place in the outer layers of the annulus fibrosus itself, resulting in bridging of the intervertebral spaces; the disc height is preserved. In (*B*) DISH, the typical diffuse flowing paravertebral ossifications are seen with relative preservation of disc height. In (*C*) DDD, osteophyte formation is typically triangular shaped, horizontally directed, and combined with intervertebral disc space narrowing.

imaging of the spine, this can be seen at the sites of previous inflammation, the vertebral corners, or discovertebral erosions, and ossifications anterior to the vertebral body, the vertebral squaring, the vertebral bony outgrowths (**Fig. 24**), and in spinal ankylosis[42,43] (**Fig. 25**). Discrimination between small syndesmophytes and fibrous tissue on MR imaging might be difficult unless focal bone marrow edema or fatty deposition is present[43,44] (see **Fig. 24**). CT is superior in detailed imaging of bone, if needed, for example, in the preoperative setting.

Degeneration of the Spine: Radiograph and MR Imaging Correlation

Spondylosis deformans
Spondylosis deformans refers to the osteophyte formation seen on radiographs, which are typically triangular in shape, a few millimeters from the corner of the vertebral body, and may bridge the intervertebral space. This horizontal direction is typical for a degenerative origin. Remarkable is the normal height of the intervertebral disc (see **Fig. 19**). Schmorl's concept of pathogenesis of spondylosis deformans is generally accepted.[4] A tear in the attachment of the annulus fibrosus to the vertebral endplate, including Sharpey fibers, facilitates protrusion

anterior and anterolateral of the disc material. A normal hydrated disc stretches the ligament, and a bony outgrowth is formed at the ligament insertion site[4] (see **Fig. 1**).

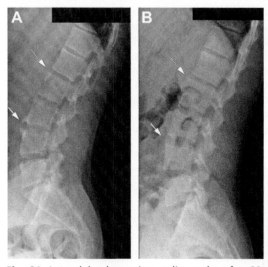

Fig. 21. Lateral lumbar spine radiographs of a 29-year-old male patient with axSpA (*A*) at present and (*B*) 3 years earlier. Development of a shiny corner at L2 (*dotted arrow*) and syndesmophyte at level L3-4 (*arrow*). Note the normal intervertebral disc spaces.

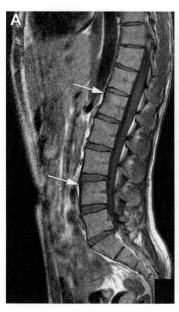
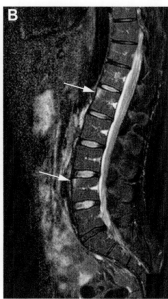

Fig. 22. (*A, B*) Sagittal lumbar spine MR imaging: (*A*) T1 TSE and (*B*) short tau inversion recovery (STIR) images. At the anterior corner of endplate L1 and L4, a focal area of high-signal intensity on STIR is appreciated (*arrow*), moderately low of signal on T1 TSE (*arrow*). This is consistent with focal bone marrow edema (same patient as **Fig. 21B** at baseline).

Degenerative Disc Disease

Degenerative disc disease is not an actual disease, but part of a physiologic process with aging.[45] Degenerative changes in the spine are seen as early as 16 years of age, without clinical correlation.[1] Disc space loss in the lower lumbar spine and Schmorl nodes at the thoracolumbar level are most frequently observed. However, degenerative disc disease may be accelerated by, for example, osteosynthesis in the spine, an artificial disc replacement, or vertebral fracture (**Fig. 26**). Degenerative disc disease is most commonly seen adjacent to the immobilized or fracture level owing to change in mechanical loading. Osteophyte development is likely to be secondary to changes in the biomechanics as well.[46,47]

The term degenerative disc disease is used in both radiographic and MR imaging reporting. On MR imaging, a classification system for lumbar disc degeneration is developed.[48] Classification is done on routine T2-weighted images using MR imaging signal intensity, disc structure, distinction between nucleus and annulus, and disc height. In addition, the vertebral endplates react to the disc space loss.[49] Changes in the vertebral body marrow in both endplates adjacent to a degenerative intervertebral disc are characterized by the (three) types that Modic and colleagues[50] suggested. Modic types are based on the presence of bone marrow edema (type 1), fatty change (type 2), and sclerosis (type 3), respectively. In addition, developing osteophytes may become large and bridge far laterally from the intervertebral disc space. The combination of endplate changes on both sides of the intervertebral disc space may help to differentiate these findings from AxSpA.[51]

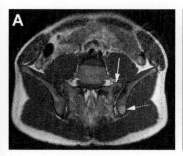
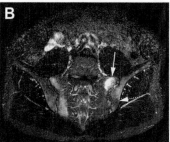

Fig. 23. Coronal oblique (*A*) T1 TSE and (*B*) STIR images of the sacroiliac joints show bilateral sacroiliitis with active and chronic components. Bilateral bone marrow edema; the more intense area on the left (*arrow*) is accompanied by fluid/synovial hypertrophy in the sacroiliac joint. Some erosions are seen. The focal area at the left iliac side (*dotted arrow*) shows high signal on T1 and low on STIR consistent with fat, a sign of repair.

656

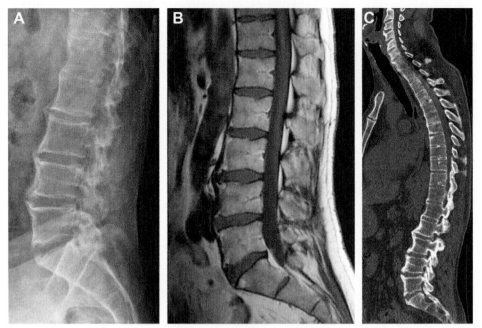

Fig. 24. Patient with axSpA. (*A*) Lateral lumbar spine radiograph, (*B*) sagittal T1TSE MR image, (*C*) sagittal reconstructed whole spine CT image. (*A*) The radiograph shows syndesmophytes, normal intervertebral disc spaces. On MR imaging, fatty replacement is seen at the vertebral corners. At the thoracolumbar level, the syndesmophytes are better appreciated on radiograph (*A*) and CT (*C*). Note the fat anterior in the ossification of vertebral body L3, vertebral squaring.

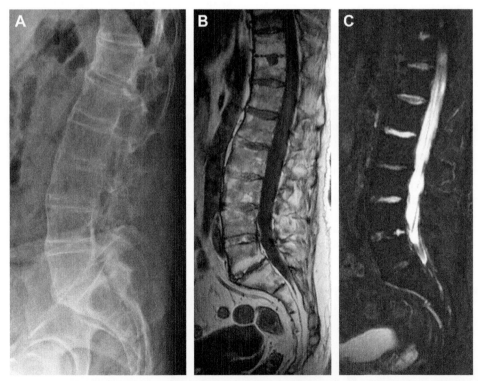

Fig. 25. Ankylosis of the lumbar spine. (*A*) Lateral lumbar spine radiograph sagittal MR imaging, (*B*) T1 TSE, and (*C*) STIR. Syndesmophytes in addition to ankylosis of vertebral bodies and posterior elements are appreciated. The inhomogeneous high-signal intensity on T1 TSE is homogenously suppressed on STIR. There is a combination of fatty replacement secondary to inflammation and fatty bone marrow owing to osteoporosis. The intervertebral disc heights are only slightly decreased, and intervertebral discs still show water content on STIR. Modic type 2 is present at L5-S1.

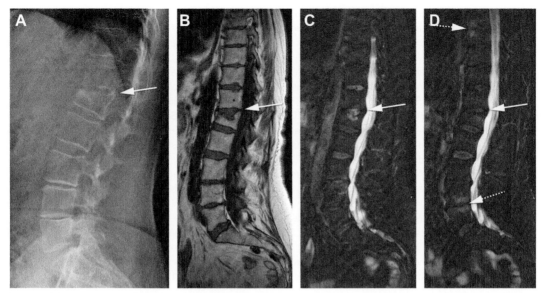

Fig. 26. Old posttraumatic fracture vertebra L1 without bone marrow edema. (*A*) Radiograph, (*B*) sagittal T1 TSE, and (*C, D*) T2 TSE fat-saturated images. Intervertebral space loss Th12-L1 and posterior osteophytes (*arrows*). Sclerosis and bony fragments anterior. Degenerative disc disease at multiple levels with prominent Modic type 1 changes at Th10-11 anterior and L5-S1 (*dotted arrows*).

SUMMARY

Knowledge of the vertebral spine anatomy and underlying processes of disease may help to characterize paravertebral ossifications. Incidental findings of ligamentous calcifications increase with aging; however, they can have clinical impact. The exuberant flowing ossifications in the cervical spine in DISH may lead to swallowing problems, and small ligamentous ossifications lining the spinal canal can cause neurologic symptoms. Knowledge of imaging findings in calcific tendinitis in the longus colli muscle may prevent unnecessary medical interventions and is self-limiting.

The vertebral body may form a bony outgrowth secondary to inflammation and degeneration. Based on its origin and growth direction, a vertebral phyte may be classified and linked to an underlying cause. Appreciation of the intervertebral disc space might be of help.

Imaging rheumatology patients has shifted toward the early detection of disease because effective medication for axSpA has become available. On MR imaging of the spine, focal bone marrow edema or fatty lesions can be detected and may increase the suspicion of axSpA. Differentiation from degenerative disc disease is possible using the correct parameters. Additional MR imaging of the sacroiliac joints might help to diagnose these patients with confidence.

It is important to recognize the early signs of paravertebral ossifications on both radiographs and MR imaging, in order to prevent incorrect or late diagnosis and delayed treatment.

ACKNOWLEDGMENTS

The author thanks her colleagues HM Kroon, MD PhD and BM Verbist, MD PhD, for their help in collecting cases and Gerrit Kracht for preparing the drawings and images.

REFERENCES

1. De Bruin F, ter Horst S, Bloem JL, et al. Prevalence of degenerative changes of the spine on magnetic resonance images and radiographs in patients aged 16-45 years with chronic back pain of short duration in the Spondyloarthritis Caught Early (SPACE) cohort. Rheumatology 2016;55(1):56–65.
2. Lambert RG, Bakker PA, van der Heijde D, et al. Defining active sacroiliitis on MRI for classification of axial spondyloarthritis: update by the ASAS MRI working group. Ann Rheum Dis 2016;75:1958–63.
3. Netter FH. Vertebral column. In: Netter FH, editor. The Ciba collection of medical illustrations, vol. 8. Musculoskeletal system. Part 1. Anatomy, physiology and metabolic disorders. New Jersey: Ciba-Geigy Corporation; 1987. p. 9–18.
4. Resnick D. Degenerative disease of the spine. In: Resnick D, editor. Diagnosis of bone and joint disorders, vol. 2, 4th edition. Philadelphia: Saunders; 2002. p. 1382–475.

5. Cattell HS, Filtzer DL. Pseudosubluxation and other normal variations in the cervical spine in children: a study of one hundred and sixty children. J Bone Joint Surg Am 1965;47:1295.

6. Woo TD, Tony G, Charran A, et al. Radiographic morphology of normal ring apophyses in the immature cervical spine. Skeletal Radiol 2018;47(9):1221–8.

7. Keats TE, Anderson MW. The spine. In: Keats TE, Anderson MW, editors. Atlas of normal roentgen variants that may simulate disease. 9th edition. Philadelphia: Elsevier Saunders; 2013. p. 197.

8. Smith CF, Pugh DG, Polley HF. Physiologic vertebral ligamentous calcification: an aging process. Am J Roentgenol 1955;74:1049–58.

9. Ehara S, Shimamura T, Nakamura R, et al. Paravertebral ligamentous ossification: DISH, OPLL and OLF. Eur J Radiol 1998;27:196–205.

10. Resnick D, Pineda C. Vertebral involvement in calcium pyrophosphate dihydrate crystal deposition disease. Radiology 1984;153:55–60.

11. Hirao Y, Chikuda H, Oshima Y, et al. Extensive ossification of the paraspinal ligaments in a patient with vitamin D-resistant rickets: case report with literature review. Int J Surg Case Rep 2016;27:125–8.

12. Resnick D, Niwayama G. Radiographic and pathologic features of spinal involvement in diffuse idiopathic skeletal hyperostosis (DISH). Radiology 1976;119:559–68.

13. Resnick D, Shaul SR, Robins JM. Diffuse idiopathic skeletal hyperostosis (DISH) Forestier's disease with extraspinal manifestations. Radiology 1975;115:513–24.

14. Forestier J, Rotes-Wuerol J. Senile ankylosing hyperostosis of the spine. Ann Rheum Dis 1950;9:321–30.

15. Kuperus JS, de Gendt EEA, Oner CF. Classification criteria for diffuse idiopathic skeletal hyperostosis: a lack of consensus. Rheumatology 2017;56:1123–34.

16. Resnick D. Diffuse idiopathic skeletal hyperostosis. In: Resnick D, editor. Diagnosis of bone and joint disorders, vol. 2, 4th edition. Philadelphia: Saunders; 2002. p. 1476–503.

17. Ono K, Ota H, Tada K, et al. Ossified posterior longitudinal ligament: a clinicopathologic study. Spine 1977;2:126.

18. Baysal T, Baysal O, Kutlu R, et al. The crowned dens syndrome: a rare form of calcium pyrophosphate deposition disease. Eur Radiol 2000;10:1003.

19. Resnick D, Guerra J Jr, Robinson CA, et al. Association of diffuse idiopathic skeletal hyperostosis (DISH) and ossification of the posterior longitudinal ligament. AJR Am J Roentgenol 1978;131:1049.

20. Newmark H, Forrester DM, Brown J, et al. Calcific tendinitis of the neck. Radiology 1978;128:355–8.

21. Zibis AH, Giannis D, Malizos KN, et al. Acute calcific tendinitis of the longus colli muscle: case report and review of the literature. Eur Spine J 2013;22(Suppl 3):S434–8.

22. Tsukimoto H. An autopsy report of syndrome of compression of spinal cord owing to ossification within spinal canal of cervical spine. Arch Jpn Chir 1960;29:1003.

23. Tsuyama N. The ossification of the posterior longitudinal ligament of the spine (OPLL). J Jpn Orthop Assoc 1981;55:425.

24. Matsunaga S, Sakou T. Ossification of the posterior longitudinal ligament of the cervical spine: etiology and natural history. Spine (Phila Pa 1976) 2012; 37(5):E309–14.

25. McAfee PC, Regan JJ, Bohlman HH. Cervical cord compression from ossification of the posterior longitudinal ligament in non-orientals. J Bone Joint Surg Br 1987;69:569–75.

26. Boody BS, Lendner M, Vaccaro AR. Ossification of the posterior longitudinal ligament in the cervical spine: a review. Int Orthop 2018. https://doi.org/10.1007/s00264-018-4106-5.

27. Resnick D. Calcification and ossification of the posterior spinal ligaments and tissues. Articular diseases. In: Resnick D, editor. Diagnosis of bone and joint disorders, vol. 2, 4th edition. Philadelphia: WB Saunders; 2002. p. 1504–16.

28. Tsuyama N. Ossification of the posterior longitudinal ligament of the spine. Clin Orthop Relat Res 1984; 184:71–84.

29. Hukuda S, Mochizuki T, Ogata M, et al. The pattern of spinal and extraspinal hyperostosis in patients with ossification of the posterior longitudinal ligament and the ligamentum flavum causing myelopathy. Skeletal Radiol 1983;10:79–85.

30. Kotani Y, Takahata M, Abumi K, et al. Cervical myelopathy resulting from combined ossification of the ligamentum flavum and posterior longitudinal ligament: report of two cases and literature review. Spine J 2013;13(1):e1–6.

31. D'Angostino MA, Olivieri I. Enthesitis. Best Pract Res Clin Rheumatol 2006;20:473–86.

32. Sieper J, van der Heijde D, Landewe R, et al. New criteria for inflammatory back pain in patients with chronic back pain: a real patient exercise by experts from the Assessment in SpondyloArthritis international Society (ASAS). Ann Rheum Dis 2009;68:784–8.

33. Resnick D. Hyperostosis and ossification in the cervical spine. Arthritis Rheum 1984;27:564–9.

34. Resnick D. Ankylosing spondylitis. In: Resnick D, editor. Diagnosis of bone and joint disorders, vol. 2, 4th edition. Philadelphia: Saunders; 2002. p. 1023–81.

35. Bywaters EGL, Dixon AStJ. Paravertebral ossification in psoriatic arthritis. Ann Rheum Dis 1965;24:313.

36. de Bruin F, de Koning A, van den Berg R, et al. Development of the CT syndesmophyte score (CTSS) in patients with ankylosing spondylitis: data from the SIAS cohort. Ann Rheum Dis 2018;77(3):371–7.

37. Kahn MA. Update on spondyloarthropathies. Ann Intern Med 2002;136:896–907.

38. Rudwaleit M. New approaches to diagnosis and classification of axial and peripheral spondyoarthritis. Curr Opin Rheumatol 2010;22:375–80.

39. Hermann KG, Baraliakos X, van der Heijde DM, et al. Descriptions of spinal MRI lesions and definition of a positive MRI of the spine in axial spondyloarthritis: a consensual approach by the ASAS/OMERACT MRI study group. Ann Rheum Dis 2012;71:1278–88.

40. Weber U, Zhao Z, Rufibach K, et al. Diagnostic utility of candidate definitions for demonstrating axial spondyloarthritis on magnetic resonance imaging of the spine. Arthritis Rheumatol 2015;67: 924–33.

41. Maksymowych WP, Chiowchanwisawakit P, Clare T, et al. Inflammatory lesions of the spine on magnetic resonance imaging predict the development of new syndesmophytes in ankylosing spondylitis: evidence of a relationship between inflammation and new bone formation. Arthritis Rheum 2009;60(1): 93–102.

42. Jurik AG. Imaging the spine in arthritis—a pictorial review. Insights Imaging 2011;2:177–91.

43. Madsen KB, Jurik AG. MRI grading method for active and chronic spinal changes in spondyloarthritis. Clin Radiol 2009;65:6–14.

44. Braun J, Baraliakos X, Golder W, et al. Analysing chronic spinal changes in ankylosing spondylitis: a systematic comparison of conventional x rays with magnetic resonance imaging using established and new scoring systems. Ann Rheum Dis 2004; 63(9):1046–55.

45. Sokoloff L. Pathology and pathogenesis of osteoarthritis. Degenerative disease of the spinal column. In: Hollander JL, editor. Arthritis and allied conditions. Philadelphia: Lea & Febiger; 1966. p. 855–7.

46. Kong L, Ma Q, Meng F, et al. The prevalence of heterotopic ossification among patients with artificial disc replacement: a systematic review and meta-analysis. Medicine 2017;96(24):e7163.

47. Tian W, Han X, Liu B, et al. Generation and development of paravertebral ossification in cervical artificial disk replacement: a detailed analytic report using coronal reconstruction CT. Clin Spine Surg 2017; 30(3):E179–88.

48. Pfirrmann CW, Metzdorf A, Zanetti M, et al. Magnetic resonance classification of lumbar intervertebral disc degeneration. Spine 2001;26:1873–8.

49. Pearce RH, Thompson JP, Bebault GM, et al. Magnetic resonance imaging reflects the chemical changes of aging degeneration in the human intervertebral disk. J Rheumatol Suppl 1991;27: 42–3.

50. Modic MT, Steinberg PM, Ross JS, et al. Degenerative disk disease: assessment of changes in vertebral body marrow with MR imaging. Radiology 1988;166:193–9.

51. de Bruin F, Treyvaud MO, Feydy A, et al. Prevalence of degenerative changes and overlap with spondyloarthritis-associated lesions in the spine of patients from the DESIR cohort. RMD Open 2018; 4:e000657.

Conventional Radiography of the Hip Revisited
Correlation with Advanced Imaging

Charbel Mourad, MD[a,b], Patrick Omoumi, MD, PhD[c],
Jacques Malghem, MD[d], Bruno C. Vande Berg, MD, PhD[b,d],*

KEYWORDS

• Hip • Osteonecrosis • Osteoarthritis • Bone marrow edema • Radiography • MR imaging

KEY POINTS

- Conventional radiographs continue to play an important role in the first-line evaluation of symptomatic hip joints despite the advent of MR imaging.
- Comparative anteroposterior and off-lateral views of the hips enable an accurate evaluation of the joint space.
- Radiographs have limited sensitivity in detecting bone changes.
- Radiographs cannot detect joint effusion and bone marrow changes.

INTRODUCTION

Conventional radiography is frequently used as the initial imaging modality to assess hip disorders.[1–4] The aim of this review article is to provide a structured approach to analyze conventional radiography of normal and abnormal adult hips. We will focus on changes in radiological bone density and contours of the femoral head and alterations of the joint space observed in common hip disorders, which include osteoarthritis, femoral head osteonecrosis, transient osteoporosis, and subchondral insufficiency fractures. The findings at radiography are correlated with MR imaging and computed tomography (CT). Pediatric, metabolic, neoplastic, and postoperative hip disorders will not be addressed. Conditions in which correlation with cross-sectional imaging does not bring added value for the understanding of conventional radiography will be out of the scope of this review.

ANATOMY OF THE HIP AND CHALLENGES IN HIP DISORDERS

The hip is a deeply located highly congruent diarthrodial joint. A nearly spherical femoral head articulates with the acetabular cavity, which is reinforced by an acetabular labrum, and the capsular ligaments (the medial and lateral arms of the iliofemoral ligament, the pubofemoral ligament, and the ischiofemoral ligament) (Fig. 1). Hip radiographs only demonstrate bone contours to which the x-ray beam is tangent[5,6] (Fig. 2).

Disclosure Statement: The authors do not have any relationship with a commercial company that has a direct financial interest in subject matter or materials discussed in article or with a company making a competing product.

[a] Department of Radiology, Hôpital Libanais Geitaoui HLG-CHU, 1100 Achrafieh, PO BOX: 175086, Beyrouth, Lebanon; [b] Institut de Recherche Expérimentale et Clinique (IREC), Université Catholique de Louvain, Brussels, Belgium; [c] Department of Diagnostic and Interventional Radiology, Lausanne University Hospital, Centre Hospitalier Universitaire, University of Lausanne, Rue du Bugnon 46, Lausanne 1011, Switzerland; [d] Department of Radiology, Cliniques Universitaires Saint Luc, 10 Avenue Hippocrate, 1200 Woluwe-Saint-Lambert, Brussels, Belgium

* Corresponding author. Department of Radiology, Cliniques Universitaires Saint Luc, 10 Avenue Hippocrate, 1200 Woluwe-Saint-Lambert, Brussels, Belgium.
E-mail address: bruno.vandeberg@uclouvain.be

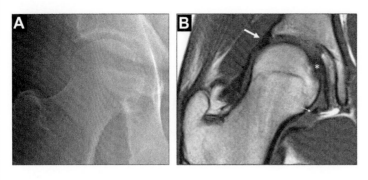

Fig. 1. (*A*) AP radiograph of the right hip with (*B*) corresponding coronal T1-weighted MR image. Only the bony components of the hip are adequately depicted on the radiograph whereas the MR image clearly demonstrates the non mineralized components of the hip: the acetabular labrum (*thick white arrow*), the transverse ligament (*thin white arrow*), the articular capsule (*black arrow*), and the ligamentum teres (*asterisk*).

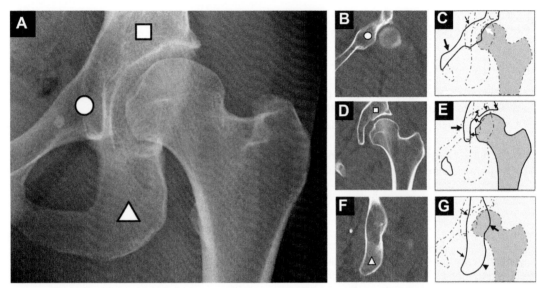

Fig. 2. Radiographic anatomy of the hip. (*A*) AP radiograph of a left hip and (*B, D, F*) corresponding coronal CT reformats with (*C, E, G*) schematic drawings. (*B, C*) Anterior column of the hip: the iliopectineal line (*thin black arrow*), the iliopubic ramus (*thick black arrow*), and the anterior acetabular wall (*white arrow*). (*D, E*) Acetabular fossa with the acetabular sourcil, the weight-bearing surface of the acetabulum (*arrowheads*), the acetabular fossa (*thin arrows*), and the quadrilateral surface (*thick arrow*). (*F, G*) Posterior column of the hip with the ilio-ischiatic line (*thin arrows*), the ischial tuberosity (*arrowhead*), and the posterior acetabular wall (*thick arrow*). Circle (in *A* and *B*): anterior column of the hip. Square (in *A* and *D*): acetabular fossa with acetabular sourcil. Triangle (in *A* and *F*): posterior columns of the hip.

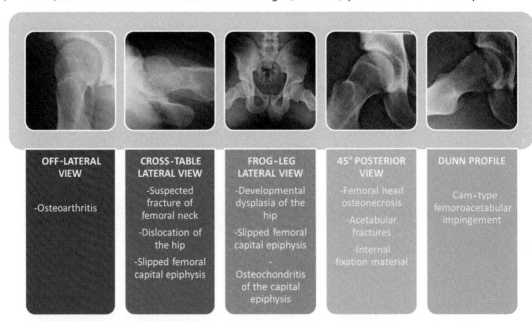

OFF-LATERAL VIEW	CROSS-TABLE LATERAL VIEW	FROG-LEG LATERAL VIEW	45° POSTERIOR VIEW	DUNN PROFILE
-Osteoarthritis	-Suspected fracture of femoral neck -Dislocation of the hip -Slipped femoral capital epiphysis	-Developmental dysplasia of the hip -Slipped femoral capital epiphysis -Osteochondritis of the capital epiphysis	-Femoral head osteonecrosis -Acetabular fractures -Internal fixation material	Cam-type femoroacetabular impingement

Fig. 3. Lateral radiographic projections of the hip and their common indications.

Medical imaging plays a major role in the work-up of patients with suspected hip disorders because the deeply located hip is not amenable to direct palpation and the clinical examination may be restricted to evaluating the range of motion.[7,8]

RADIOLOGICAL WORK-UP OF THE HIP

Radiological work-up of the hip includes an anteroposterior (AP) radiograph of the pelvis and a lateral radiograph of the symptomatic hip. The pelvic radiograph allows the assessment of the entire pelvic girdle, providing an overview of the entire region. Moreover, by allowing the comparative analysis of both hips, it enhances the detection of subtle bone and joint abnormalities. The AP pelvic radiograph should be obtained with the patient lying supine, the lower limbs medially rotated (20 degrees).[4,9,10] When obtained in a standing position, it enables detecting leg length discrepancy but provides a less satisfactory analysis of the bone structure. Standing hip radiograph does not provide additional information on the joint space except in severe hip dysplasias, opposite to the knee joint, for which proper assessment of the joint space width requires weight-bearing radiographs.[11,12]

Table 1
Lateral radiographic projections of the hip joint

Radiographic Projection	Value	Limitation	Common Indication
Off lateral view (Lequesne false profile)	• Acetabular morphology • Evaluation of the anterior and posterior joint space	Poor evaluation of the femoral neck	• Osteoarthritis
Lateral both hips (frog-leg projection)	• Allows a comparison with the contralateral side • Profiles the head-neck junction adequately	• Anterior and posterior aspects of the joint space are not evaluated • Femoral neck is not adequately evaluated	• Developmental dysplasia of the hip • Slipped femoral capital epiphysis • Osteochondritis of the capital epiphysis
45° posterior oblique, (Lauenstein projection)	• Evaluation of the ilioischial column and anterior acetabular rim • Lateral view of the upper third of femur		• Femoral head osteonecrosis • Acetabular fractures • Internal fixation material
30° anterior oblique (Judet projection)	• Evaluation of the posterior acetabular rim and the iliopubic column	• Anterior and posterior aspects of the joint space are not evaluated • The greater trochanter can obscure the head-neck anatomy.	• Acetabular fractures • Internal fixation material
True lateral neck of femur (cross-table lateral view)	• Evaluation of the proximal femur	• Not for evaluation of joint space and acetabulum • Poor image quality	• Suspected fracture of femoral neck • Dislocation of the hip • Slipped femoral capital epiphysis
Urethral profile	• Same as Lauenstein projection • Evaluation of femoral neck	• Anterior and posterior aspects of the joint space are not evaluated	• Femoral head osteonecrosis • Acetabular fractures • Internal fixation material
Dunn profile	• To evaluate the proximal femur • Profiles the head-neck junction	• Poor evaluation of acetabulum and joint space	• Cam-type femoroacetabular impingement

The added value of an AP hip radiograph to complement pelvic radiograph is open to debate except after total hip replacement. In the authors' institution, an AP hip radiograph usually is obtained because of the high quality of the bony details secondary to beam collimation. Several different lateral views of the hip can be obtained, the choice of which may depend on the clinical situation (**Fig. 3, Table 1**).[2] Most of the lateral radiographs are obtained with different degrees of hip abduction and flexion providing a lateral view of the proximal femur.[9,13] The off-lateral view (also called false profile of Lequesne) is a unique radiograph that provides an evaluation of the hip joint in a near sagittal plane, with the femur in an anatomic position[14] (**Fig. 4**). It allows analyzing the most anterior and posterior aspects of the joint space that are not depicted on the AP and the other lateral radiographs, at the expense of a decrease in the overall quality of the image.

Conventional radiography yields a high spatial resolution that enables detecting subtle changes in cortical contours and joint space width. Because conventional radiography corresponds to a bidimensional projection of 3-D structures, however, it can only detect cortical changes to which the x-ray beam is tangent[5] (see **Figs. 1** and **4**). Other limitations of conventional radiography of the hip include limited sensitivity for the detection of trabecular bone and medullary changes and the inability to show joint effusion[6] (**Fig. 5**).

RADIOLOGICAL DENSITY OF THE FEMORAL HEAD

Normal Radiological Density of the Femoral Head

The physician interpreting conventional hip radiographs should first focus on alterations in radiological bone density. The radiographic appearance of the hip joint is largely influenced by its anatomy. The femoral head varies in thickness due to its spherical shape and it contains a thin sclerotic line that corresponds to the remnant of the physis (also called the physeal scar). The head is partially covered by the

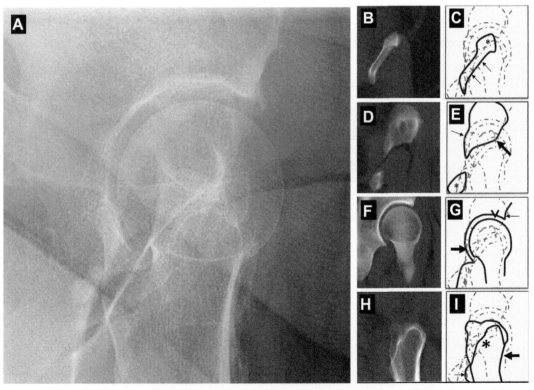

Fig. 4. Radiographic anatomy of the hip. (*A*) Off-lateral view (Lequesne false profile) of the left hip and (*B, D, F, H*) corresponding sagittal CT reformats with (*C, E, G, I*) schematic drawings, from anterior to posterior. (*B, C*) Pubic bone (*asterisk*) and the iliopubic ramus (*arrows*). (*D, E*) The anterior acetabular wall (*thick arrow*), acetabular fossa (*thin arrow*), and the ischiopubic ramus (*asterisk*). (*F, G*) Anterior acetabular rim (*thin arrow*). The posterior (*thick arrow*) and the anterosuperior (*arrowhead*) aspects of the joint space are adequately depicted. (*H, I*) Greater trochanter (*asterisk*) superimposed on the femoral neck (*thick arrow*); the lesser trochanter (*thin arrow*) also is seen.

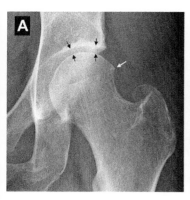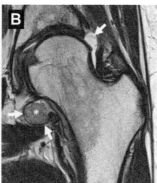

Fig. 5. (A) Conventional radiography does not demonstrate joint effusion. Note the preserved joint space (*black arrows in A*) and early osteophyte formation (*white arrow in A*). (B) The coronal T2-weighted MR image shows distended joint recesses of variable signal intensity (*thick arrows and asterisk* in a case of synovial chondromatosis of the hip [*B*]).

acetabulum, which is obliquely oriented in the coronal and axial planes. The radiological density of the femoral head can be divided into 3 zones, reflecting the superimposition of the anterior and posterior acetabular walls and their oblique orientation (**Fig. 6**). The upper medial zone shows the highest bone density due to the superimposition of both acetabular walls on the upper femoral head. It is delimited by the upper limit of the femoral head superiorly and the anterior acetabular wall inferiorly. The intermediate zone shows intermediate density and is delineated by the projection of the anterior acetabulum medially and by the posterior acetabulum laterally. The lower and lateral zone of the femoral head shows the lowest density and corresponds to the lateral aspect of the femoral head projecting outside the acetabular borders. The relative importance of these 3 zones is largely dependent on the anatomy and the position of the body relative to the direction of the x-ray beam. Any deviation from this normal zonal description may reflect an alteration of the bone density, the only exception being the physeal scar. The apparent radiological density of the femoral head also may depend on technical factors, acetabular changes and other superimposing structures.

Increased Radiological Density of the Femoral Head

Femoral head osteonecrosis

Femoral head osteonecrosis can be associated with increased radiological density of the femoral head (**Table 2**). Bone hyperostosis is mainly due to trabecular bone apposition at the margin of or within the osteonecrotic lesion.[15–19] Therefore,

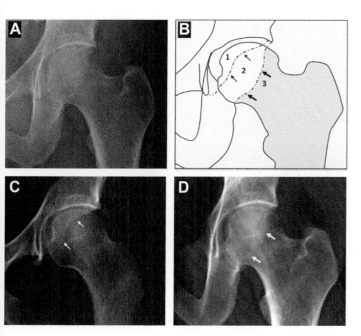

Fig. 6. Normal zonal pattern of the radiological density of the femoral head on an (A) AP radiograph and (B) corresponding schematic representation. The anterior (*thin arrows* [B, C]) and posterior (*thick arrows* [B, D]) acetabular walls delineate 3 zones of variable density depending on the superposition of the femoral head and both acetabular walls. 1: femoral head + anterior and posterior walls. 2: femoral head + posterior wall. 3: femoral head (B). Coronal thick multiplanar reformats in the (C) anterior and (D) posterior aspects of the hip joint demonstrating the anterior acetabular wall (*arrows* [C]) and posterior acetabular wall (*arrows* [D]), respectively.

Table 2
Focal increase in radiological density of the hip

Examples	Histologic Correlation	Radiological Features
Osteoarthritis	• Apposition of trabecular bone and thickening of subchondral bone plate	• Sclerosis occurs in subchondral bone • Joint space narrowing • Geodes • Osteophytes
Femoral head osteonecrosis	• Apposition of trabecular bone at the margin of necrotic territory • Mineral deposits in necrotic bone	• Dense concave sclerotic rim • Preserved joint space (early stages) • Horseshoe subchondral sclerosis on lateral view
Subchondral insufficiency fracture	• Microcallus formation in subchondral trabecular bone	• Sclerosis is faint and predominates in subchondral trabecular bone • Preserved joint space • Occasional subtle alteration of head contour

the radiological hallmark of osteonecrosis is the presence of a sharply delineated sclerotic lesion in the femoral head that represents the sclerotic interface that separates the subchondral necrotic segment of the epiphysis from the normal adjacent bone when the x-ray beam is tangent to it[18–20] (**Fig. 7**). Occasionally, the sclerotic zone may appear ill defined, without sclerotic line, on the AP radiograph. The sclerotic bone margin may become more conspicuous on the oblique projection of the femoral head (**Fig. 8**). When the lesion is extensive it may involve the entire femoral head with a horseshoe pattern and it becomes difficult to detect the real margins of the necrotic lesion on the radiographs (**Fig. 9**).

Subchondral insufficiency fracture

In patients with subchondral insufficiency fracture, a subtle increase in bone density in the subchondral area can be observed, usually late in the

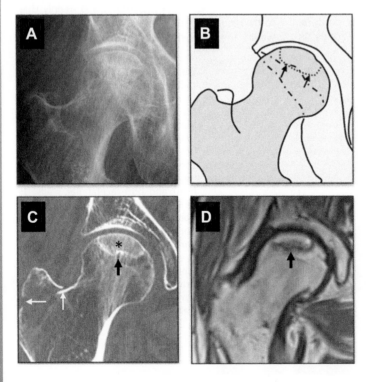

Fig. 7. Focal increased density in osteonecrosis of the femoral head in a 69-year-old woman. (*A*) AP radiograph of the right hip with (*B*) corresponding schematic representation show a wedge-shaped area in the femoral head demarcated by a sclerotic line (*arrows* [*B*]). (*C*) Coronal CT reformat shows a thin sclerotic line (*black arrow*) delineating a territory with focal increased density (*asterisk*); note the fracture lines (*white arrows*) on that CT performed in the context of a low-energy trauma. (*D*) Coronal T1-weighted MR image showing the necrotic territory delineated by a low T1 line (*arrow*).

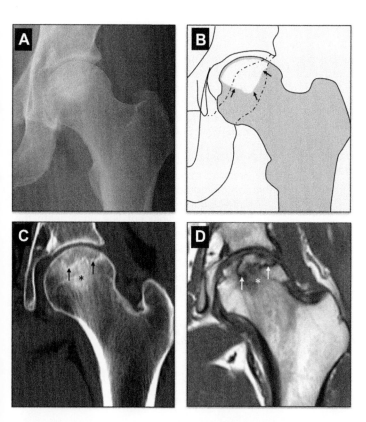

Fig. 8. A 36-year-old man with left hip pain. (*A*) AP radiograph of the left hip and (*B*) corresponding schematic representation show a wedge-shaped sclerotic area (*arrows* [*B*]) in the femoral head that is not related to the acetabular wall. (*C*) Coronal reformat of a CT scan of the same hip shows a thin sclerotic line (*arrows*) delineating the necrotic territory, surrounded by ill-defined trabecular bone sclerosis (*asterisk*). (*D*) On the coronal T1-weighted MR image, the sclerotic margin is seen as a linear low signal intensity band (*arrows*) surrounded by ill-defined low signal intensity area (*asterisk*) corresponding to the trabecular sclerosis.

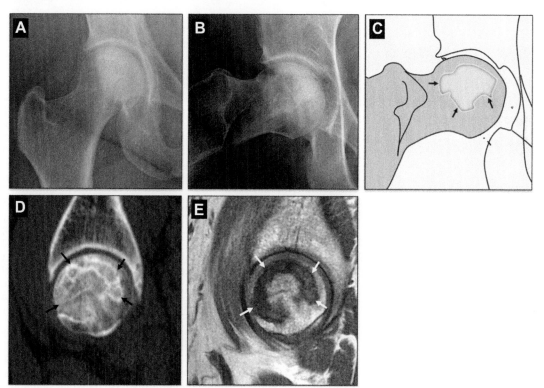

Fig. 9. Focal increased density of the femoral head. A 42-year-old man with osteonecrosis of the right femoral head. (*A*) AP radiograph shows a subtle ill-defined increased density of the femoral head. (*B*) The Lauenstein view increases the conspicuity of the osteonecrotic lesion since the sclerotic line becomes tangent to the margins of the lesion (*arrows* [*C*], corresponding schematic representation). On the (*D*) sagittal CT reformat and the (*E*) sagittal T1-weighted MR image, the osteonecrotic territory has a horseshoe pattern, occupying a large volume of the femoral head (*arrows* [*D*, *E*]).

course of the disease (**Fig. 10**). These subtle sclerotic changes are probably due to callus formation in the subchondral area.[21,22]

Osteoarthritis

In advanced hip osteoarthritis, increased radiological bone density can be seen in association with important joint space narrowing. These changes, related to the thickening of the subchondral bone plate and/or of the trabecular bone network, can occur on either or both sides of the joint[23] (**Fig. 11**).

Decreased Radiological Density of the Femoral Head

Femoral head osteonecrosis

Several patterns of decreased bone density can be observed in femoral head osteonecrosis[24]

(**Table 3**). The first pattern of radiological lucency consists of predominant bone resorption within the necrotic lesion[25] (**Fig. 12**). It usually involves the peripheral zones of the necrotic tissue and, possibly, leads to progressive resorption of necrotic tissue, a phenomenon that has been denominated "creeping substitution" by Phemister.[26] Extensive resorption of the necrotic bone is more conspicuous on CT than on radiographs.

Another pattern of bone lucency is the presence of a thin radiolucent line underneath the subchondral bone plate (**Fig. 13**). This radiolucent pattern has been called the radiological crescent sign[27] and corresponds to a delaminating fracture of the trabecular bone underneath the subchondral bone.[28–31] A real vacuum

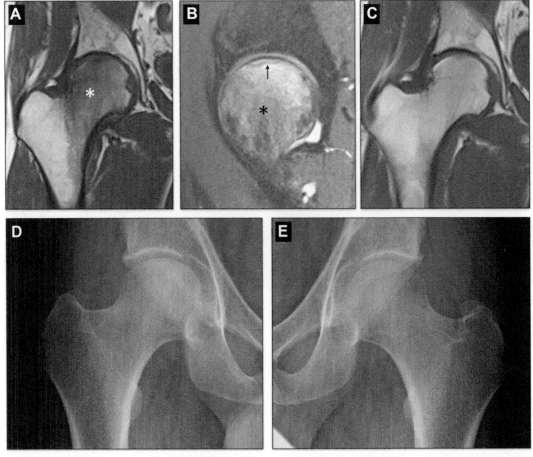

Fig. 10. Increased bone density in subchondral insufficiency fracture. A 40-year-old man with right hip pain. (*A*) Coronal T1-weighted and (*B*) sagittal intermediate-weighted image with fat saturation show an ill-defined area with low signal intensity on T1 (*asterisk* [*A*]) and high signal intensity on intermediate weighted fat saturation (*asterisk* [*B*]) corresponding to bone marrow edema involving the femoral head and extending to the femoral neck. A subtle linear low signal intensity band is seen in the subchondral bone (*arrow* [*B*]) corresponding to trabecular microimpaction, consistent with subchondral insufficiency fracture. (*C*) Follow-up coronal T1-weighted MR image 3 months later was normal. (*D, E*) Follow-up comparative radiographs obtained 10 months later show a subtle increase in bone density of the right femoral head in comparison to the left hip.

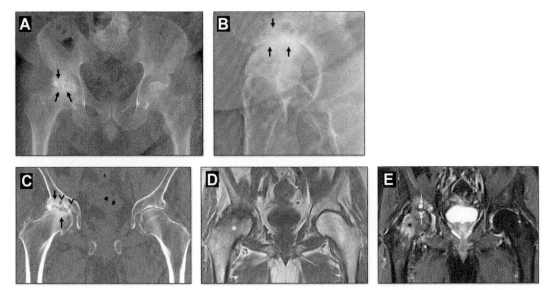

Fig. 11. Focal femoral head sclerosis in a 73-year-old man with right hip osteoarthritis. (*A*) AP radiograph of the pelvis and (*B*) off-lateral view of the right hip showing severe joint space narrowing associated with sclerotic subchondral changes of the femoral head and acetabulum (*arrows [A, B]*). (*C*) Coronal CT reformat demonstrates sclerotic (*arrows*) and cystic changes (*arrowheads*) in the right hip. (*D*) Coronal T1-weighted and (*E*) short tau inversion recovery MR images show an ill-delimited low T1-weighted and high short tau inversion recovery area (*asterisk [D, E]*) involving the right femoral head and extending to the femoral neck, corresponding to bone marrow edema. Subchondral cystic changes also are seen (*arrows [E]*).

phenomenon can be seen when traction is applied on the femoral head during hip abduction and the lucent line is usually better seen on the lateral radiograph than on the AP view. The presence of the crescent sign indicates failure of the subchondral bone and is a turning point in femoral head osteonecrosis, because it is associated with progressive collapse of the articular surface and subsequent osteoarthritis.

A final pattern of bone resorption is caused by cystic changes that develop near the surface or within the deep layers of the osteonecrotic femoral head (**Fig. 14**). This condition differs from the previous one by the presence of more clearly defined and round lucent areas in the femoral head. These cystic changes could be associated with a more chronic pattern of femoral head failure.[32–34]

Transient osteoporosis
A specific condition named transient or migratory osteoporosis of the femoral head can be

Table 3
Focal decrease in radiological density of the hip

Examples	Histologic Correlation	Radiological Features
Osteoarthritis	• Subchondral geodes due to cartilage loss	• Joint space narrowing • Subchondral sclerosis • Osteophytes
Femoral head osteonecrosis	• Bone resorption at the reactive interface outside necrosis • Formation of cysts • Delamination fracture of the subchondral trabecular bone	• Marginal lucency around necrotic area • Heterogeneous density of the femoral head • Resorption and cysts are better seen on CT • Crescent sign (Lauenstein view increases its conspicuity due to vacuum phenomenon)
Transient osteoporosis	• Unbalanced bone metabolism with increased bone resorption and delayed bone formation • Fibrovascular connective tissue	• Blurring/disappearance of subchondral bone plate • Normal joint space, no osteophytes • Return to normal at 6-mo follow-up

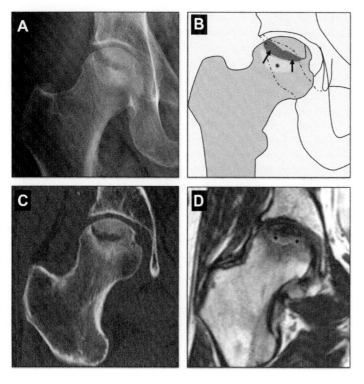

Fig. 12. Focal decreased density of the femoral head. A 32-year-old man with femoral head osteonecrosis. (A) AP radiograph of the right hip and (B) schematic representation showing a band of decreased density in the right femoral head (arrows [B]) corresponding to bone resorption at the margin of the osteonecrotic lesion on the (C) coronal CT reformat. It is surrounded by trabecular bone sclerosis (asterisk [B]). On the (D) coronal T2-weighted MR image, the area of bone resorption has intermediate signal intensity (asterisks [D]).

encountered, mainly in middle-aged men in association with the spontaneous onset of acute hip pain relieved by bed rest and worsened by weight-bearing.[35–38] It also is referred to as transient bone marrow edema syndrome when seen on MR imaging.[39–41] Careful comparison with the contralateral side or with previous radiographs may help to detect subtle alterations of the bone architecture, including focal fading of the subchondral bone plate of the femoral head

(Fig. 15). The joint space should be preserved in transient osteoporosis, a distinctive feature from that observed in septic hip arthritis in which joint space thinning progressively appears. On MR imaging, a regional moderate and ill-delimited decrease in signal intensity can be seen on fat-sensitive (T1 intermediate weighted) sequences that convert to high signal intensity on fat-suppressed fluid-sensitive sequences. As a distinctive feature, marrow changes

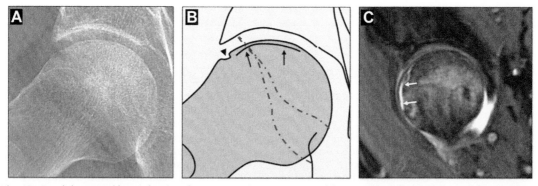

Fig. 13. Focal decreased bone density: the crescent sign. A 47-year-old man with right hip pain and femoral head osteonecrosis. (A) Lauenstein lateral view of the right hip and (B) corresponding schematic representation showing a linear subchondral lucency in the anterior and lateral aspect of the femoral head (arrows [B]). Also note the subtle focal depression of the articular surface (arrowhead [B]). (C) Sagittal intermediate-weighted MR image with fat saturation demonstrates a high signal intensity subchondral line corresponding to subchondral fracture (arrows).

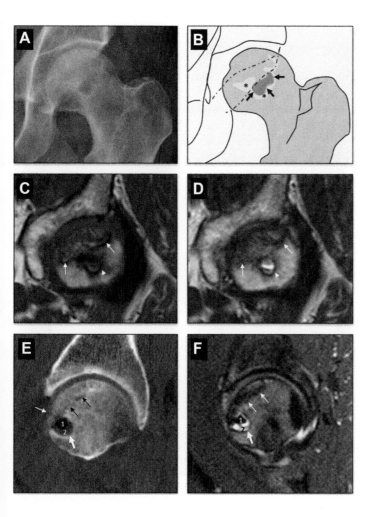

Fig. 14. Cystic changes in femoral head osteonecrosis. A 37-year-old man with left hip pain. (*A*) AP radiograph of the left hip and (*B*) corresponding schematic representation show a cystic lucency (*arrows*) surrounded by a rim of trabecular sclerosis (*asterisks*). (*C*) Coronal T1-weighted and (*D*) T2-weighted MR images show a cystic lesion with heterogeneous signal intensity (*arrowhead*) at the margin of the osteonecrotic lesion (*arrows*). (*E*) Sagittal CT reformat and (*F*) proton-density MR image with fat suppression show the cystic lesion (*thick white arrow*) with 2 distinct components: the first is very hypodense on CT and has a low signal intensity on MR image (1) corresponding to gas. The second (2) has an intermediate density on CT and fluidlike signal intensity on MR image. Note the focal deformity of the anterior aspect of the femoral head (*thin white arrow* [*E*]) and the fracture line at the margin of osteonecrosis (*black arrows* [*E*] and *thin arrows* [*F*]).

predominate in the subchondral area of the femoral head and the acetabular marrow remains normal.[40] Its transient character can be demonstrated only on subsequent follow-up MR imaging. In a vast majority of cases, marrow edema predominates in the anterior aspect of the femoral head and migrates posteriorly with involvement of the posterior aspect of the acetabulum in approximately 15% of cases at 3 months' follow-up MR imaging (**Fig. 16**). The presence of a subchondral low T2 intensity line can sometimes be observed and is thought to

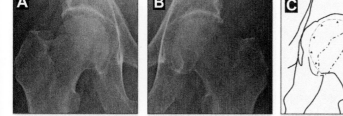
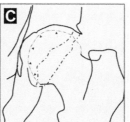
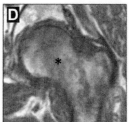

Fig. 15. Decreased bone density of the left femoral head in a 54-year-old woman with left hip pain. Comparative AP radiographs show decreased bone density of the left femoral head compared with the right, with fading of the subchondral bone plate (Arrowheads in [*C*], corresponding schematic representation) well depicted (*A*) and not seen (*B*). (*D*) Coronal T1-weighted image of the left hip shows bone marrow edema (*asterisk*) of the femoral head extending to the intertrochanteric area. MR image was normal at 3-month follow-up (not shown) confirming the transient nature of bone marrow edema.

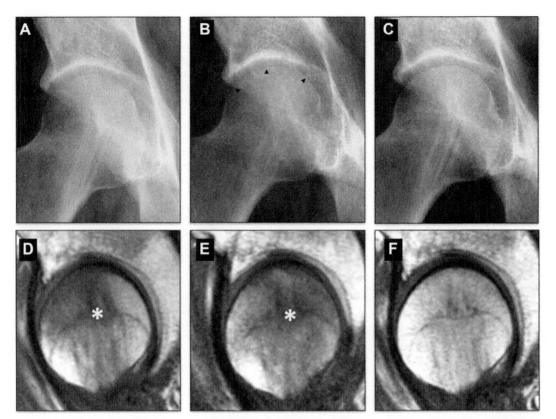

Fig. 16. Evolution of transient osteoporosis and bone marrow edema in a 62-year-old woman with right hip pain. (A) AP radiograph of the right hip on presentation was normal. At 3-month follow-up, (B) the radiograph showed decreased bone density of the femoral head with fading of the subchondral bone plate (*arrowheads*). At 6-month follow-up, (C) the radiograph was normal. (D) Sagittal T1-weighted MR image of the right hip on presentation showed ill-defined low signal intensity in the anterior and superior aspect of the femoral head (*asterisk*) with high signal intensity on short tau inversion recovery (not shown) corresponding to bone marrow edema. At 3 months' follow-up, the sagittal image showed partial regression of the marrow edema in the anterior aspect of the femoral head and appearance of edema in the posterior aspect (*asterisk* [*E*]). (*F*) At 6-month follow-up, MR image of the femoral head returned to normal.

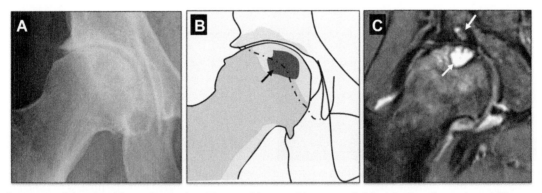

Fig. 17. Focal decreased bone density in a 74-year-old man with osteoarthritis. (A) AP radiograph and (B) corresponding schematic representation show ill-defined areas of decreased bone density (*arrow*) in the subchondral area of the femoral head. (C) Coronal short tau inversion recovery MR image shows round areas of fluidlike signal intensity indicating cystic changes on both articular margins (*arrows*).

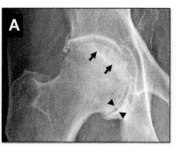
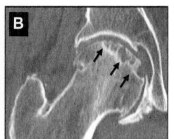

Fig. 18. Focal decreased bone density in the femoral head. 64-year-old man with right hip osteoarthritis and calcium pyrophosphate deposition disease. (*A*) AP radiograph and (*B*) coronal CT reformat of the right hip demonstrate cystic changes in the subchondral area of the femoral head (*arrows*). Also note narrowing of the inferomedial aspect of the joint space (*arrowheads*) with osteophyte formation.

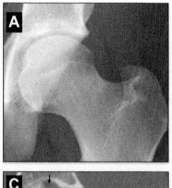
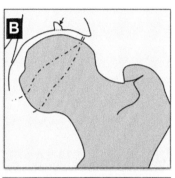
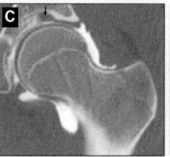
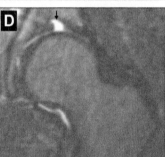

Fig. 19. Supraacetabular fossa; a normal variant in a 17-year-old woman. (*A*) AP radiograph of the left hip and (*B*) corresponding schematic representation showing a subtle focal subchondral lucency in the acetabular roof (*arrow*) with fading of the overlying subchondral bone plate. (*C*) On a coronal reformat of a CT arthrogram, the defect (*arrow*) contains a low attenuating tissue. (*D*) On the coronal short tau inversion recovery image, the defect has a fluidlike signal intensity (*arrow*).

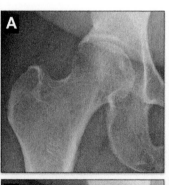
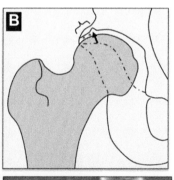
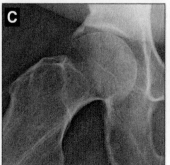
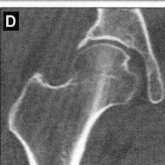

Fig. 20. Labral ossification in a 56-year-old woman. (*A*) AP radiograph of the right hip and (*B*) corresponding schematic illustration show an ossified labrum (*bracket* [*B*]) responsible for the pseudo-narrowing of the lateral radiological joint space (*asterisks* [*B*]) that should not to be misinterpreted as osteoarthritis. A diagnostic clue is the presence of a notch (*arrow* [*B*]) at the interface between the acetabulum and the ossified labrum (the previous chondrolabral recess). It is also visualized on the (*C*) Lauenstein lateral view. (*D*) Coronal CT reformat demonstrates the same features.

Table 4
Depression of the femoral head contours

Examples	Histologic Correlation	Radiological Features
Osteoarthritis	• In rapidly destructive osteoarthritis, eburnation and sclerosis of subchondral bone plate • Microfractures of trabecular bone and failure of subchondral bone plate • In cases of large subchondral geodes (calcium pyrophosphate deposition disease), fractures of the subchondral bone plate due to weakened support	• In rapidly destructive osteoarthritis, joint space narrowing on serial radiographs • Joint space narrowing out of proportion to osteophyte formation • Subchondral sclerosis • Large cyst formation • Chondrocalcinosis
Femoral head osteonecrosis (systemic and spontaneous osteonecrosis)	• Failure of subchondral bone plate and trabecular bone	• Fracture generally starts in the lateral or anterior aspect of the necrotic territory • Preserved joint space until late in the disease course
Subchondral insufficiency fracture	• Trabecular microfractures • Eventually leads to a focal form of subchondral necrosis (spontaneous osteonecrosis of the hip) similar to spontaneous osteonecrosis of the knee	• Decreased bone mineral density • Radiographic aspect may sometimes be difficult to differentiate from systemic osteonecrosis but both pathologies occur in different age groups. • A small crescent sign may be present

be related to subchondral trabecular microfractures, making the distinction between subchondral fracture and transient osteoporosis impossible on MR imaging.[41]

Osteoarthritis
Hip osteoarthritis can be associated with osseous cysts that are large, round, well-delimited areas of bone resorption located in the acetabulum or in the

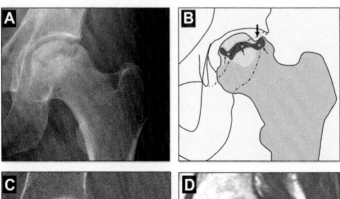
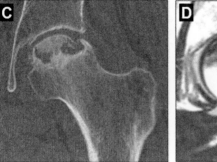
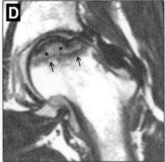

Fig. 21. Focal deformity of the femoral head in a 42-year-old man with left hip pain and femoral head osteonecrosis. (*A*) AP radiograph of the left hip with (*B*) corresponding schematic presentation show a focal depression in the superolateral aspect of the femoral head (*thick arrow* [*B*]). The osteonecrotic lesion is delineated by a sclerotic rim (*thin arrows*). Also note the lucent area (*asterisks*) corresponding to bone resorption at the margin of the necrotic lesion. These changes are better demonstrated on the (*C*) coronal CT reformat. (*D*) Coronal T2-weighted MR image shows the thin low intensity band (*arrows*) delineating the osteonecrosis. The area corresponding to bone resorption has an intermediate signal (*asterisks*) and is less conspicuous at MR image than at CT.

femoral head.[25,42] They usually occur underneath the areas of predominant cartilage abrasion (**Fig. 17**). Subchondral cysts, also referred to as geodes, are a hallmark of osteoarthritis. In cases of osteoarthritis of the hip associated with calcium pyrophosphate deposition disease, larger cysts occasionally are observed, even in the absence of joint space narrowing on the radiographs (**Fig. 18**).

RADIOLOGICAL CONTOURS OF THE HIP
Normal Radiological Contours of the Hip

The femoral head and the acetabulum show important variations in shape among individuals but there is limited intraindividual variation.[43] The shape of the femoral head is rarely a perfect sphere and rather is oval-shaped. The weight-bearing area of the acetabulum also can have a variable morphology on AP radiographs, including an excessively arched roof, an excessively flat roof, and an angular roof with a prominent intermediate segment.[44] It also may demonstrate a focal defect in cortical continuity that is typically located at its apex and is called the supra-acetabular fossa.[43] On radiographs, there is focal blurring of the acetabular subchondral bone plate (**Fig. 19**).[45] This osseous defect can contain cartilage-like tissue or articular fluid and is seen at MR imaging in approximately 10% of individuals. Ossification of the labrum is frequently encountered in asymptomatic individuals and is associated with narrowing of the most lateral joint space width that should not be confused with osteoarthritis[46] (**Fig. 20**). The ossified labrum is frequently separated from the acetabular roof by a small sulcus and, unlike acetabular osteophytes associated with osteoarthritis, is not associated with pericephalic or perifoveal femoral osteophytes.

Depression of the Femoral Head

Femoral head osteonecrosis
Femoral head deformity may occur in femoral head osteonecrosis as a result of biomechanical failure, probably due to a fracture of the subchondral bone plate and of the trabecular bone of the epiphysis[28,33] (**Table 4**). On conventional radiographs, changes in sphericity of the articular surface can

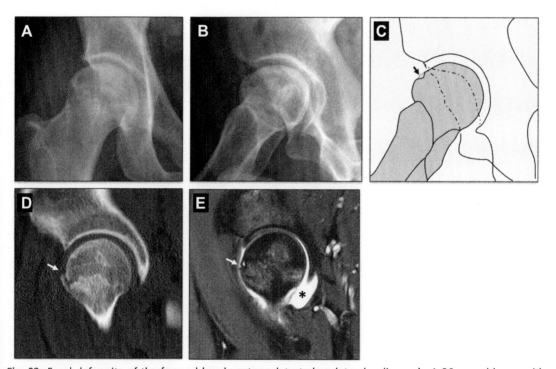

Fig. 22. Focal deformity of the femoral head contour detected on lateral radiograph. A 36-year-old man with right hip pain and femoral head osteonecrosis on MR image (not shown). (*A*) AP radiograph of the right hip shows abnormal bone structure in the femoral head with preserved femoral head contours. (*B*) Lateral view of the right hip and (*C*) corresponding schematic representation show a focal deformity of the anterior aspect of the femoral head (*arrow*). (*D*) Sagittal CT reformat and (*E*) intermediate-weighted MR image with fat saturation image show a focal depression of the anterior aspect of the femoral head (*arrows* [*D, E*]). Also note joint effusion (*asterisk* [*E*]).

be either abrupt or smooth and it usually involves the lateral aspect of the femoral head, underneath the acetabular margin (**Fig. 21**). Sometimes, it is more conspicuous either on the radiographs or on the MR images[31] (**Fig. 22**).

Osteoarthritis

In advanced stages of osteoarthritis, eburnation of the bone surface can occur, which may lead to a progressive flattening of the femoral head. In cases of rapidly progressive osteoarthritis, the destruction of the articular surface occurs early in the disease course and leads to a severe flattening of the femoral head (**Fig. 23**).

Subchondral insufficiency fracture

In a subset of patients with subchondral insufficiency fracture, progression of the fracture can occur in the subchondral bone, which leads to a focal flattening of the overlying articular surface (**Fig. 24**). Sometimes, a focal crescent sign can also occur in the subchondral area, as in osteonecrosis. This progression of insufficiency fracture may not heal, leading to early osteoarthritis.[22]

Osseous Prominence of the Femoral Head

An osseous bump at the femoral head-neck junction has been described as a causative factor of cam-type femoroacetabular impingement[47] (**Table 5**). It consists of a bony prominence that is in continuity with the epiphysis, without intervening lamellar bone plate (**Fig. 25**). It generally develops during growth in young active boys, particularly associated with high impact sports, and its pathologic significance is debated.[48]

Osseous bumps can be differentiated from osteophytes, which are bony proliferations growing on the epiphysis,[49,50] with intervening lamellar bone plate (opposite to cam-type morphotype).

RADIOLOGICAL JOINT SPACE OF THE HIP
Normal Radiological Joint Space

On an AP radiograph, the hip joint space corresponds to the distance between the acetabular roof and the femoral head; it reflects the

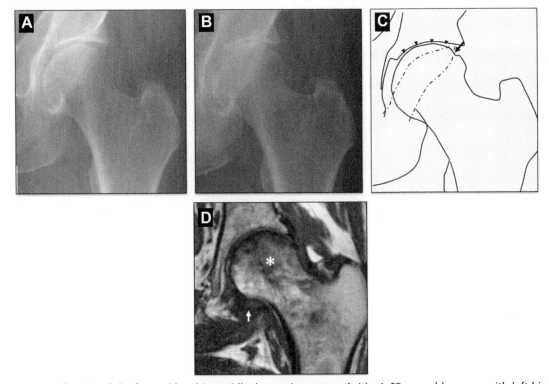

Fig. 23. Deformity of the femoral head in rapidly destructive osteoarthritis. A 65-year-old woman with left hip pain. (*A*) Initial AP radiograph of the left hip is unremarkable. (*B*) AP radiograph obtained at 3 months follow-up and (*C*) corresponding schematic representation show significant narrowing of the joint space (*arrowheads* [*C*]) keeping with the diagnosis of rapidely destructive osteoarthritis. A focal depression of bone contours (*arrow* [*C*]) has appeared in the lateral aspect of the femoral head indicative of a fracture of the subchondral bone plate. (*D*) Corresponding coronal T1-weighted MR image show bone marrow edema of the femoral head extending to the femoral neck (*asterisk*) and joint fluid effusion (*arrow*). Joint space narrowing is more conspicuous on conventional radiography than on MR image (compare [*B*] to [*D*]).

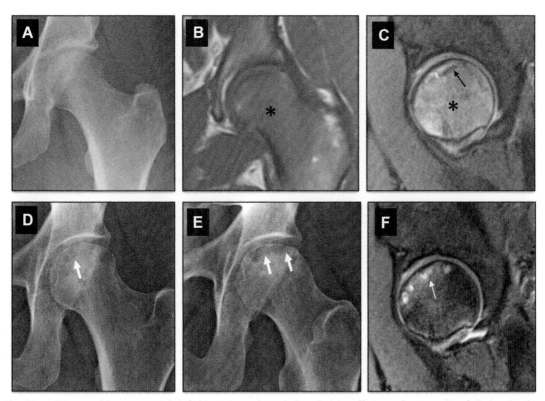

Fig. 24. A 36-year-old woman with left hip pain and a subchondral insufficiency fracture that failed to heal at follow up. (*A*) AP radiograph of the left hip is normal. (*B*) Coronal T1-weighted and (*C*) sagittal intermediate-weighted image with fat suppression show extensive bone marrow edema in the proximal femur (*asterisks*). A thin low signal intensity line is seen in the subchondral area (*arrow* [*C*]) compatible with an insufficiency fracture. Follow-up after 6 months: (*D*) AP and (*E*) lateral views show heterogeneous density of the femoral head with microcystic changes in the subchondral bone (*arrows* [*D, E*]) and flattening of the femoral head. (*F*) Sagittal intermediate weighted fat-suppressed image shows edema and focal fluid like signal intensity changes (*arrow*). Total hip replacement was performed 1 year later due to further collapse of the femoral head and subsequent osteoarthritis.

combined thickness of the acetabular and femoral head cartilage[51] (see **Fig. 1**). The acetabular fossa is devoid of articular cartilage; therefore, any change in the distance between the fovea capitis and the teardrop does not reflect alterations in the articular cartilage thickness.[5] On AP radiographs, the lateral aspect of the joint space width is larger than its medial aspect in 85% of cases, whereas in the remaining 15%, the radiological joint space has a uniform width.[44] There is an important interindividual variation in the joint space width among normal hips, ranging from 2 mm to 7 mm, but there is limited variability (<1 mm) between both hips of

Table 5
Osseous prominence of the proximal femur

Examples	Histologic Correlation	Additional Radiological Features
Osteophyte	• Fibrocartilage-capped bony outgrowth caused by endochondral ossification	• Bone proliferation covers the native lamellar bone that remains visible • Features of osteoarthritis • En miroir changes in the acetabulum
Bump	• Smooth deformity at the femoral head-neck junction • Association with stress overload during skeletal maturity	• Bone proliferation in continuity with the epiphysis without residual lamellar bone plate underneath • Young, male, active sports.

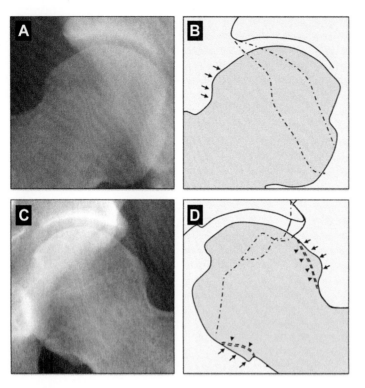

Fig. 25. Altered bone contours at the femoral head-neck junction in two different patients. (A) AP radiograph of the right hip and (B) corresponding schematic representation showing a bump at the lateral aspect of the femoral head-neck junction (*arrows*). There is no normal subchondral bone plate underneath the bump indicating that the deformity occurred during growth. (C) AP radiograph of the left hip in another patient and (D) corresponding schematic representation showing an osteophyte at the lateral aspect of the femoral head-neck junction (*arrows*). In contrary to the previous case (A, B), the original subchondral bone plate can still be seen (*arrowheads*) underneath the osteophyte.

the same individual.[44] The added value of the AP pelvic radiograph in comparison with the AP radiograph of a presumed symptomatic hip will never be emphasized enough.

The off-lateral (Lequesne false profile) view of the hip is used to assess the hip joint width in a profile view similar to the of the sagittal MR images or CT images of the hip. It enables the assessment of the anterosuperior and posteroinferior aspects of the joint space when the femoral head is placed in a more physiologic conditions than on the lateral views of the femur[14] (see Table 1). In individuals with normal hip radiographs, the anterosuperior joint width is larger than the posteroinferior joint width (see **Fig. 4**).

Decreased Joint Space

Osteoarthritis

Focal narrowing of the joint space is the radiographic hallmark of osteoarthritis (**Table 6**). On the AP radiograph, joint space narrowing more frequently involves the lateral aspect of the joint and less frequently the medial or the superomedial region. Therefore, 3 patterns of femoral head

Table 6
Joint space narrowing and patterns of migration in hip disorders

Migration Patterns	Associations	Additional Features
Superomedial narrowing	• Inflammatory (Aseptic or septic) arthritis • Chondrocalcinosis • Rapidly destructive osteoarthritis • Osteoarthritis in elderly	• Decreased bone density • No osteophyte formation • Elderly patients
Superolateral narrowing	• Osteoarthritis in young men • Association with cam- type femoroacetabular impingement is debated	• Signs of hip dysplasia, epiphysiolysis • Anterior narrowing on off-lateral view
Posteromedial narrowing	• Osteoarthritis in middle-age women • Association with pincer-type femoroacetabular impingement is debated	• Association with acetabular protrusion • Posterior narrowing on off-lateral view

migration have been described according to the direction of the head displacement subsequent to the area of predominant cartilage loss[52,53] (**Fig. 26**). On the off-lateral view, osteoarthritis with lateral or medial femoral head migration is associated with anterior or posterior head migration, respectively (**Fig. 27**).

Hip osteoarthritis is generally a slowly progressive disease with associated bony changes that develop in the area adjacent to the chondropathy (bone sclerosis and cysts) or at the margins of the articular surfaces (osteophytes). Occasionally, hip osteoarthritis is a rapidly progressive disease and is associated with extensive medullary and synovial changes mimicking septic arthritis[54–56] (see **Fig. 23**). Conversely, hip osteoarthritis can be associated with obvious bone and medullary changes despite no or little change in radiological joint space width (**Fig. 28**).

Arthritis (septic/aseptic)

In inflammatory and infectious arthritis, there is a more uniform cartilage loss due to the inflammatory mediators, leading to global joint space narrowing (**Fig. 29**). Homogeneous cartilage loss can be easily overlooked at MR imaging and comparative assessment of both joint space widths on a pelvic radiograph may contribute to detect cartilage damage.

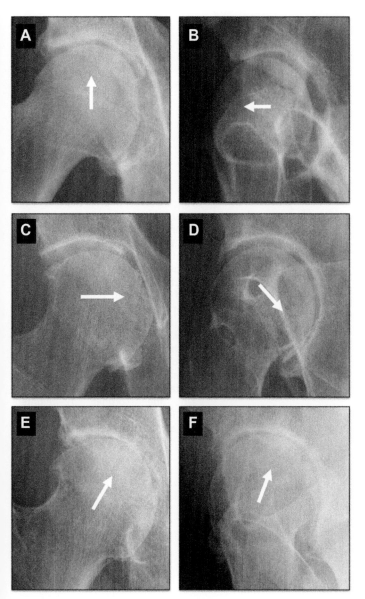

Fig. 26. Patterns of joint space narrowing in osteoarthritis of the hip in three different patients. Arrows indicate the predominant direction of migration of the femoral head in the acetabular cavity secondary to focal joint space narrowing. Anteroposterior (*A*) and off-lateral view (*B*) of the right hip in a 75 year-old man showing a focal narrowing of the anterior and superior joint space. Anteroposetrior (*C*) and off-lateral view (*D*) of the right hip in a 68 year-old woman showing a focal narrowing of the medial and posterior joint space. Anteroposterior (*E*) and off-lateral view (*F*) of the right hip in a 72 year-old woman showing a focal narrowing of the superomedial joint space.

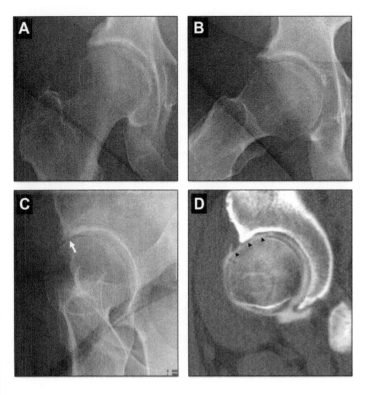

Fig. 27. The added value of the off-lateral view of the hip in osteoarthritis in a 51-year-old woman with right hip pain. (A) AP and (B) Lauenstein lateral views of the right hip show an almost normal joint space. (C) Off-lateral view demonstrates severe joint space narrowing in the anterior aspect of the joint (*arrow* in C) that is not visible in (A) and (B). (D) Sagittal reformat of a CT arthrogram obtained in the same patient demonstrates a full-thickness focal cartilage defect at the anterosuperior aspect of the femoral head (*arrowheads*) and acetabulum.

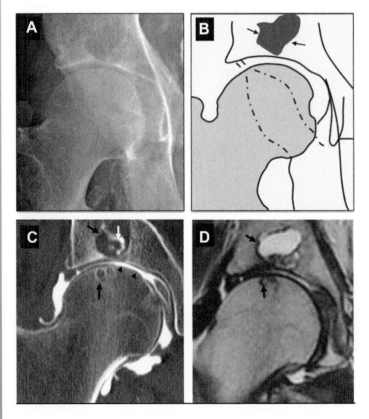

Fig. 28. Subchondral changes with preserved joint space width in osteoarthritis. A 78-year-old man with right hip pain. (A) AP radiograph of the right hip and (B) corresponding schematic representation show a large subchondral cyst in the acetabular roof (*arrows* in B); note the preserved joint space. (C) Coronal reformat of a CT arthrogram shows large full-thickness en miroir cartilage defects of the femoral head and acetabulum (*arrowheads*). Iodinated contrast material (*white arrow*) partially fills the acetabular cyst (*black arrows*). (D) On the coronal T2-weighted MR image, the cyst has a high fluid-like signal intensity (*arrows*).

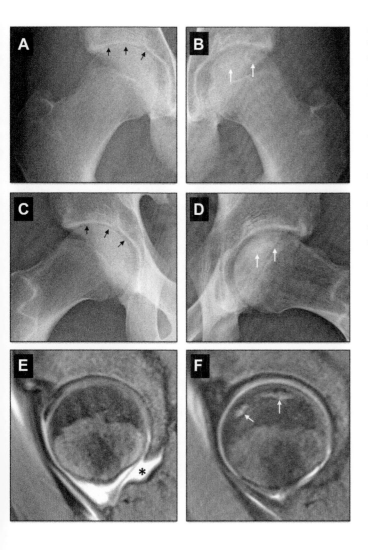

Fig. 29. Diffuse joint space narrowing of the right hip in inflammatory arthritis. A 17-year-old boy with juvenile rheumatoid arthritis and right hip pain. AP radiographs of the (*A*) right and (*B*) left hips with ([*C*] and [*D*], respectively) corresponding Lauenstein lateral projections show diffuse joint space narrowing of the right hip (*black arrows* in *A* and *C*) in comparison with the left hip. Incidentally, note a small osteonecrotic lesion of the left femoral head (*white arrows* in *B* and *D*). (*E, F*) On the corresponding sagittal fat-saturated proton density–weighted images, joint space narrowing of the right hip is barely visible. Note right hip effusion (*asterisk*) and left hip osteonecrosis (*arrows*).

SUMMARY

Conventional radiographs continue to play an important role in the first evaluation of symptomatic hip joints. It enables a rapid evaluation of the articular joint space, despite its lack in sensitivity in the detection of soft tissue changes and its limited sensitivity in the detection of bony changes.

REFERENCES

1. Expert Panel on Musculoskeletal Imaging, Mintz DN, Roberts CC, et al. ACR appropriateness criteria® chronic hip pain. J Am Coll Radiol 2017;14(4S): S90–102.
2. Clohisy JC, Carlisle JC, Beaule PE, et al. A systematic approach to the plain radiographic evaluation of the young adult hip. J Bone Joint Surg Am 2008; 90(Suppl 4):47–66.
3. Taljanovic MS, Hunter TB, Fitzpatrick KA, et al. Musculoskeletal magnetic resonance imaging: importance of radiography. Skeletal Radiol 2003; 32(7):403–11.
4. Clohisy JC, Keeney JA, Schoenecker PL. Preliminary assessment and treatment guidelines for hip disorders in young adults. Clin Orthop Relat Res 2005;441:168–79.
5. Armbuster TG, Guerra J Jr, Resnick D, et al. The adult hip: an anatomic study. Part I: the bony landmarks. Radiology 1978;128(1):1–10.
6. Guerra J Jr, Armbuster TG, Resnick D, et al. The adult hip: an anatomic study. Part II: the soft-tissue landmarks. Radiology 1978;128(1):11–20.
7. Byrd JW. Evaluation of the hip: history and physical examination. N Am J Sports Phys Ther 2007;2(4):231–40.
8. Chong T, Don DW, Kao MC, et al. The value of physical examination in the diagnosis of hip osteoarthritis. J Back Musculoskelet Rehabil 2013;26(4):397–400.

9. Manaster BJ. From the RSNA Refresher courses. Radiological Society of North America. Adult chronic hip pain: radiographic evaluation. Radiographics 2000;20(Spec No):S3–25.

10. Godefroy D, Chevrot A, Rousselin B, et al. Plain films of pelvis. J Radiol 2008;89(5):679–90 (article in french).

11. Fuchs-Winkelmann S, Peterlein CD, Tibesku CO, et al. Comparison of pelvic radiographs in weight-bearing and supine positions. Clin Orthop Relat Res 2008;466(4):809–12.

12. Troelsen A, Jacobsen S, Rømer L, et al. Weightbearing anteroposterior pelvic radiographs are recommended in DDH assessment. Clin Orthop Relat Res 2008;466(4):813–9.

13. Eijer H, Leunig M, Mahomed MN, et al. Cross-table lateral radiographs for screening of anterior femoral head-neck offset in patients with femoro-acetabular impingement. HIP Int 2018;11(1):37–41.

14. Lequesne M, de SEZE. False profile of the pelvis. A new radiographic incidence for the study of the hip. Its use in dysplasias and different coxopathies. Rev Rhum Mal Osteoartic 1961;28:643–52 [in French].

15. Catto M. Ischaemia of bone. J Clin Pathol Suppl (R Coll Pathol) 1977;11:78–93.

16. Glimcher MJ, Kenzora JE. Nicolas Andry award. The biology of osteonecrosis of the human femoral head and its clinical implications. 1. Tissue biology. Clin Orthop 1979;138:284–309.

17. Glimcher MJ, Kenzora JE. The biology of osteonecrosis of the human femoral head and its clinical implications. III. Discussion of the etiology and genesis of the pathological sequelae; comments on treatment. Clin Orthop 1979;140:273–312.

18. Maldague BM. Le diagnostic radiologique précoce de la nécrose aseptique post-traumatique de a tête fémorale. J Acta Orthop Belg 1984;50:324–42.

19. Fondi C, Franchi A. Definition of bone necrosis by the pathologist. Clin Cases Miner Bone Metab 2007;4(1):21–6.

20. Sugano N, Kubo T, Takaoka K, et al. Diagnostic criteria for non-traumatic osteonecrosis of the femoral head. A multicentre study. J Bone Joint Surg Br 1999;81-B:590–5.

21. Yamamoto T, Schneider R, Bullough PG. Subchondral insufficiency fracture of the femoral head: histopathologic correlation with MRI. Skeletal Radiol 2001;30(5):247–54.

22. Yamamoto T. Subchondral insufficiency fractures of the femoral head. Clin Orthop Surg 2012;4(3):173.

23. Xu L, Hayashi D, Guermazi A, et al. The diagnostic performance of radiography for detection of osteoarthritis-associated features compared with MRI in hip joints with chronic pain. Skeletal Radiol 2013;42(10):1421–8.

24. Gao F, Han J, He Z, et al. Radiological analysis of cystic lesion in osteonecrosis of the femoral head. Int Orthop 2018;42(7):1615–21.

25. Resnick D, Niwayama G, Coutts RD. Subchondral cysts (geodes) in arthritic disorders: pathologic and radiographic appearance of the hip joint. AJR Am J Roentgenol 1977;128(5):799–806.

26. Phemister DB. The classic: repair of bone in the presence of aseptic necrosis resulting from fractures, transplantations, and vascular obstruction. Clin Orthop Relat Res 2008;466(5):1021–33.

27. Norman A, Bullough P. The radiolucent crescent line–an early diagnostic sign of avascular necrosis of the femoral head. Bull Hosp Joint Dis 1963;24:99–104.

28. Kenzora JE, Glimcher MJ. Pathogenesis of idiopathic osteonecrosis: the ubiquitous crescent sign. Orthop Clin North Am 1985;16(4):681–96.

29. Pappas JN. The musculoskeletal crescent sign. Radiology 2000;217(1):213–4.

30. Murphey MD, Foreman KL, Klassen-Fischer MK, et al. From the radiologic pathology archives imaging of osteonecrosis: radiologic-pathologic correlation. Radiographics 2014;34(4):1003–28.

31. Stevens K, Tao C, Lee SU, et al. Subchondral fractures in osteonecrosis of the femoral head: comparison of radiography, CT, and MR imaging. AJR Am J Roentgenol 2003;180(2):363–8.

32. Sugano N, Atsumi T, Ohzono K, et al. The 2001 revised criteria for diagnosis, classification, and staging of idiopathic osteonecrosis of the femoral head. J Orthop Sci 2002;7(5):601–5.

33. Hamada H, Takao M, Sakai T, et al. Subchondral fracture begins from the bone resorption area in osteonecrosis of the femoral head: a micro-computerised tomography study. Int Orthop 2018;42(7):1479–84.

34. Sugano N, Ohzono K. Natural course and the JIC classification of osteonecrosis of the femoral head. Berlin: Springer; 2014. p. 207–10.

35. Lequesne M. Transient osteoporosis of the hip. A nontraumatic variety of Südeck's atrophy. Ann Rheum Dis 1968;27(5):463–71.

36. Hunder GG, Kelly PJ. Roentgenologic transient osteoporosis of the hip. Ann Intern Med 1968;69(3):633.

37. Longstreth PL, Malinak LR, Hill CS Jr. Transient osteoporosis of the hip in pregnancy. Obstet Gynecol 1973;41(4):563–9.

38. Crespo E, Sala D, Crespo R, et al. Current concepts review: transient osteoporosis. Acta Orthop Belg 2001;67(4):330–7.

39. Malizos KN, Zibis AH, Dailiana Z, et al. MR imaging findings in transient osteoporosis of the hip. Eur J Radiol 2004;50(3):238–44.

40. Vande Berg BC, Lecouvet FE, Maldague B, et al. Osteonecrosis and transient osteoporosis of the femoral head. Imaging of the hip & bony pelvis. Berlin: Springer; 2006. p. 195–216.

41. Vande Berg BC, Lecouvet FE, Koutaïssoff S, et al. Le syndrome d'œdème médullaire de la tête fémorale. J Radiol 2011;92(6):557–66.

42. Rhaney K, Lamb DW. The cysts of osteoarthritis of the hip; a radiological and pathological study. J Bone Joint Surg Br 1955;37-B(4):663–75.

43. Vande Berg BC, Omoumi P. Hip imaging: normal variants and asymptomatic findings. Semin Musculoskelet Radiol 2017;21(05):507–17.

44. Lequesne M, Malghem J, Dion E. The normal hip joint space: variations in width, shape, and architecture on 223 pelvic radiographs. Ann Rheum Dis 2004;63(9):1145–51.

45. Dietrich TJ, Suter A, Pfirrmann CWA, et al. Supraacetabular Fossa (Pseudodefect of Acetabular Cartilage): frequency at MR arthrography and comparison of findings at MR arthrography and arthroscopy. Radiology 2012;263(2):484–91.

46. Ninomiya S, Shimabukuro A, Tanabe T, et al. Ossification of the acetabular labrum. J Orthop Sci 2000; 5(5):511–4.

47. Peelle MW, Della Rocca GJ, Maloney WJ, et al. Acetabular and femoral radiographic abnormalities associated with labral tears. Clin Orthop Relat Res 2005;441:327–33.

48. Agricola R, Waarsing JH, Arden NK, et al. Cam impingement of the hip—a risk factor for hip osteoarthritis. Nat Rev Rheumatol 2013;9(10):630–4.

49. Resnick D. Osteophytosis of the femoral head and neck. Arthritis Rheum 1983;26(7):908–13.

50. Wong SH, Chiu KY, Yan CH. Review article: osteophytes. J Orthop Surg (Hong Kong) 2016;24(3): 403–10.

51. Fredensborg N, Nilsson BE. The joint space in normal hip radiographs. Radiology 1978;126(2): 325–6.

52. Resnick D. Patterns of migration of the femoral head in osteoarthritis of the hip. Am J Roentgenol 1975; 124(1):62–74.

53. Solomon L. Patterns of osteoarthritis of the hip. J Bone Joint Surg 1976;58-B(2):176–83.

54. Boutry N, Paul C, Leroy X, et al. Rapidly destructive osteoarthritis of the hip: MR imaging findings. AJR Am J Roentgenol 2002;179(3):657–63.

55. Flemming DJ, Gustas-French CN. Rapidly progressive osteoarthritis: a review of the clinical and radiologic presentation. Curr Rheumatol Rep 2017;19(7):42.

56. Hart G, Fehring T. Rapidly destructive osteoarthritis can mimic infection. Arthroplast Today 2016;2(1):15–8.

Joint Effusion and Bone Outlines of the Knee
Radiographic/MR Imaging Correlation

Thibaut Jacques, MD, MSc[a,b,c],*, Sammy Badr, MD, MSc[a,b,c],
Paul Michelin, MD, MSc[d,e], Guillaume Lefebvre, MD[a,c], Julien Dartus, MD[b,f,g],
Anne Cotten, MD, PhD[a,b,c]

KEYWORDS

- Knee radiograph • Patellar dislocation • Segond fracture • Trochlear dysplasia

KEY POINTS

- Joint effusion, lipohemarthrosis, and exuberant subsynovial frondlike fatty proliferation in lipoma arborescens can be depicted on a lateral view.
- Normal femoral notches should be differentiated from the lateral femoral notch sign associated with anterior cruciate ligament tears.
- Trochlear dysplasia and features reflecting its severity should be systematically sought after.
- Patella alta, patellar tilt, and complete lateral patellar dislocation can be associated with trochlear dysplasia.
- Analysis of the bone outlines can allow depiction of small avulsion fractures.

Knee radiographs are still widely used in clinical practice. Many features can be depicted when a systematic analysis of the different views is performed. In this article, after discussing different types of joint effusion, we focus on the analysis of the bone outlines of the knee, particularly on the lateral view. Systematic analysis of these bone outlines and knowledge of several key points are particularly useful for the depiction of abnormal bone morphology or positioning, and of several injuries.

JOINT EFFUSION

Whatever the clinical context, the presence of a joint effusion should be systematically looked for on a lateral knee radiograph. This increased intra-articular amount of fluid is not specific of a particular disorder, as can occur in a variety of settings. However, it draws attention to the presence of a joint disorder. It leads to the separation between the suprapatellar and prefemoral fat pads by a well-defined rounded suprapatellar recess (**Fig. 1**).[1] Loss of normal posterior fat plane of the quadriceps tendon and anterior displacement of the latter and of the patella are only seen in large joint effusions.

In trauma, a fat-fluid level related to lipohemarthrosis can be seen when a lateral knee view with horizontal ray is performed (**Fig. 2**) or

Disclosure Statement: The authors have nothing to disclose.
[a] Department of Musculoskeletal Radiology, Lille University Hospital, Rue du Professeur Emile Laine, 59037 Lille CEDEX, France; [b] Lille University School of Medicine, Faculté de Médecine Henri Warembourg, F-59045 Lille CEDEX, France; [c] Service de Radiologie et Imagerie Musculosquelettique, Centre de Consultations et d'Imagerie de l'Appareil Locomoteur (C.C.I.A.L.), Rue du Professeur, Emile Laine, 59037 Lille CEDEX, France; [d] Department of Radiology, Rouen University Hospital, 1 Rue de Germont, 76031 Rouen Cedex 1, France; [e] Imagerie de l'Appareil Locomoteur, CHU Rouen Normandie, 1 Rue de Germont, 76031 Rouen Cedex 1, France; [f] Department of Orthopedic Surgery, Lille University Hospital, Rue du Professeur Emile Laine, 59037 Lille CEDEX, France; [g] Service d'Orthopédie D, Hopital Roger Salengro, CHRU de Lille, Rue du Professeur Emile Laine, 59037 Lille CEDEX, France
* Corresponding author. Service de Radiologie et Imagerie Musculosquelettique, Centre de Consultations et d'Imagerie de l'Appareil Locomoteur (C.C.I.A.L.), Rue du Professeur Emile Laine, 59037 Lille CEDEX, France.
E-mail address: thibaut.jacques@chru-lille.fr

Magn Reson Imaging Clin N Am 27 (2019) 685–699
https://doi.org/10.1016/j.mric.2019.06.001
1064-9689/19/© 2019 Elsevier Inc. All rights reserved.

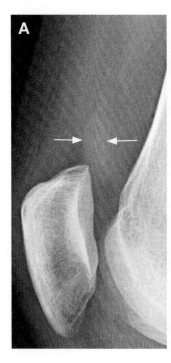
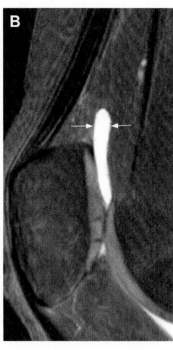

Fig. 1. Joint effusion. Well-defined rounded suprapatellar recess (*arrows*) on (*A*) lateral knee radiograph and on (*B*) sagittal proton density (PD)-weighted image.

on a lateral knee view performed in a standing patient[2]; it is specific for the existence of an intra-articular fracture, allowing bone marrow fat to leak into the joint via the fracture and to float on top of the blood. The detection of this sign is particularly useful when the intra-articular extent of a fracture is not obvious on plain films, as it should lead to additional imaging assessment.

Sometimes, fatty lucencies that seem to be entrapped in a distended suprapatellar pouch can be detected on radiographs (**Fig. 3**). They are related to extensive subsynovial frondlike fatty proliferation in lipoma arborescens and can be depicted radiographically when exuberant. This latter disorder is typically associated with chronic arthropathies, such as osteoarthritis or rheumatoid arthritis.[3]

LATERAL FEMORAL NOTCH SIGN
Normal Anatomy

On a true lateral view, the 2 femoral condyles are superimposed, particularly their posterior border.

However, analysis of their shape allows differentiating them: the middle third of the lateral condyle is flat and may demonstrate a mild notch, whereas the medial condyle is more rounded. When the superposition of the 2 condyles is not perfect, which is frequently the case, a large notch also can be recognized at the junction between the anterior and middle third of the medial condyle. These normal notches, also known as condylopatellar sulcus, represent the junction zone on the femoral condyles where the tibiofemoral and patellofemoral radii of curvature meet (**Fig. 4**).

Lateral Femoral Notch Sign

Normal notches should be differentiated from the lateral femoral notch sign, which results from the impaction between the lateral femoral condyle and the posterior aspect of the tibial plateau during anterior cruciate ligament tears (**Fig. 5**). This inconstant osteochondral fracture involves the middle to anterior portion of the lateral femoral condyle; it can be recognized radiographically

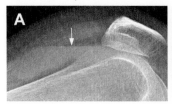
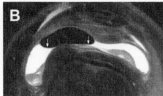

Fig. 2. Lipohemarthrosis with a fat-fluid level on a (*A*) lateral knee view with horizontal ray (*arrow*) and on an (*B*) axial PD-weighted image (*arrows*).

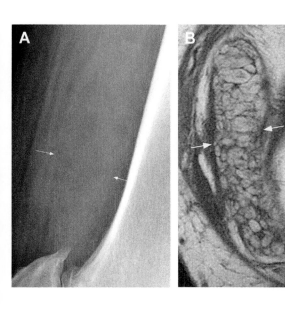

Fig. 3. Lipoma arborescens. Fatty lucencies depicted in a distended suprapatellar pouch (*arrows*) on a (*A*) lateral radiograph; (*B*) sagittal T1-weighted image confirms the extensive frondlike fatty proliferation.

when it is deeper (>1.5 mm) and/or has sharper angulation than the normal lateral notch (see **Fig. 5**).[4]

TROCHLEAR DYSPLASIA

This developmental anomaly is one of the most important risk factors for lateral patellar dislocation. Its depiction relies on the analysis of the proximal part of the trochlea on a true lateral radiograph, as it has been demonstrated that this view is more reliable for the diagnosis of trochlear dysplasia than axial radiographs obtained at 30° of flexion of the knee.[5] Thus, it is crucial for diagnostic accuracy of trochlear dysplasia to have a correct lateral radiograph with superimposition of

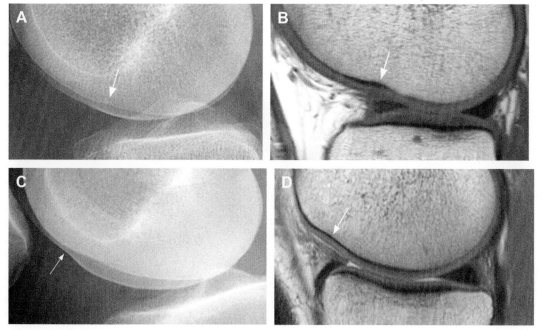

Fig. 4. Normal femoral condyle outlines. The middle third of the lateral condyle is flat and shows a mild notch (*arrow*) on a (*A*) lateral view and on a (*B*) sagittal T1-weighted image. The medial condyle is more rounded and shows a large notch at the junction between its anterior and middle thirds on a (*C*) lateral view and on a (*D*) sagittal PD-weighted image.

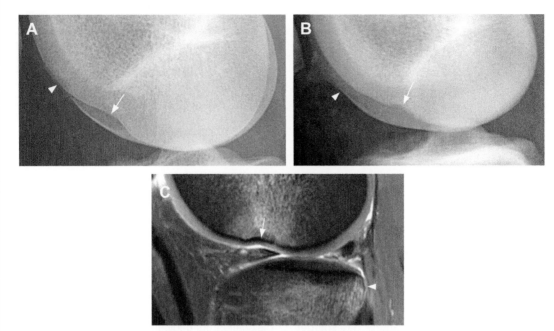

Fig. 5. Lateral femoral notch sign (*arrow*). (*A*) Deep (>1.5 mm) depression and (*B*) depression with sharp angulation of the middle third of the lateral femoral condyle on a lateral view. Note the normal medial femoral notch (*arrowheads*). (*C*) Deep depression of the lateral femoral condyle with surrounding bone marrow contusion, associated with contusion of the posterior aspect of the lateral tibial plateau on a sagittal PD-weighted image.

the femoral condyles posteriorly, as a rotational deviation of at least 5° can cause false-positive or false-negative diagnosis of trochlear dysplasia.[6]

Normal Anatomy

Normally, the ventral outline of both femoral condyles projects at a distance from the tangent to the deepest part of the trochlear groove and should not cross it, as both condyles continue with the ventral cortical bone of the femoral metaphysis. This means there is a normal shape and depth of the proximal trochlea (**Fig. 6**). The depth of the proximal trochlea can be assessed 1 cm below the proximal end of the trochlear groove and should be more than 5 mm (see **Fig. 6**). This

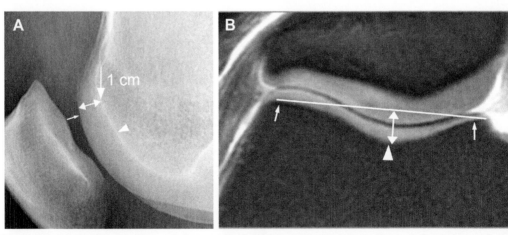

Fig. 6. Normal depth and shape of the proximal trochlea. The ventral outline of the 2 femoral condyles (*small arrow*) are superimposed and project anteriorly to the tangent to the deepest part of the trochlear groove (*arrowhead*) on a (*A*) lateral view. (*A*) The depth of the proximal trochlea (*double arrow*) measured 1 cm below the proximal end of the trochlear groove (*large arrow*) is more than 5 mm. (*B*) The corresponding axial PD-weighted image shows normal shape and depth of the proximal trochlea.

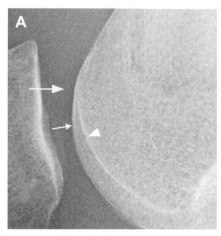
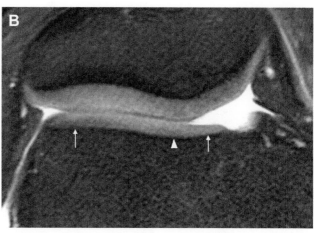

Fig. 7. Trochlear dysplasia: crossing sign (*large arrow*). (*A*) The tangent to the deepest part of the trochlear groove (*arrowhead*) crosses the ventral outline of the 2 femoral condyles (*small arrow*). (*B*) On the corresponding level on axial PD-weighted image, the trochlea is flat.

measure is rarely performed in clinical practice, but it constitutes a good landmark for normal anatomy in cases of doubt.

Trochlear Dysplasia

Trochlear dysplasia is defined by the presence of the crossing sign, when the tangent to the deepest part of the trochlear groove crosses the ventral outline of the lateral condyle (**Fig. 7**).[7] At this level, the trochlea becomes flat, which may lead to patellar instability, as the patella cannot engage normally in the trochlea.

It is important to keep in mind that in a normal knee, the lateral femoral condyle extends higher anteriorly than the medial condyle. This feature can be used to differentiate the 2 condyles, but it also explains that, quite frequently, the ventral outline of the medial condyle joins the tangent to the trochlear groove, as the proximal part of the medial trochlear facet can be in a frontal plane. This is a normal and frequent feature; this is not a crossing sign (**Fig. 8**). The crossing sign must involve at least the lateral condyle. This feature should be kept in mind to avoid overdiagnosis of trochlear dysplasia.

Features Reflecting the Severity of the Trochlear Dysplasia

Once the crossing sign has been recognized, other features reflecting the severity of the

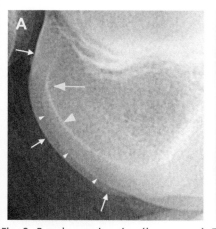
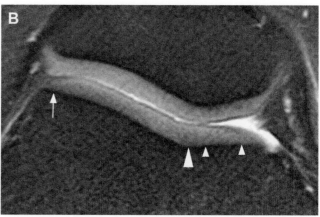

Fig. 8. Pseudo crossing sign (*large arrow*). The proximal ventral outline of the medial femoral condyle (*small arrowheads*) can join the tangent to the trochlear groove (*large arrowhead*) when it has a frontal direction (*large arrow*) on a (*A*) lateral view. The lateral femoral condyle (*small arrows*) extends higher anteriorly than the medial condyle. (*B*) The corresponding axial PD-weighted image shows that the proximal aspect of the medial trochlear facet is in a frontal plane (same plane as the proximal trochlear groove).

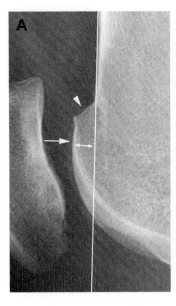
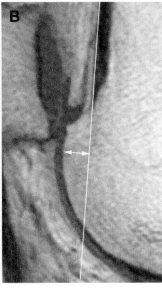

Fig. 9. Ventral prominence of the trochlea, which is more than 3 mm (*double arrow*) on this (*A*) lateral view. Note the associated crossing sign (*arrow*) and the spur (*arrowhead*). Spur and ventral prominence of the trochlea in another patient on a (*B*) sagittal T1-weighted image.

trochlear dysplasia should be systematically sought out[8]:

- *A supratrochlear spur or bump*, which plays a role similar to a ski jump when the patella engages in the trochlea (**Fig. 9**). This feature usually indicates ventral prominence of the trochlea, which can be measured by the distance between a line drawn through the ventral cortical bone of the femoral shaft and a parallel line tangent to the most ventral point of the trochlear floor. This measure is approximately 0 to 2 mm in normal knees but can be more than 3 mm in severe trochlear dysplasia (**Fig. 10**). The trochlea is usually markedly flattened or even convex in this region.

- *The double contour sign.* A double line can be depicted at the anterior aspect of femoral metaphysis above the trochlea; this is a common feature, as the anterolateral metaphysis is usually more developed and prominent than the medial one. This double line is abnormal, and called the "double contour sign" if it continues and ends below the level of the crossing sign, thus indicating that the medial femoral condyle is hypoplastic (see **Fig. 10**). This leads to a pronounced asymmetry of the height between trochlear facets, with a hypoplastic medial trochlear facet. A cliff

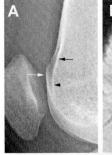
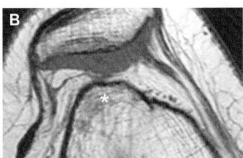
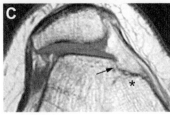

Fig. 10. Double contour sign. (*A*) The double line depicted at the anterior aspect of femoral metaphysis above the trochlea (*black arrow*) means the anterolateral metaphysis is more prominent than the medial one. There is a double contour sign (*black arrowhead*) as this double line continues and ends below the level of the crossing sign (*white arrow*). This feature means that the medial femoral condyle is hypoplastic. Note the associated patellar tilt. Axial PD images show the (*B*) prominent anterolateral metaphysis (no covering cartilage) (*white star*) (level of the *black arrow* in A) and the (*C*) hypoplastic medial condyle (*black star*) with a cliff pattern between the 2 condyles (*arrow*) (level of the *black arrowhead* in A).

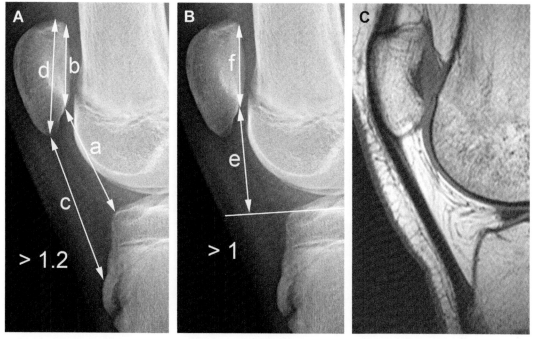

Fig. 11. Patella alta on a lateral view with (*A, B*) 30° of flexion and on a (*C*) sagittal T1-weighted image. (*A*) The Caton-Deschamps index is the ratio of the distance between the distal aspect of patellar articular surface and the anterosuperior aspect of the tibia (a) to the length of patellar articular surface (b); the Insall-Salvati index is the ratio between the patellar tendon length (c) to the length of the patella (d). (*B*) The Blackburne-Peel index is the ratio of the distance between the inferior aspect of the patellar articular surface and a line tangent to the surface of the tibial plateau (e) to the length of patellar articular surface (patella alta >1 for this index) (f). (*C*) Patella alta in another patient.

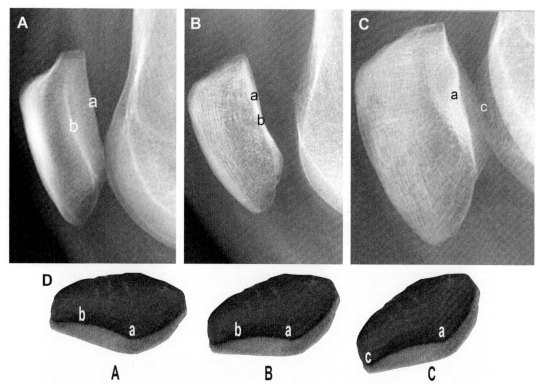

Fig. 12. Detection of a patellar tilt on a lateral view. (*A*) Normally, the tangent to the vertical ridge between the 2 patellar facets (a) is posterior to the tangent to the lateral facet (b). (*B*) An overlapping of these lines means that there is a mild tilt of the patella. (*C*) A convex posterior border of the patella (c) means that there is a severe tilt. (*D*) Corresponding diagram of the previous radiographs.

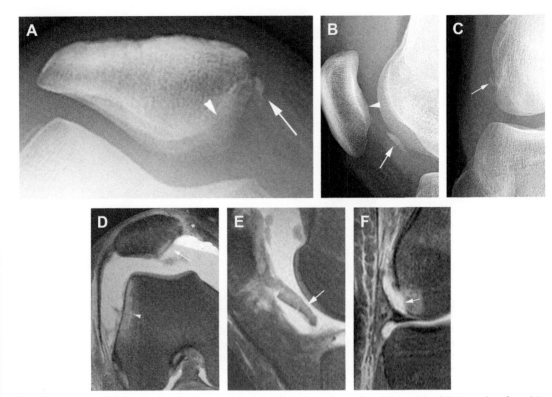

Fig. 13. Radiographic features indicating a prior complete lateral patellar dislocation. (*A*) Sequela of avulsion fracture of the medial ligamentous patellar stabilizers (*arrow*) associated with an ill-defined tangent to the medial facet (*arrowhead*). (*B*) Intra-articular linear bone fragments (sliver sign) (*arrow*) arising from the patellar vertical ridge and the medial facet (*arrowhead*). (*C*) Impaction fracture of the anterolateral aspect of the lateral femoral condyle (*arrow*). (*D*) Corresponding images on PD-weighted images with avulsion of the medial ligamentous patellar stabilizers (*star*) with patellar osteochondral avulsion (*arrow*) and impaction of the lateral femoral condyle (*arrowhead*). Note the shallow trochlea and the fluid level related to hemarthrosis. (*E*) Osteochondral fragment (*arrow*) arising from the patella. (*F*) Osteochondral fracture of the anterolateral aspect of the lateral femoral condyle (*arrow*).

pattern usually separates the 2 condyles in the axial plane.

Associated Disorders

When trochlear dysplasia is depicted, 3 other types of radiographic features should be systematically sought out, as they are frequently associated (although they can be seen in isolation):

- *A patella alta.* A patella alta means that the patella is located too high. As a consequence, the degree of flexion required for the patella to engage in the trochlea tends to be higher, as compared with a normal knee. This increases the risk of patellar instability and dislocation in shallow degrees of flexion. Several indexes have been described on a true lateral view with a knee flexed at 30°. Patella alta is present when the Caton-

Deschamps or Insall-Salvati index is >1.2, or when the Blackburne-Peel index is >1 (**Fig. 11**).[9–11]

- *A patellar tilt.* Patellar tilt, which is a rotation of the patella in the axial plane, is favored by the presence of a patella alta, a trochlear dysplasia, and a lateralization of the tibial tuberosity. It is more obvious and frequent on a true lateral view with a knee extended, as the patella is not yet engaged, but it also may be seen in flexion at 30°. Normally, 2 lines are seen at the posterior part of the patella. The most posterior one, which is straight or slightly concave backward, is a tangent to the vertical ridge located between the 2 patellar facets (**Fig. 12**). The anterior line is a tangent to the lateral facet. An overlapping of these lines means that there is a mild tilt of the patella; a posterior border of the patella becoming convex backward means that there

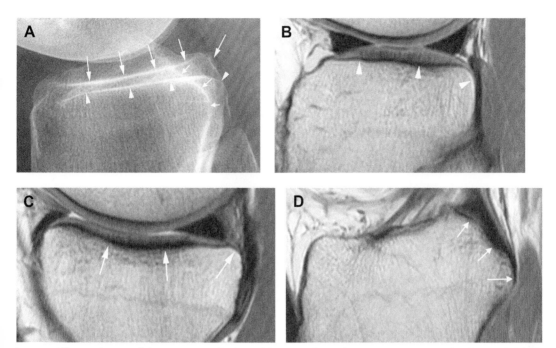

Fig. 14. Different shapes of the posterior tibial condyles. On a lateral view, 3 tangents can be depicted. (A) The tangent to the lateral plateau is mildly convex upward (*arrowheads*), whereas the tangent to the medial one is concave (*large arrows*). The third posterior sloping line is tangent to the posterior intercondylar area (*small arrows*). (B-D) Corresponding sagittal PD-weighted images.

is a severe patellar tilt, the lateral border of the patella then projects behind the tangent to the vertical ridge (see **Fig. 12**).[12]

- *Radiographic features indicating a prior complete lateral patellar dislocation.* They include avulsion fracture or ossification of the medial ligamentous patellar stabilizers, and osteochondral fractures resulting from

impaction of the inferomedial aspect of the patella on the anterolateral aspect of the lateral femoral condyle (**Fig. 13**). These features are usually better demonstrated on the skyline and anteroposterior views than on the lateral view. Intra-articular linear or curvilinear bone fragments (sliver sign), arising from the patella or lateral femoral

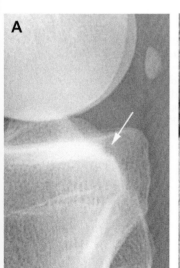
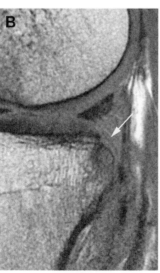

Fig. 15. Impaction fracture of the posterior aspect of the lateral tibial condyle (*arrow*) after ACL injury on a (A) lateral radiographic view and on a (B) sagittal T1-weighted image.

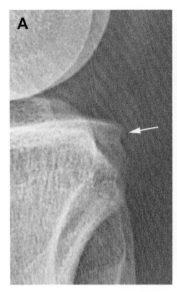
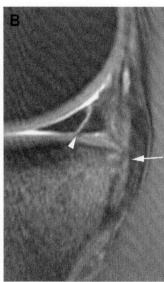

Fig. 16. Impaction fracture of the posterior aspect of the medial tibial condyle (*arrow*) after ACL injury on a (*A*) lateral radiographic view and on a (*B*) sagittal T1-weighted image. Note the associated tear of the posterior horn of the medial meniscus (*arrowhead*).

condyle, can be present and might be quite specific of acute lateral patellar dislocation (see **Fig. 13**).[13]

DETECTION OF POSTERIOR TIBIAL FRACTURES
Normal Anatomy

The tibial condyles also have different shapes (**Fig. 14**). The lateral one is mildly convex upward, whereas the medial one is concave, facing the round-shaped medial femoral condyle. The third posterior sloping line is tangent to the posterior intercondylar area, where the posterior cruciate ligament (PCL) inserts.

Posterior Tibial Fractures

In trauma, analysis of the 3 posterior tibial lines can allow the depiction of impaction fractures (**Fig. 15**). Fractures of the posterior medial condyle are less common than those of the lateral condyle but better demonstrated, as the medial condyle projects posteriorly to the lateral one (**Fig. 16**). Such lesions are typically associated with anterior cruciate ligament (ACL) injury and highly associated with damage of the adjacent structures, including the tibial insertion of the central tendon of the semimembranous muscle, and the posterior horn of the medial meniscus. Detection of a fracture involving the tangent to the

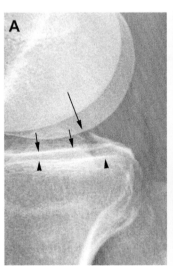
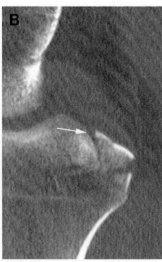

Fig. 17. (*A*) Fracture interrupting the tangent to the posterior intercondylar area (*large arrow*) on a lateral view. The tangents to the lateral (*arrowheads*) and medial (*small arrows*) tibial condyles are not involved. (*B*) Sagittal computed tomography image confirms the PCL tibial avulsion fracture (*arrow*).

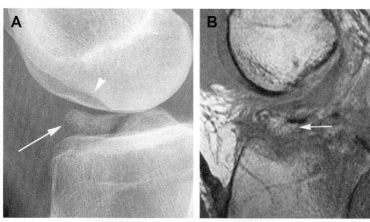

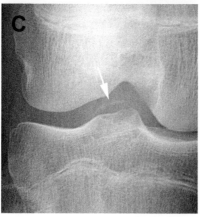

Fig. 18. Avulsion of the tibial attachment of the ACL. Large fragment (*arrow*) detected on the (*A*) lateral view and on a (*B*) sagittal T1-weighted image. Note the associated lateral femoral notch sign (*arrowhead*). (*C*) Small bone avulsion depicted on an AP view.

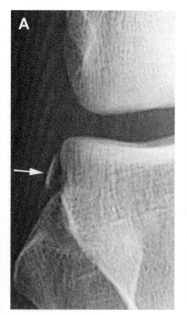
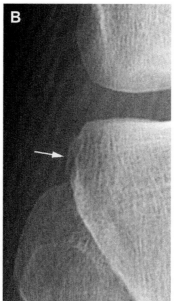
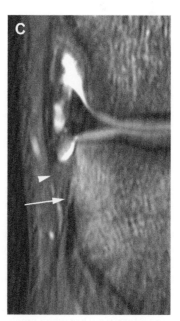

Fig. 19. Segond fracture. (*A*) Thick and (*B*) thin vertical bone fragments (*arrow*) parallel to the lateral aspect of the tibial plateau. (*C*) Coronal PD-weighted image of case B showing the tibial avulsion (*arrow*) of the anterolateral ligament (*arrowhead*). Note the adjacent bone marrow edema.

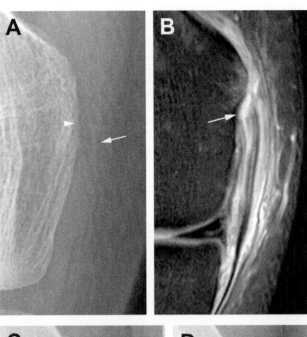

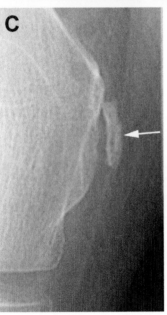

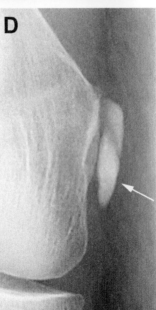

Fig. 20. Lesions of the proximal aspect of the superficial MCL. (*A*) Thin femoral bone avulsion (*arrow*) in the acute phase; note the irregular femoral epicondyle outline (*arrowhead*). (*B*) Corresponding PD-weighted image (*arrow*). (*C*) Thick ossification 6 months after superficial MCL avulsion (*arrow*). (*D*) Amorphous apatite calcification of the superficial MCL (*arrow*).

posterior intercondylar area means that there is a PCL tibial avulsion fracture (**Fig. 17**).

Avulsion of the tibial attachment of the ACL also can be detected on the lateral view (**Fig. 18**). This is typically encountered in children and adolescents due to the relative weakness of incompletely ossified bone and increased elasticity of ligament at those ages. A bone fragment of variable size, more or less displaced, is usually well depicted on the lateral view but when small, it may be better demonstrated on the anteroposterior (AP) view (see **Fig. 18**).

OTHER FRACTURES

Many other avulsion fractures can be depicted on the lateral and AP view of the knee. Their depiction on plain films is particularly important, as these thin bone fragments can be missed on MR imaging. We have a look at only the most frequent ones:

- *Segond fracture*, related to the tibial avulsion of the anterolateral ligament and typically associated with ACL tears.[14] The classic appearance of this fracture is that of a

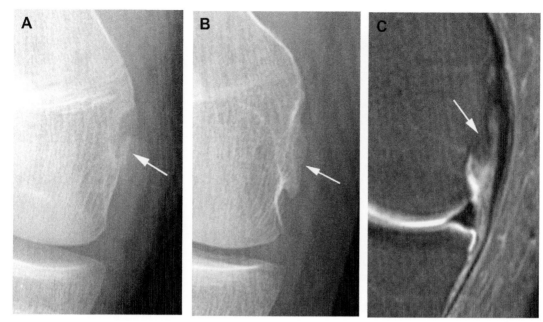

Fig. 21. Bone avulsion (*arrow*) of the deep portion of the MCL in the (*A*) acute and (*B*) chronic phases on AP radiographs. (*C*) Corresponding image on PD-weighted image.

curvilinear or elliptical vertical bone fragment projected parallel to the lateral aspect of the tibial plateau on AP view (**Fig. 19**). Sometimes, only a defect of the tibial outline is apparent on radiographs, which will be missed if this region is not systematically assessed in trauma.

- *Bone avulsion of the medial collateral ligament (MCL).* The avulsion of the proximal aspect of the superficial MCL is sometimes very difficult to detect in the acute phase (**Fig. 20**), and may be missed if the medial epicondyle outline is not systematically carefully analyzed on AP radiographs in trauma. A few weeks later, an ossification can develop in this area and is more or less extensive proximally due to the close proximity among the MCL, adductor tendons, and medial ligamentous stabilizers of the knee (see **Fig. 20**). This Pellegrini-Stieda lesion, which may or may not be associated with symptoms, is not to be confused with apatite calcifications, which are amorphous (see **Fig. 20**). The deep portion of the MCL also can be avulsed, with ossifications located more inferiorly (**Fig. 21**). This lesion is isolated or associated with a lesion of the superficial MCL. Finally, the tibial insertion of the deep portion of the MCL also can be avulsed, and is called the reverse Segond fracture. This lesion is frequently associated with PCL and medial meniscus tears.

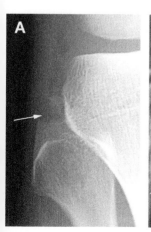
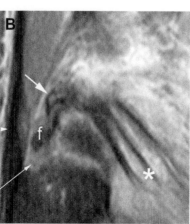

Fig. 22. Avulsion fracture involving the styloid process of the fibula (*arrow*) on (*A*) AP radiograph. The fragment is mildly displaced superiorly. (*B*) On the corresponding coronal PD-weighted image, the fragment (f) is displaced superiorly by the popliteofibular ligament (*large arrow*). Injury of the popliteal musculotendinous junction is also demonstrated (*star*). The fracture (*thin arrow*) does not involve the BFT (*arrowhead*) inserted on the lateral aspect of the fibular head.

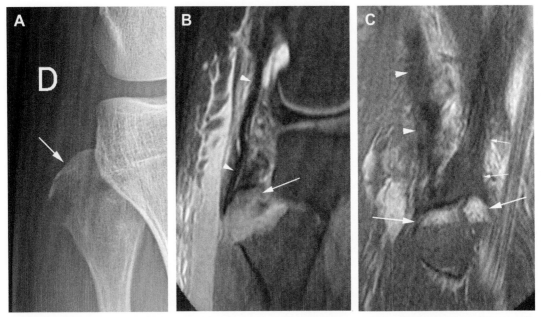

Fig. 23. Avulsion fracture (*arrow*) involving the lateral and medial aspects of the fibular head on (*A*) AP radiograph. The fragment is mildly displaced superiorly. (*B*) On the corresponding coronal PD-weighted and (*C*) sagittal T1-weighted images, the LCL (*arrowheads*) and the BFT (*thin arrows*) are attached to the bone fragment (*large arrows*).

- *Bone avulsion of the proximal aspect of the fibular head.* Depiction of such fractures is important, as they are considered to be a sign of injury to the posterior lateral corner (PLC) of the knee, frequently associated with cruciate ligament injury. Indeed, many components of the PLC insert on it, including the lateral collateral ligament (LCL), the biceps femoris tendon (BFT), and the arcuate complex, which consists of the popliteofibular ligament, the arcuate ligament, and the variably

present fabellofibular ligament. Failing to identify injury of the PLC can lead to chronic posterolateral instability of the knee.

Originally described as an avulsed fibular styloid fragment at the insertion site of the arcuate ligament complex,[15] the arcuate sign is often applied broadly to include small fractures of the fibular head. The shape, size, and location of the avulsed fragment vary according to which structures of the PLC are involved (**Figs. 22 and 23**).[16–18] When any avulsion

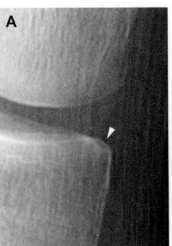
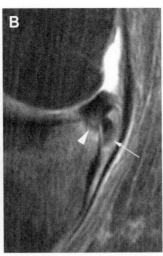

Fig. 24. Impaction fracture of the medial margin of the tibia (*arrowhead*) on (*A*) AP view. (*B*) Corresponding PD-weighted image showing the meniscal flap displaced in the medial meniscotibial recess (*arrow*). Note the associated edema of the adjacent bone and soft tissues.

fracture in this region is depicted, even in the absence of significant bone fragment displacement, one should perform an MR imaging examination of the PLC, particularly when the fracture involves the lateral aspect of the fibular head (LCL and BFT bone insertion). As such bone avulsions can be subtle, this region should be systematically carefully analyzed in trauma, particularly on the AP view.

Chronic tibial impaction fracture, highly suggestive of a meniscal tear, is sometimes depicted on the AP view of the knee. It typically involves the medial margin of the tibia and is related to a chronic horizontal or parrot beak meniscal tear, with a flap displaced in the meniscotibial recess. The meniscal fragment can be depicted on MR imaging or ultrasound,[19] but MR imaging also can show edema of the adjacent bone and soft tissues, particularly in the presence of pain (**Fig. 24**).

SUMMARY

Despite increased use of advanced imaging modalities, plain films remain the most available and affordable diagnostic test for an efficient analysis of the knee. Through a systematic evaluation of the knee views, a great deal of information can be obtained. This is all the more important because minor radiographic features can be missed on MR images.

REFERENCES

1. Hall FM. Radiographic diagnosis and accuracy in knee joint effusions. Radiology 1975;115(1):49–54.

2. Lee JH, Weissman BN, Nikpoor N, et al. Lipohemarthrosis of the knee: a review of recent experiences. Radiology 1989;173(1):189–91.

3. Ryu KN, Jaovisidha S, Schweitzer M, et al. MR imaging of lipoma arborescens of the knee joint. AJR Am J Roentgenol 1996;167(5):1229–32.

4. Pao DG. The lateral femoral notch sign. Radiology 2001;219(3):800–1.

5. Malghem J, Maldague B. Depth insufficiency of the proximal trochlear groove on lateral radiographs of the knee: relation to patellar dislocation. Radiology 1989;170:507–10.

6. Koëter S, Bongers EM, de Rooij J, et al. Minimal rotation aberrations cause radiographic misdiagnosis of trochlear dysplasia. Knee Surg Sports Traumatol Arthrosc 2006;14(8):713–7.

7. Maldague B, Malghem J. Significance of the radiograph of the knee profile in the detection of patellar instability. Preliminary report. Rev Chir Orthop Reparatrice Appar Mot 1985;71(Suppl 2):5–13 [in French].

8. Dejour H, Walch G, Nove-Josserand L, et al. Factors of patellar instability: an anatomic radiographic study. Knee Surg Sports Traumatol Arthrosc 1994; 2(1):19–26.

9. Caton J, Deschamps G, Chambat P, et al. Les rotules basses (Patellæ inferæ). À propos de 128 observations. Rev Chir Orthop Reparatrice Appar Mot 1982;68:317–25.

10. Insall J, Salvati E. Patella position in the normal knee joint. Radiology 1971;101(1):101–4.

11. Blackburne JS, Peel TE. A new method of measuring patellar height. J Bone Joint Surg Br 1977;59(2): 241–2.

12. Maldague B, Malghem J. The true lateral view of the patellar facets. A new radiological approach of the femoro-patellar joint (author's transl)]. Ann Radiol (Paris) 1976;19(6):573–81.

13. Haas JP, Collins MS, Stuart MJ. The "sliver sign": a specific radiographic sign of acute lateral patellar dislocation. Skeletal Radiol 2012;41(5):595–601.

14. Claes S, Luyckx T, Vereecke E, et al. The Segond fracture: a bony injury of the anterolateral ligament of the knee. Arthroscopy 2014;30(11):1475–82.

15. Shindell R, Walsh WM, Connolly JF. Avulsion fracture of the fibula: the 'arcuate sign' of posterolateral knee instability. Nebr Med J 1984;69:369–71.

16. Cohen BH, DeFroda SF, Hodax JD. Johnson D, Kristopher Ware J, Fadale PD. The arcuate fracture: a descriptive radiographic study. Injury 2018;49(10): 1871–7.

17. Lee J, Papakonstantinou O, Brookenthal KR, et al. Arcuate sign of posterolateral knee injuries: anatomic, radiographic, and MR imaging data related to patterns of injury. Skeletal Radiol 2003; 32:619–27.

18. Strub WM. The arcuate sign. Radiology 2007;244(2): 620–1.

19. Moraux A, Khalil C, Demondion X, et al. Inferiorly displaced flap tear of the medial meniscus: sonographic diagnosis. J Ultrasound Med 2008;27(12): 1795–8.

Anteroposterior Radiograph of the Ankle with Cross-Sectional Imaging Correlation

Dana J. Lin, MD[a], Erin F. Alaia, MD[a], Ignacio Martín Rossi, MD[b],
Jonathan Zember, MD[c], Zehava Sadka Rosenberg, MD[a,d,*]

KEYWORDS

• AP radiograph • MR imaging • Ankle • Correlation • Fracture • Injury • Variant

KEY POINTS

- Several characteristic locations should be scrutinized on the AP radiograph of the ankle so as to detect various disease entities which may otherwise remain undetected.
- Small ossific densities, protuberances, or abnormal interfaces on the AP radiograph of the ankle can be the harbingers of more extensive underlying soft tissue injury, better characterized on cross-sectional imaging.
- Given the clinical overlap of many of the entities described in this article with lateral ankle sprains, they may be clinically misdiagnosed and thus, the radiologist can play a crucial role by helping avoid delayed diagnosis and patient morbidity.

INTRODUCTION

Radiographic evaluation of the ankle is exceedingly common, fast, and relatively inexpensive. Often obtained to evaluate for fractures in the setting of trauma, ankle radiographs can reveal several other types of traumatic and nontraumatic lesions that may overlap clinically with lateral ankle sprain or may be unsuspected by the referring clinician at the time of injury.

The purpose of this article is to illustrate several pathologic entities and variants heralding disease about the ankle that can be initially diagnosed on anteroposterior (AP) radiograph of the ankle alone, with correlative findings on MR imaging. Many of these entities can be detected only on the AP ankle radiograph, particularly if foot films are not available, and if not recognized may lead to delayed diagnosis and persistent morbidity to the patient. However, the vigilant radiologist, equipped with the knowledge of the characteristic appearance and typical locations of the imaging findings, will often be able to make the crucial initial diagnosis and surmise additional pathologic conditions, which, if necessary, can be confirmed on cross-sectional imaging.

The article is subdivided into 2 major sections: lateral entities and medial entities. Lateral entities include extra-articular lateral hindfoot impingement, superior peroneal retinaculum (SPR) avulsion, fracture of the lateral process of the talus, fracture of the anterior process of the calcaneus, enlarged peroneal tubercle (PT), with associated

Disclosure: The authors have nothing to disclose.
[a] Department of Radiology, Division of Musculoskeletal Radiology, NYU Langone Health, 301 East 17th Street, 6th Floor, New York, NY 10003, USA; [b] Centro Rossi, Arenales 2777, C1425BEE, Buenos Aires, Argentina; [c] Childrens National Medical Center, DC, 111 Michigan Avenue NW, Washington, DC 20010, USA; [d] Department of Orthopaedic Surgery, Division of Musculoskeletal Radiology, NYU Langone Health, 301 East 17th Street, 6th Floor, New York, NY 10003, USA
* Corresponding author. Departments of Orthopedic Surgery and Radiology, NYU Langone Health, 301 East 17th Street, 6th Floor, New York, NY 10003.
E-mail address: zehava.rosenberg@nyulangone.org

Magn Reson Imaging Clin N Am 27 (2019) 701–719
https://doi.org/10.1016/j.mric.2019.07.001

peroneal tendon disease, and peroneus longus tendon tear, associated with os peroneum retraction. Medial entities include deltoid ligament injury, talar body fractures, and extra-articular (posteromedial) talocalcaneal coalition. In addition to emphasis on key radiographic and cross-sectional imaging features for each topic, the relevant anatomy, mechanism of injury, clinical features, and management are also briefly discussed.

LATERAL ENTITIES
Extra-articular Lateral Hindfoot Impingement

Severe flatfoot and hindfoot valgus deformity can predispose to extra-articular, lateral hindfoot impingement, composed of talocalcaneal and subfibular impingements.[1,2] With progressive hindfoot valgus alignment, the weight-bearing forces are shifted laterally from the talar dome to the lateral talus and fibula and talocalcaneal joint subluxation may develop. Despite the pathologic condition being medial, typically in the setting of posterior tibial tendon dysfunction, patients can present with lateral ankle pain because of impingement between the lateral talus and calcaneus (talocalcaneal impingement) and, as the valgus deformity progresses, between the lateral

calcaneus and the distal fibula (subfibular impingement). Secondary lateral soft tissue entrapment can further contribute to pain.[2,3]

On a weight-bearing AP view of the ankle, the presence of hindfoot valgus and lateral extra-articular impingement can be surmised when there is lateral tilting of the normal calcaneal axis (**Fig. 1**) relative to the tibial axis. As impingement develops, there will be greater proximity of the fibular tip to the calcaneus (**Fig. 2**), eventual direct contact and even a pseudofacet between the 2 bones. Imaging findings of extra-articular impingement may be delineated in greater detail with computed tomography (CT) and MR imaging, where there is compromise of the sinus tarsi space, subluxation at the subtalar joint, and apposing subcortical sclerosis, cyst formation and, in the case of MR imaging, marrow edema, at the sites of contact between the lateral talus and calcaneus and between the fibular tip and lateral calcaneus. A fibulocalcaneal pseudofacet may also be noted. MR imaging may further depict soft tissue abnormalities such as entrapment and thickening of the calcaneofibular ligament and peroneal tendon subluxation in the later stages of the disease (see **Figs. 1 and 2**).

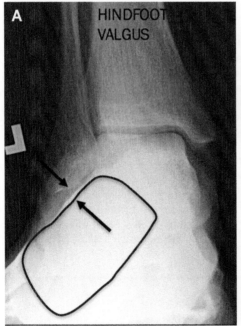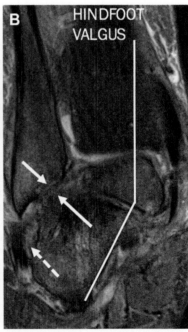

Fig. 1. Flatfoot deformity and extra-articular lateral hindfoot impingement. (*A*) Extra-articular impingement in an 83-year-old woman with rheumatoid arthritis and acquired flatfoot deformity. Ankle AP radiograph demonstrates valgus tilt of the calcaneus (*black outline*) and close proximity of the fibula to the calcaneus (*arrows*), suggesting calcaneofibular impingement. (*B*) Extra-articular impingement in a 45-year-old man with lateral ankle pain for 2 years. Coronal proton-density fat-suppressed MR imaging demonstrates valgus tilt of the calcaneus relative to the tibial axis (*white lines*), subfibular (calcaneofibular) impingement (*solid arrows*), and lateral displacement of the peroneal tendons (*dashed arrow*).

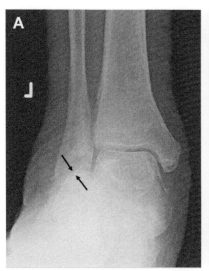
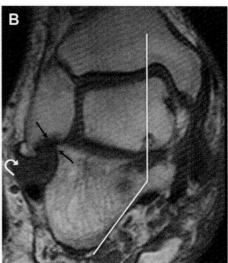

Fig. 2. Flatfoot deformity and extra-articular lateral hindfoot impingement in an 82-year-old man. (*A*) Ankle AP radiograph shows valgus tilt of the calcaneus, and close apposition of the fibula to the calcaneus (*arrows*), suggesting calcaneofibular impingement. (*B*) Coronal T1 ankle MR imaging demonstrates valgus tilt of the calcaneus relative to the tibial axis (*white lines*), and confirms calcaneofibular impingement (*arrows*). There is also soft tissue entrapment with obliteration of soft tissue fat (*curved arrow*).

Management of hindfoot deformity usually begins with conservative measures such as physical therapy and orthotics. Advanced osseous deformity, with the development of extra-articular impingement, typically requires calcaneal osteotomy or arthrodesis in the most severe cases.

Superior Peroneal Retinaculum Avulsion

The SPR is a band of fibrous tissue that acts as the primary restraint to peroneal tendon subluxation out of the retromalleolar groove of the distal fibula. The retinaculum originates from the posterolateral aspect of the fibula, spanning across the superficial margin of the peroneal tendons, and most commonly inserting onto the calcaneus and Achilles tendon sheath.[4,5]

Often misdiagnosed as an ankle sprain in the acute setting, SPR injury, with peroneal tendon dislocation, occurs as a result of sudden, strong, reflexive peroneal muscle contraction during ankle dorsiflexion, and is most commonly seen in young adults because of sports activity.[6] Numerous predisposing factors to SPR injuries have been described, including, but not limited to, variations in the morphology of the retromalleolar groove.[7]

Avulsion fractures of the SPR are only noted on AP and possibly oblique radiographs of the ankle. A vertical avulsion fracture fragment, off the lateral margin of the distal fibula, is nearly pathognomonic for SPR avulsion, with or without associated peroneal tendon dislocation.[8] The SPR avulsion fracture is easily distinguishable from a distal

fibular fracture, because it occurs superior and lateral to the fibular tip, with the fragment typically linear in shape, conforming to the lateral fibular cortex (**Figs. 3 and 4**).

Acute SPR injuries leading to peroneal tendon instability can be readily assessed on axial MR imaging and graded according to the classification first described by Eckert and Davis.[4] According to this classification, the most common injuries include stripping of the SPR from its fibular attachment (see **Fig. 4**), with formation of a subperiosteal pouch into which the peroneal tendons can dislocate, and bony avulsions at the SPR attachment to the fibula. A recent classification, with surgical implications,[9] describes a large lateral fracture fragment, with an intact SPR and dislocation of the peroneal tendons between the fracture fragment and fibula.

Both MR imaging and CT allow for assessment of retro-malleolar groove morphology, because flat, convex, or irregular grooves can predispose to injuries of the SPR and peroneal tendon dislocation. MR imaging also allows for evaluation of concomitant lateral collateral ligament or peroneal tendon tears, whereas periosteal stripping and small avulsion fractures may be better characterized on radiographs or CT (see **Fig. 3**). Given their association with other types of ankle fractures, typically intra-articular calcaneal fractures, SPR injuries may, on occasion, be detected on ankle CT obtained for fracture characterization elsewhere.[10,11] The SPR can be also be assessed with ultrasound, with

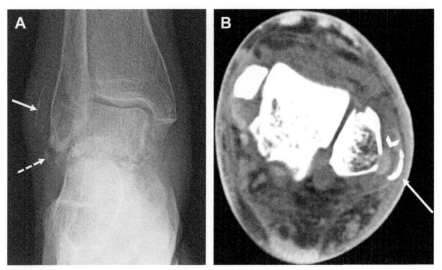

Fig. 3. Superior peroneal retinacular avulsion fracture in a 71-year-old woman. (*A*) Ankle AP radiograph shows a laterally displaced linear avulsion fracture (*solid arrow*), along the superior peroneal retinacular attachment site. More distally, there is a fracture fragment (*dashed arrow*) originating from a talar body fracture. (*B*) Axial CT image in the same patient redemonstrates superior peroneal retinacular avulsion fracture (*solid arrow*), with resultant anterior dislocation of the peroneal tendons (*arrowhead*), which are now interposed between the lateral malleolus and the displaced avulsion fracture.

the particular advantage of demonstrating transient peroneal tendon subluxation or dislocation with dynamic resisted dorsiflexion-eversion of the ankle.[12]

Conservative management in a short leg cast with the foot in neutral to slight inversion for 6 weeks may be recommended for acute type I and possibly type III injuries.[13] Although several

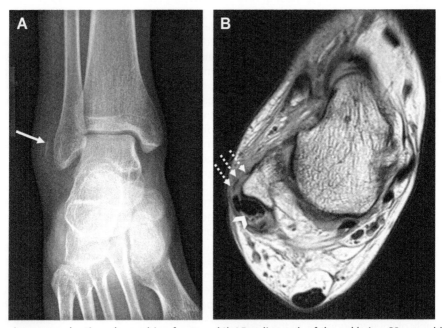

Fig. 4. Superior peroneal retinacular avulsion fracture. (*A*) AP radiograph of the ankle in a 32-year-old man with ankle pain after fall, showing a longitudinally oriented superior peroneal retinacular avulsion fracture (*arrow*) paralleling the lateral malleolus. (*B*) Axial proton-density image of the ankle in a 33-year-old woman with lateral ankle pain demonstrates ossification and stripping off the superior peroneal retinaculum and periosteum from the lateral malleolus, with formation of a pouch (*dashed arrows*). The peroneal tendons are in normal position (*arrowhead*).

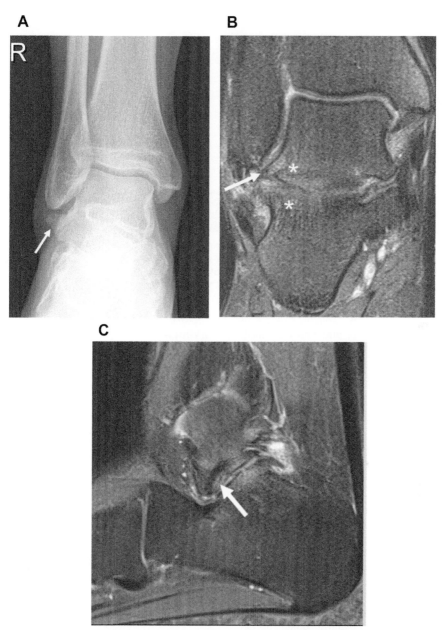

Fig. 5. Deformity of the lateral talar process in a 42-year-old woman following fracture 2 years previous to presentation. (*A*) AP radiograph of the ankle demonstrates focal bony protuberance (*arrow*) due to a healed fracture deformity of the lateral talar process. (*B*) Coronal proton-density fat-suppressed image demonstrates fracture deformity of the lateral talar process (*arrow*) and degenerative changes at the opposing surfaces of the posterior subtalar joint (*asterisks*). (*C*) Sagittal proton-density fat-suppressed image demonstrates the V sign with deformity and asymmetry of the wedge-shaped morphology of the lateral talar process (*arrow*).

other procedures exist, surgical management most commonly includes anatomic repair of the SPR with fibular groove deepening.[13]

Fracture of the Lateral Process of the Talus

The lateral process of the talus is part of the posterior subtalar and talofibular joints. Although relatively uncommon, fractures of the lateral process of the talus (LTPFs) account for up to 20% of talar fractures.[14] The mechanism of injury is axial loading and dorsiflexion of the foot with external rotation, most commonly associated with snowboarding.[15] LTPFs can also be seen in patients after motor vehicle accidents and falls

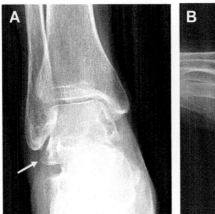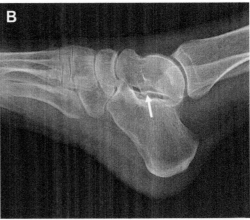

Fig. 6. Posttraumatic deformity of the lateral talar process in a 50-year-old woman. (*A*) The AP view depicts bony protuberance (*arrow*) of the lateral talar process. (*B*) The V sign (*arrow*), seen on the lateral view, reflects disruption and asymmetry of the normal wedge-shaped morphology of the lateral talus.

from height. These fractures clinically present as persistent lateral ankle pain and can be initially misdiagnosed as lateral ankle sprain, with secondary significant morbidity and subtalar arthritis.[16]

Fractures of the lateral process of the talus are frequently detected only on AP radiographs of the ankle, manifesting as inframalleolar bony protuberances and irregularities of the lateral talus (**Fig. 5**). Secondary subtalar arthritis may depict additional changes in the opposing calcaneus. LTPFs, although difficult to detect, may be noted on the lateral ankle view using the V sign, which is an interruption or asymmetry of the normal V-shaped contour of the lateral process of the talus (**Fig. 6**). Recent literature, however, suggests that the presence of the V sign varies with the extent of the fracture and foot position, and is subject to interobserver variability.[17] CT is usually required for confirmation of LTPFs in suspected cases and for further characterization of the fracture.[18] Given the often delayed clinical presentation or misdiagnosis as lateral ankle sprain, LTPFs may be seen subacutely or even remotely on MR imaging with evidence of secondary posterior subtalar arthritis (see **Fig. 5**).

Small or nondisplaced LTPFs can be managed nonoperatively with immobilization and progressive weight-bearing, whereas larger and displaced fractures require fixation with lag screws or a miniplate.[19] Significantly comminuted fractures are treated with excision.[20] Nonunited fractures with a late presentation can be excised if small and internally fixed if large.[20] In cases that have progressed to malunion or nonunion, pseudoarthrosis[18] and even lateral hindfoot impingement have been reported.[21]

Fracture of the Anterior Process of the Calcaneus

The anterior process of the calcaneus projects distal to the calcaneal sulcus, articulating with both the talus, via the middle and anterior subtalar joints, and with the cuboid.

Fractures of the anterior process of the calcaneus (APCFs) occur as a result of 2 proposed mechanisms of injury. The more common mechanism involves avulsion fractures of the dorsal calcaneocuboid ligament, the bifurcate ligament, and/or the extensor digitorum brevis muscle during inversion of a plantarflexed ankle.[22] A less common mechanism is shearing/compression during forced dorsiflexion and eversion (nutcracker fracture).[23] Clinically, APCFs present as ecchymosis and tenderness approximately 2 cm distal and 1 cm inferior to the anterior talofibular ligament.[24] As the fractures often coexist with lateral collateral ligament tears, the injury is often mistaken for ankle sprain, with a delayed diagnosis of an average of 22 weeks.[25]

On radiographs, APCFs may only be detected on AP radiographs of the ankle, particularly if radiographs of the foot are not available. Depending on the size of the fracture fragment they are often discerned on lateral and oblique views of the foot or a lateral view of the ankle (**Fig. 7**). On AP view of the ankle, APCFs are detected by presence of a subfibular bone fragment. In the setting of ankle inversion injury, soft tissue swelling, distal, rather than at the level of the fibula, can be a clue to the presence of this fracture (see **Fig. 7**).[26] Smaller APCFs are thought to be due to avulsion of the dorsal calcaneocuboid and/or bifurcate ligaments, whereas larger avulsion fractures may be due to

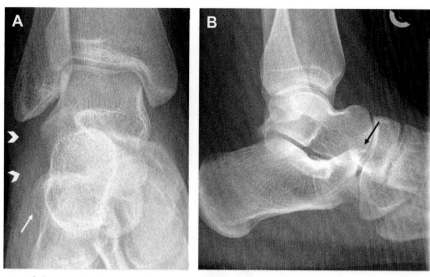

Fig. 7. Fracture of the anterior process of the calcaneus in a 24-year-old woman following inversion injury. (*A*) Ankle AP radiograph demonstrates a small fracture fragment (*arrow*) along the lateral aspect of the calcaneus with overlying soft tissue swelling (*arrowheads*). Note the absence of soft tissue swelling adjacent to the fibula. (*B*) Lateral radiograph of the ankle confirms a small fracture fragment at the anterior process of the calcaneus (*arrow*).

avulsion at the origin of the extensor digitorum brevis muscle.

APCFs often reflect a component of Chopart joint disruption, or midtarsal sprain, with additional fractures at the talonavicular joints (**Fig. 8**).[27,28] Thus, whereas inversion-related distraction forces at the calcaneocuboid joint produce avulsion fractures, typically of the dorsal calcaneocuboid

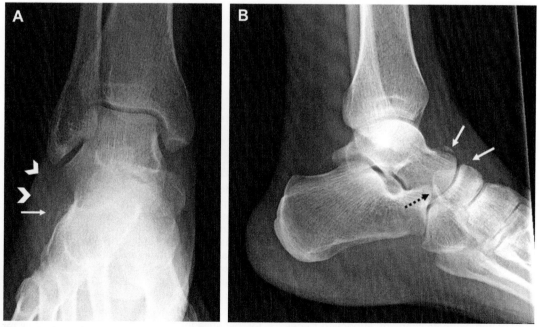

Fig. 8. Avulsion fractures associated with midtarsal joint injury in a 34-year-old man. (*A*) AP radiograph of the ankle demonstrating a small avulsion fracture (*arrow*) along the lateral aspect of the calcaneus with swelling of the overlying soft tissues (*arrowheads*). Note again the absence of soft tissue edema adjacent to the fibula. (*B*) Lateral radiograph of the ankle depicts small avulsion fractures along the dorsal talar head and navicular bone at the dorsal talonavicular ligament attachment sites (*solid arrows*). An additional avulsion fracture is present at the anterior process of the calcaneus (*dashed arrow*).

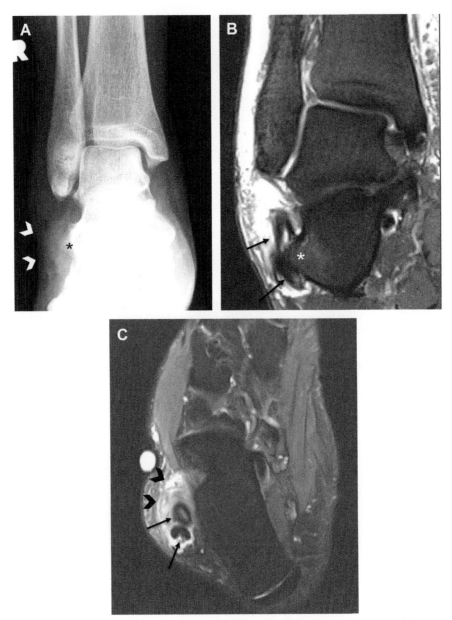

Fig. 9. Enlarged peroneal tubercle and secondary peroneal tendon disease in a 51-year-old man with lateral ankle pain. (A) Ankle AP radiograph demonstrates a large osseous protuberance (*asterisk*) along the lateral calcaneus, compatible with an enlarged peroneal tubercle. Note extensive soft tissue swelling (*arrowheads*). (B) Coronal proton-density fat-suppressed image of the ankle demonstrates reactive marrow edema in an enlarged peroneal tubercle (*asterisk*) as well as tenosynovitis and longitudinal split tearing of the peroneus brevis and longus tendons (*arrows*). (C) Axial proton-density fat-suppressed image demonstrates a marker denoting the patient's site of pain and corresponding to the marked tenosynovitis and longitudinal split tearing of both tendons (*arrows*). Note the marked soft tissue reactive changes (*arrowheads*).

ligament and bifurcate ligament, impaction forces can result in fractures of the navicular and talar head. Concomitant avulsion of the dorsal talonavicular ligament is secondary to simultaneous foot plantarflexion. Therefore, in the setting of APCFs, additional fractures should be scrutinized for, because they indicate a more significant injury of the Chopart joint.

CT and MR imaging are helpful when the APCFs are radiographically occult or nondisplaced, by further characterizing fracture morphology, displacement, and intra-articular extension. The

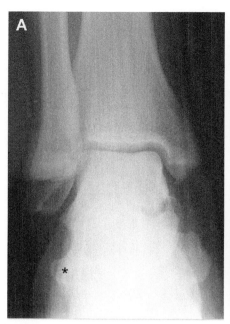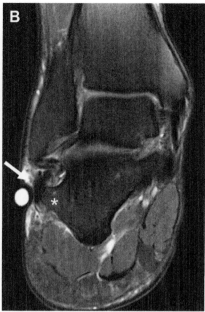

Fig. 10. Enlarged peroneal tubercle and secondary peroneal tendinosis in a 42-year-old man with lateral ankle pain. (*A*) Ankle AP radiograph demonstrates a large osseous protuberance (*asterisk*) originating from the lateral calcaneus, compatible with an enlarged peroneal tubercle. (*B*) Coronal proton-density fat-suppressed image of the ankle confirms an enlarged peroneal tubercle (*asterisk*) deep to the marker denoting the patient's site of pain, displacement of the peroneal tendons (*arrow*), and surrounding edema.

fractures are best visualized in the sagittal plane and are most often vertical in orientation.[28]

MR imaging is useful also for detecting concurrent injuries to the lateral collateral ligament complex, the medial aspect of the Chopart joint, and for assessing the integrity of the dorsal talonavicular, dorsal calcalcaneocuboid, and bifurcate ligaments.

Minimally displaced APCFs can be treated conservatively but may require longer immobilization and nonweight-bearing when compared with ankle sprains.[23,24] In patients with displaced fractures or with refractory pain, open reduction internal fixation of larger fragments and surgical excision of smaller fragments have both shown satisfactory outcomes.[25]

Enlarged Peroneal Tubercle

The PT, also known as the trochlear process, is an osseous protuberance, located along the lateral calcaneal wall, with commonly reported prevalence of approximately 40%, although higher prevalence of up to 97% has been reported.[29,30] The PT serves as the attachment site of the inferior peroneal retinaculum, divides the peroneus longus and brevis tendon sheaths, and acts as a pulley or fulcrum for the peroneus longus tendon as it turns toward the cuboid.[31] The peroneus brevis and longus tendons course superior/anterior and inferior/posterior to the PT, respectively.

The mean width of the PT is 3 mm, with 5 mm often used as a cutoff to diagnose an enlarged PT.[32] The reported prevalence of an enlarged PT is approximately 21%.[33] Morphologic variations of the PT have also been described.[34] An enlarged PT displaces the peroneus longus tendon posterolaterally and effectively increases the acuity of the angle that the tendon must take toward the cuboid, predisposing it to increased tension and secondary disease such as tendinosis and tearing. Peroneus brevis disease is less common in the setting of hypertrophied PT.

The PT may only be detected on AP view of the ankle, if no foot films are available, as a lateral osseous protuberance, arising from the calcaneus (**Fig. 9**). The PT is optimally seen on cross-sectional imaging, with either ultrasonography, CT, or MR imaging of the ankle. On MR imaging, an enlarged PT may demonstrate reactive marrow edema with adjacent tendinosis, tenosynovitis, and longitudinal split tearing of the peroneus longus tendon, and, less commonly, concomitant involvement of the peroneus brevis tendon (see **Figs. 9** and **10**).

Conservative management for a symptomatic enlarged PT includes shoe modifications, orthotics, and immobilization.[35] If conservative treatment fails, operative excision of the tubercle can be carried out with peroneal tendon repair as necessary.[30]

Peroneus Longus Tendon Tear Associated with Os Peroneum Retraction

Complete tears of the peroneus longus tendon most commonly occur at the cuboid tunnel, at the level of, proximal to, or distal to an os peroneum.[7,36] Less common than peroneus brevis tendon tears, peroneus longus tendon tears typically occur after acute, direct trauma or sports-related, inversion injury.[12] Underlying disease of the tendon, however, often precedes the acute trauma. Complete tears of the peroneus longus tendon, although optimally diagnosed on MR imaging, can sometimes be surmised on an AP radiograph of the ankle, based on proximal migration of the os peroneum.

The os peroneum is a unipartite or multipartite sesamoid bone, located in close proximity to the cuboid tunnel, along the lateral aspect of the cuboid.[7,36] An ossified os peroneum is seen in 30% of foot radiographs and is bilateral in almost 60% of people.[12,37]

The presence of an os peroneum has been associated with the painful os peroneum syndrome, with predisposition to plantar lateral ankle pain, os peroneum fractures, and peroneus longus tendon tears.[38] Fracture of the os peroneum or distraction of a bipartite or multipartite os peroneum is a useful marker of peroneus longus tendon tear.[39] The distance between the components of a multipartite os peroneum has been reported to be less than 2 mm, and a distance greater than or equal to 6 mm suggests an os peroneum fracture or diastasis of a multipartite os peroneum.[40,41] Furthermore, a distance of greater than 10 mm between a proximal os peroneum fragment and the calcaneocuboid joint on a lateral foot radiograph has been reported to be highly suggestive of peroneus longus tendon rupture and retraction.[41]

On an AP radiograph of the ankle, a peroneus longus tendon tear can be surmised by a proximally retracted os peroneum (**Figs. 11 and 12**), noted as a well-corticated ossification, to be distinguished from a distal fibular fracture, along the lateral soft tissues of the ankle. MR imaging can confirm the diagnosis, and further assess the extent of tendon retraction and degree of underlying tendon disease (see **Fig. 12**).

Peroneus longus tendon ruptures, with or without os peroneum fracture, can be treated conservatively or with fracture fixation, excision of the os peroneum with direct tendon repair,

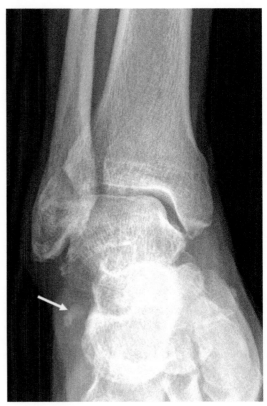

Fig. 11. Displaced os peroneum in a 42-year-old man with lateral ankle pain. Ankle AP radiograph demonstrates a large, corticated ossific fragment (*arrow*) along the lateral hindfoot, representing a proximally migrated os peroneum and indicating a tear and proximal retraction of the peroneus longus tendon.

tenodesis of the peroneus longus to the peroneus brevis, or anchoring of the proximal peroneus longus tendon segment to the cuboid or calcaneus.[42,43]

MEDIAL ENTITIES
Deltoid Ligament Injury

The deltoid ligament is a strong ligamentous complex, serving as the primary medial stabilizer to the ankle.[44] It also limits external rotation, abduction, and pronation of the talus. Commonly accepted nomenclature subdivides the deltoid ligament into superficial and deep components with varying prevalence of multiple bands originating from the medial malleolus and inserting on the talus, calcaneus, and navicular.[45]

The primary mechanism of acute deltoid ligament injury is eversion or external rotation of the ankle, seen in athletes or in the setting of complex ankle fractures and dislocations.[44] Secondary medial ankle instability may develop depending on the location and severity of ligament injury.[46]

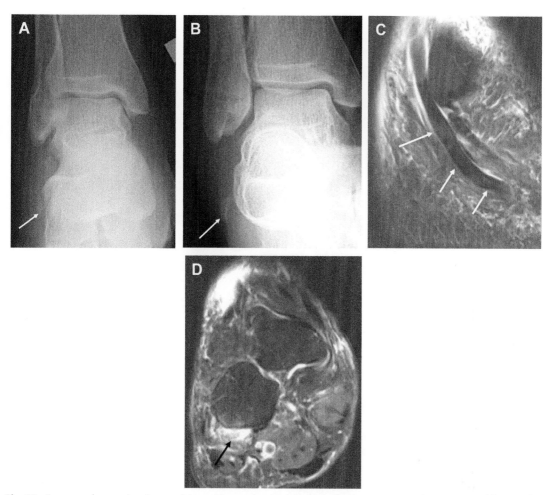

Fig. 12. Peroneus longus tendon avulsion with proximal migration of an os peroneum in a 59-year-old man after twisting injury. (*A*) Ankle AP radiograph demonstrates an ill-defined ossific density (*arrow*) along the inferolateral margin of the ankle, with overlying soft tissue swelling. The findings may be mistaken for a fracture of the anterior process of the calcaneus. (*B*) Mortise view better demonstrates the well-corticated margins of the ossicle (*arrow*). (*C*) Sagittal proton-density fat-suppressed image of the ankle demonstrates proximal retraction, waviness and thickening of the torn peroneus longus tendon (*arrows*). The os peroneum is better visualized on the radiographs. (*D*) Coronal proton-density fat-suppressed image demonstrates absence of the peroneus longus tendon at the cuboid tunnel (*arrow*), consistent with retracted tear, and cuboid reactive marrow edema.

An AP radiograph of the ankle may demonstrate both acute and remote superficial or deep deltoid ligament injuries. In the acute setting, a small avulsion fracture can be seen either proximally, along the superomedial margin of the medial malleolus, at the origin of the superficial component, or distally along the medial talar surface, where the deep fibers of the deltoid ligament attach (**Figs. 13 and 14**). A smooth, osseous protuberance along the superomedial margin of the medial malleolus, on either AP or oblique ankle radiographs, indicates old, superficial deltoid ligament injury and is consistent with healed detachment of the fascial sleeve of the medial malleolus, implying previous stripping of the periosteum at the attachment of the superficial deltoid origin.[47] MR imaging will depict osseous remodeling along the superficial medial malleolus, with or without marrow edema, depending on the acuity of injury (**Fig. 15**).

Management of deltoid ligament injuries depends on the stability of the ankle. Acute, stable deltoid ligament injury is generally treated conservatively and allowed to heal on its own. Patients with more complex ankle fractures or mortise instability require surgical management.[44]

Talar Body Fractures

Fractures of the talar dome, lateral and posterior processes, and shear or crush injuries of the talar body are all considered talar body fractures.[18,48] High-energy trauma causes talar body proper

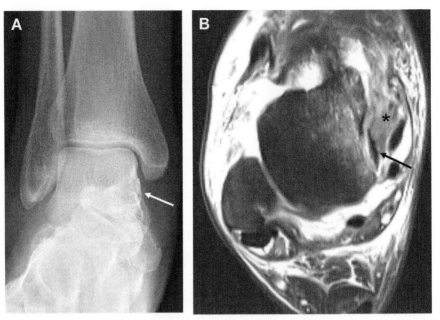

Fig. 13. Acute deep deltoid ligament avulsion in a 40-year-old woman with acute ankle pain. (*A*) Ankle AP radiograph demonstrates osseous irregularity along the medial talus (*arrow*), with small avulsion fragment overlapping the talus. (*B*) Axial proton-density fat-suppressed MR imaging of the ankle confirms talar avulsion fracture at the deep deltoid attachment (*arrow*) and talar marrow edema. The deep deltoid (*asterisk*) depicts poor definition and edema.

fractures, which may involve the tibiotalar joint, talocalcaneal joint, or both. The typical mechanism is axial loading on a dorsiflexed foot in the setting of a high-level fall or motor vehicle trauma. The worst prognosis of all talar body injuries is associated with crush, comminuted, talar body fractures, which are frequently open fractures.[49] These fractures have a high incidence of bone loss, nonanatomic reduction, and avascular necrosis.

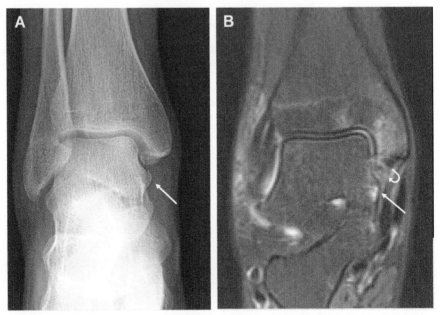

Fig. 14. Acute deep deltoid ligament avulsion in a 15-year-old girl following a twisting injury. (*A*) Ankle AP radiograph demonstrates a small talar avulsion fracture at the distal attachment of the deep deltoid fibers (*arrow*). (*B*) Coronal short tau inversion recovery image of the ankle demonstrates focal marrow edema at the site of avulsion (*straight arrow*), contusion of the medial malleolus and poor definition of the torn deep deltoid fibers (*curved arrow*).

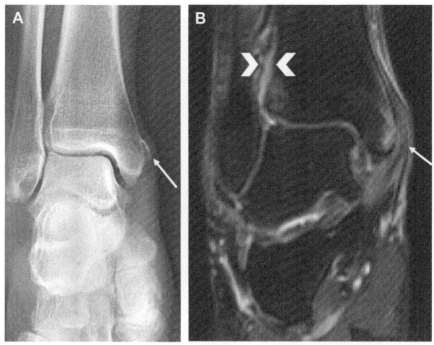

Fig. 15. Acute on chronic superficial deltoid ligament injury in a 53-year-old woman. (A) Slightly obliqued AP radiograph of the ankle demonstrates ossification (*arrow*) at the origin of the superficial fibers of the deltoid ligament complex, compatible with previous injury. (B) Coronal T2 fat-suppressed image of the ankle demonstrates thickening and loss of definition of the superficial (*arrow*) and deep deltoid fibers, associated with marrow edema at the origin of the superficial fibers, compatible with recent acute injury. Fluid and marrow edema along the distal tibiofibular syndesmosis, consistent with high ankle sprain, is also present (*arrowheads*).

When nondisplaced, true talar body fractures can be difficult to discern on ankle radiographs (**Fig. 16**). Careful study of the medial and lateral walls of the talus on the AP view may allow fracture detection. Subtle step-off in the talar dome articular surface should be vigilantly searched for in the setting of ankle trauma, on AP, lateral, and oblique radiographs of the ankle. Lateral radiographs of

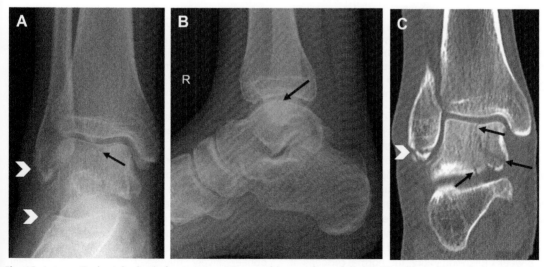

Fig. 16. Intra-articular talar body fracture in a 36-year-old man after a fall. (A) AP ankle radiograph demonstrates an intra-articular fracture of the talar dome (*arrow*). Incidentally noted are healing lateral malleolar and anterior calcaneal process avulsion fractures (*arrowheads*). (B) Lateral ankle radiograph redemonstrates intra-articular talar body fracture (*arrow*). (C) Coronal CT image better demonstrates the extent of the comminuted, intra-articular talar fracture (*arrows*). Note healing lateral malleolar fracture (*arrowhead*).

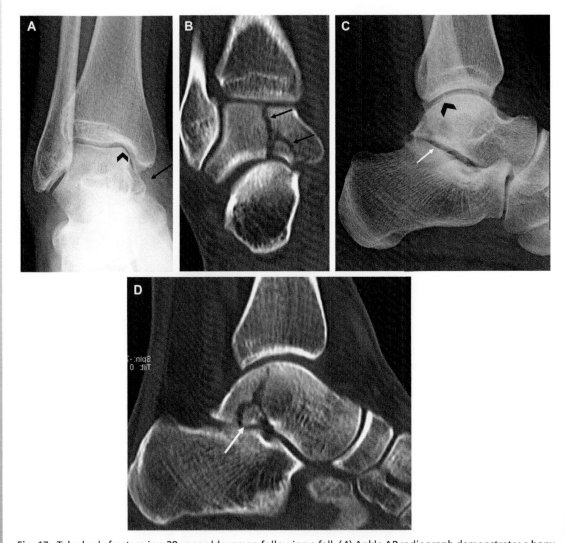

Fig. 17. Talar body fracture in a 28-year-old woman following a fall. (*A*) Ankle AP radiograph demonstrates a bony prominence along the medial talus (*arrow*). A questionable radiolucency, seen in retrospect, is also noted along the medial talar dome (*arrowhead*). (*B*) Coronal CT of the ankle demonstrates a comminuted sagittal shear type fracture of the talar body (*arrows*). (*C*) Lateral ankle radiograph demonstrates fracture fragments, overlying the posterior subtalar joint (*arrow*). Also noted is subtle step-off of the talar dome articular surface (*arrowhead*). (*D*) Sagittal CT of the ankle demonstrates a comminuted talar body fracture extending into the posterior subtalar joint (*arrow*).

either the ankle or foot may depict subtle extension of fracture lines into the subtalar joint. CT, with multiplanar reformats, offers assessment of comminution and intra-articular extension for preoperative planning (**Fig. 17**). MR imaging, obtained when there is persistent ankle pain of unknown or unclear origin, can demonstrate low signal fracture planes, with surrounding bone marrow edema.

AP and oblique views of the ankle may also provide information on perfusion of the talar body. Six to 8 weeks following injury, the normal process of bony remodeling will produce subchondral resorption of the talar dome, manifesting as thin, linear subchondral lucency known as the "Hawkin's sign," indicating a preserved talar body vascularity

(**Fig. 18**).[50] Absence of normal subchondral resorption serves as an indicator of avascular necrosis (see **Fig. 18**). Occasionally, partial avascular necrosis will occur, with interrupted talar dome subchondral resorption. Partial avascular necrosis most often involves the lateral talar dome, owing to the more robust medial-sided blood supply.[51]

The primary aim of treating talar body fractures is to restore congruity to the tibiotalar and talocalcaneal articulations. Nondisplaced fractures are conservatively managed. Because most talar body fractures are displaced, most require operative treatment of fracture fragment fixation and restoration of joint alignment. Complications include avascular necrosis and posttraumatic

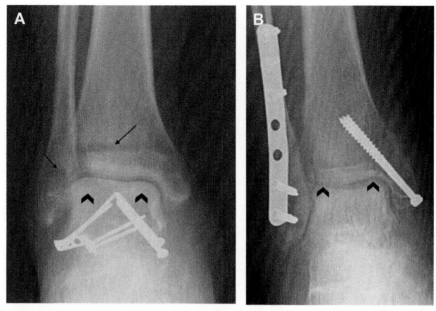

Fig. 18. Talar avascular necrosis in a 30-year-old man, after open reduction and internal fixation for talar body fracture. (*A*) Ankle AP radiograph demonstrates diffuse talar sclerosis and lack of subchondral resorption, suggesting avascular necrosis (*arrowheads*). Note expected disuse-related resorption along the metaphyses of both the distal tibia and fibula (*arrows*). (*B*) Comparison ankle AP radiograph in a 66-year-old woman following open reduction and internal fixation of distal fibular and medial malleolar fractures, showing normal disuse-related subchondral resorption along the talar dome (*arrowheads*).

arthritis, with higher likelihood of complications in talar neck and open fractures.[19,52]

Extra-articular Posteromedial Talocalcaneal Coalition

Talocalcaneal coalition, or abnormal fusion between the talus and the calcaneus, arises from a congenital failure of mesenchymal segmentation, and may be intra-articular, extra-articular, or overlap, with intra-articular and extra-articular involvement. The overwhelming majority of intra-articular talocalcaneal coalitions involve the middle subtalar joint, with anterior and posterior subtalar joint coalitions being extremely rare. Extra-articular talocalcaneal coalitions occur in the posteromedial

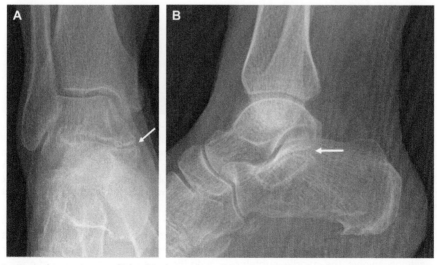

Fig. 19. Extra-articular posteromedial talocalcaneal coalition in a 65-year-old woman with ankle pain. (*A*) AP ankle radiograph demonstrates bony protuberances along the apposing medial talus and calcaneus (*arrow*), with a pseudofacet formation, compatible with nonosseous talocalcaneal coalition. (*B*) Lateral ankle radiograph demonstrates close apposition of the posterior talus and calcaneus (*arrow*).

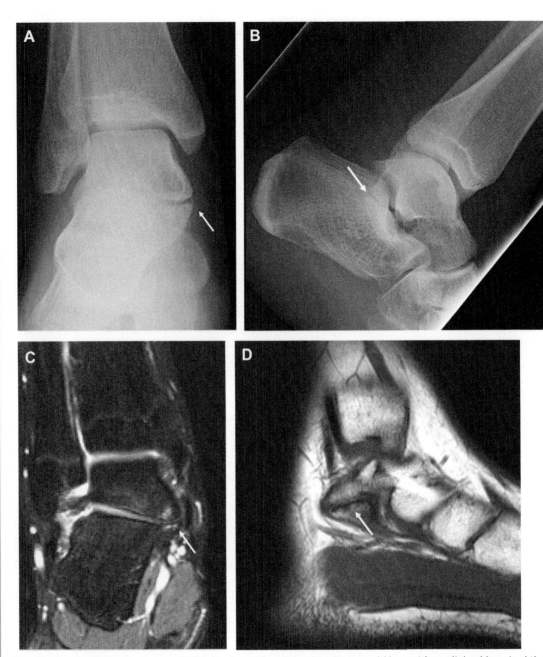

Fig. 20. Extra-articular (posteromedial) talocalcaneal coalition in a 17-year-old boy with medial ankle pain. (*A*) AP ankle radiograph demonstrates bony protuberances along the medial aspect of the hindfoot (*arrow*). (*B*) Lateral ankle radiograph demonstrates an anomalous articulation along the posterior aspect of the hindfoot (*arrow*), posterior to the middle subtalar joint. (*C*) Coronal short tau inversion recovery image of the ankle demonstrates posteromedial, nonosseous coalition, at the level of the posterior subtalar joint, with apposing marrow edema and cyst formation (*arrow*). (*D*) Sagittal T1 image of the ankle confirms a more posterior location of the coalition (*arrow*), relative to the middle subtalar joint.

hindfoot, in the interval between the sustentaculum tali and posteromedial talus. Finally, overlap talocalcaneal coalitions involve the middle subtalar joint and extend into the extra-articular interval between the sustentaculum tali and the posteromedial talus. Coalition between the talus and the calcaneus may be osseous (synostosis), fibrous (syndesmosis), or cartilaginous (synchondrosis), with the overwhelming majority of coalitions being either fibrous or cartilaginous. The more common fibrocartilaginous coalitions permit motion across the apposing talar and calcaneal bony surfaces, with gradual formation of a hypertrophic pseudoarthrosis.[53–55]

CT is the optimal modality for detecting talocalcaneal coalition. The coalition can also be easily detected on MR imaging. Radiographs of the ankle, mostly weight-bearing lateral views, demonstrate varying sensitivity and specificity when making the diagnosis of talocalcaneal coalition, using signs such as talar beak, dysmorphic sustentaculum, nonvisualization of the middle subtalar joint, and C sign.[56–59] However, the presence of talocalcaneal coalition, especially when an extra-articular component is present, can also be discerned on a well-positioned, well-penetrated AP ankle radiograph, where medial, hypertrophic bony protuberances along the posterior calcaneus and posterior talus, often with formation of a pseudofacet, are consistent with coalition (**Fig. 19**). The lateral view typically confirms the posterior location of an isolated extra-articular coalition but may demonstrate additional involvement of the middle subtalar joint in overlap coalitions (see **Figs. 19 and 20**).

MR imaging of talocalcaneal coalition, similar to radiographs, will demonstrate either osseous fusion or hypertrophic bony change at the site of coalition, with the frequent added findings of marrow edema and subchondral cystic change,[60,61] when the coalition is nonosseous (see **Fig. 20**). MR imaging may also detect abnormalities of the tarsal tunnel contents, due to mass effect by the coalition related to hypertrophic bone, affecting the medial compartment tendons, particularly the flexor hallucis longus tendon, as well as the posterior tibial nerve and its medial and lateral plantar branches.[62]

Talocalcaneal coalition, when clinically symptomatic, is typically treated with surgical resection in the pediatric and adolescent population, and with arthrodesis in the adult population.[55,63]

SUMMARY

Several characteristic locations about the ankle should be scrutinized on the AP radiograph of the ankle to detect various pathologic processes such as bony malalignment, ligamentous and retinacular avulsion injuries, tendon disease, fractures and variants predisposing to pathologic conditions. These entities are frequently only detected on the AP radiograph of the ankle, especially when foot films are not available. Small ossific densities, protuberances, or abnormal interfaces on AP ankle radiographs can also be the harbinger of more extensive underlying soft tissue injury, better characterized on MR imaging. Given the clinical overlap of some of these disease entities with lateral ankle sprain, the radiologist can help avoid delayed diagnosis or misdiagnosis by raising suspicion for these disease entities, thereby preventing patient morbidity.

REFERENCES

1. Malicky ES, Crary JL, Houghton MJ, et al. Talocalcaneal and subfibular impingement in symptomatic flatfoot in adults. J Bone Joint Surg Am 2002;84-A(11):2005–9.

2. Donovan A, Rosenberg ZS. MRI of ankle and lateral hindfoot impingement syndromes. AJR Am J Roentgenol 2010;195(3):595–604.

3. Sellon E, Robinson P. MR imaging of impingement and entrapment syndromes of the foot and ankle. Magn Reson Imaging Clin N Am 2017;25(1):145–58.

4. Eckert WR, Davis EA Jr. Acute rupture of the peroneal retinaculum. J Bone Joint Surg Am 1976;58(5):670–2.

5. Niemi WJ, Savidakis J Jr, DeJesus JM. Peroneal subluxation: a comprehensive review of the literature with case presentations. J Foot Ankle Surg 1997;36(2):141–5.

6. Heckman DS, Reddy S, Pedowitz D, et al. Operative treatment for peroneal tendon disorders. J Bone Joint Surg Am 2008;90(2):404–18.

7. Wang XT, Rosenberg ZS, Mechlin MB, et al. Normal variants and diseases of the peroneal tendons and superior peroneal retinaculum: MR imaging features. Radiographics 2005;25(3):587–602.

8. Church CC. Radiographic diagnosis of acute peroneal tendon dislocation. AJR Am J Roentgenol 1977;129(6):1065–8.

9. Wong-Chung J, Tucker A, Lynch-Wong M, et al. The lateral malleolar bony fleck classified by size and pathoanatomy: the IOFAS classification. Foot Ankle Surg 2018;24(4):300–8.

10. Crim J, Enslow M, Smith J. CT assessment of the prevalence of retinacular injuries associated with hindfoot fractures. Skeletal Radiol 2013;42(4):487–92.

11. Rosenberg ZS, Bencardino J, Astion D, et al. MRI features of chronic injuries of the superior peroneal retinaculum. AJR Am J Roentgenol 2003;181(6):1551–7.

12. Taljanovic MS, Alcala JN, Gimber LH, et al. High-resolution US and MR imaging of peroneal tendon injuries. Radiographics 2015;35(1):179–99.

13. Saragas NP, Ferrao PN, Mayet Z, et al. Peroneal tendon dislocation/subluxation - case series and review of the literature. Foot Ankle Surg 2016;22(2):125–30.

14. Summers NJ, Murdoch MM. Fractures of the talus: a comprehensive review. Clin Podiatr Med Surg 2012;29(2):187–203, vii.

15. Kirkpatrick DP, Hunter RE, Janes PC, et al. The snowboarder's foot and ankle. Am J Sports Med 1998;26(2):271–7.

16. Romeo NM, Hirschfeld AG, Githens M, et al. The significance of lateral process fractures associated with

talar neck and body fractures. J Orthop Trauma 2018;32(12):601–6.

17. Jentzsch T, Hasler A, Renner N, et al. The V sign in lateral talar process fractures: an experimental study using a foot and ankle model. BMC Musculoskelet Disord 2017;18(1):284.

18. Melenevsky Y, Mackey RA, Abrahams RB, et al. Talar fractures and dislocations: a radiologist's guide to timely diagnosis and classification. Radiographics 2015;35(3):765–79.

19. Shakked RJ, Tejwani NC. Surgical treatment of talus fractures. Orthop Clin North Am 2013;44(4):521–8.

20. Perera A, Baker JF, Lui DF, et al. The management and outcome of lateral process fracture of the talus. Foot Ankle Surg 2010;16(1):15–20.

21. Wang PH, Su WR, Jou IM. Lateral hindfoot impingement after nonunion of fracture of the lateral process of the talus. J Foot Ankle Surg 2016;55(2):387–90.

22. Berkowitz MJ, Kim DH. Process and tubercle fractures of the hindfoot. J Am Acad Orthop Surg 2005;13(8):492–502.

23. Lau BC, Moore LK, Thuillier DU. Evaluation and management of lateral ankle pain following injury. JBJS Rev 2018;6(8):e7.

24. Degan TJ, Morrey BF, Braun DP. Surgical excision for anterior-process fractures of the calcaneus. J Bone Joint Surg Am 1982;64(4):519–24.

25. Dhinsa BS, Latif A, Walker R, et al. Fractures of the anterior process of the calcaneum; a review and proposed treatment algorithm. Foot Ankle Surg 2018;25(3):258–63.

26. Walter WR, Hirschmann A, Alaia EF, et al. Normal anatomy and traumatic injury of the midtarsal (Chopart) joint complex: an imaging primer. Radiographics 2019;39(1):136–52.

27. Hirschmann A, Walter WR, Alaia EF, et al. Acute fracture of the anterior process of calcaneus: does it herald a more advanced injury to Chopart joint? AJR Am J Roentgenol 2018;210(5):1123–30.

28. Ouellette H, Salamipour H, Thomas BJ, et al. Incidence and MR imaging features of fractures of the anterior process of calcaneus in a consecutive patient population with ankle and foot symptoms. Skeletal Radiol 2006;35(11):833–7.

29. Saupe N, Mengiardi B, Pfirrmann CW, et al. Anatomic variants associated with peroneal tendon disorders: MR imaging findings in volunteers with asymptomatic ankles. Radiology 2007;242(2):509–17.

30. Boya H, Pinar H. Stenosing tenosynovitis of the peroneus brevis tendon associated with hypertrophy of the peroneal tubercle. J Foot Ankle Surg 2010;49(2):188–90.

31. Ruiz JR, Christman RA, Hillstrom HJ. 1993 William J. Stickel Silver Award. Anatomical considerations of the peroneal tubercle. J Am Podiatr Med Assoc 1993;83(10):563–75.

32. Zanetti M. Founder's lecture of the ISS 2006: borderlands of normal and early pathological findings in MRI of the foot and ankle. Skeletal Radiol 2008;37(10):875–84.

33. Laidlaw PP. The varieties of the os calcis. J Anat Physiol 1904;38(Pt 2):133–43.

34. Bruce WD, Christofersen MR, Phillips DL. Stenosing tenosynovitis and impingement of the peroneal tendons associated with hypertrophy of the peroneal tubercle. Foot Ankle Int 1999;20(7):464–7.

35. Hyer CF, Dawson JM, Philbin TM, et al. The peroneal tubercle: description, classification, and relevance to peroneus longus tendon pathology. Foot Ankle Int 2005;26(11):947–50.

36. Lee SJ, Jacobson JA, Kim SM, et al. Ultrasound and MRI of the peroneal tendons and associated pathology. Skeletal Radiol 2013;42(9):1191–200.

37. Muehleman C, Williams J, Bareither ML. A radiologic and histologic study of the os peroneum: prevalence, morphology, and relationship to degenerative joint disease of the foot and ankle in a cadaveric sample. Clin Anat 2009;22(6):747–54.

38. Sobel M, Pavlov H, Geppert MJ, et al. Painful os peroneum syndrome: a spectrum of conditions responsible for plantar lateral foot pain. Foot Ankle Int 1994;15(3):112–24.

39. Tawk S, Lecouvet F, Putineanu DC, et al. Unusual proximal fragment migration of an os peroneum fracture with associated peroneus longus tendon injury - a tree often hides a forest. Skeletal Radiol 2019;48(2):317–22.

40. Bianchi S, Abdelwahab IF, Tegaldo G. Fracture and posterior dislocation of the os peroneum associated with rupture of the peroneus longus tendon. Can Assoc Radiol J 1991;42(5):340–4.

41. Brigido MK, Fessell DP, Jacobson JA, et al. Radiography and US of os peroneum fractures and associated peroneal tendon injuries: initial experience. Radiology 2005;237(1):235–41.

42. Maurer M, Lehrman J. Significance of sesamoid ossification in peroneus longus tendon ruptures. J Foot Ankle Surg 2012;51(3):352–5.

43. Stockton KG, Brodsky JW. Peroneus longus tears associated with pathology of the os peroneum. Foot Ankle Int 2014;35(4):346–52.

44. Savage-Elliott I, Murawski CD, Smyth NA, et al. The deltoid ligament: an in-depth review of anatomy, function, and treatment strategies. Knee Surg Sports Traumatol Arthrosc 2013;21(6):1316–27.

45. Won HJ, Koh IJ, Won HS. Morphological variations of the deltoid ligament of the medial ankle. Clin Anat 2016;29(8):1059–65.

46. Hintermann B. Medial ankle instability. Foot Ankle Clin 2003;8(4):723–38.

47. Crim J, Longenecker LG. MRI and surgical findings in deltoid ligament tears. AJR Am J Roentgenol 2015;204(1):W63–9.

48. Sneppen O, Christensen SB, Krogsoe O, et al. Fracture of the body of the talus. Acta Orthop Scand 1977;48(3):317–24.
49. Ebraheim NA, Patil V, Owens C, et al. Clinical outcome of fractures of the talar body. Int Orthop 2008;32(6):773–7.
50. Hawkins LG. Fractures of the neck of the talus. J Bone Joint Surg Am 1970;52(5):991–1002.
51. Tehranzadeh J, Stuffman E, Ross SD. Partial Hawkins sign in fractures of the talus: a report of three cases. AJR Am J Roentgenol 2003;181(6):1559–63.
52. Vallier HA, Nork SE, Benirschke SK, et al. Surgical treatment of talar body fractures. J Bone Jt Surg Am 2003;85-A(9):1716–24.
53. Kumar SJ, Guille JT, Lee MS, et al. Osseous and non-osseous coalition of the middle facet of the talocalcaneal joint. J Bone Joint Surg Am 1992;74(4):529–35.
54. Harris RI. Rigid valgus foot due to talocalcaneal bridge. J Bone Joint Surg Am 1955;37-A(1):169–83.
55. Downey MS. Tarsal coalitions. A surgical classification. J Am Podiatr Med Assoc 1991;81(4):187–97.
56. Crim JR, Kjeldsberg KM. Radiographic diagnosis of tarsal coalition. AJR Am J Roentgenol 2004;182(2):323–8.
57. Resnick D. Talar ridges, osteophytes, and beaks: a radiologic commentary. Radiology 1984;151(2):329–32.
58. Brown RR, Rosenberg ZS, Thornhill BA. The C sign: more specific for flatfoot deformity than subtalar coalition. Skeletal Radiol 2001;30(2):84–7.
59. Lateur LM, Van Hoe LR, Van Ghillewe KV, et al. Subtalar coalition: diagnosis with the C sign on lateral radiographs of the ankle. Radiology 1994;193(3):847–51.
60. Wechsler RJ, Schweitzer ME, Deely DM, et al. Tarsal coalition: depiction and characterization with CT and MR imaging. Radiology 1994;193(2):447–52.
61. Nalaboff KM, Schweitzer ME. MRI of tarsal coalition: frequency, distribution, and innovative signs. Bull NYU Hosp Jt Dis 2008;66(1):14–21.
62. Alaia EF, Rosenberg ZS, Bencardino JT, et al. Tarsal tunnel disease and talocalcaneal coalition: MRI features. Skeletal Radiol 2016;45(11):1507–14.
63. Takakura Y, Sugimoto K, Tanaka Y, et al. Symptomatic talocalcaneal coalition. Its clinical significance and treatment. Clin Orthop Relat Res 1991;(269):249–56.

Pitfalls in Pediatric Trauma and Microtrauma

Sarah D. Bixby, MD

KEYWORDS

- Fracture • Pediatric • Physis • Developmental variant • MR imaging

KEY POINTS

- Pediatric fractures are subtle and may mimic other conditions.
- Growth plates in children are a common source of confusion regarding presence or absence of fracture.
- Patterns of injury in children are different from those in adults.
- MR imaging features of trauma include bone marrow and soft tissue edema, and subtle fracture lines, and help clarify equivocal plain radiographic findings.

INTRODUCTION

Osseous injuries are common in children and constitute 10% to 15% of all childhood injuries.[1] The risk of developing a fracture by age 16 years is 42% for boys and 27% for girls.[2] Fractures are more common in children than in adults following minimal trauma, related to a proportionate increase in the amount of cartilage and collagen within the pediatric skeleton[3] contributing to a reduced strength of the immature skeleton compared with adults.[4] Growth spurts represent an additional point of risk for the pediatric skeleton as bone strength and development lags behind muscle mass.[4,5] Patterns of injury in pediatric patients can subtle, and it is these subtle injuries that may elude even the most experienced reader. Radiologists and clinicians presented with skeletal radiographs in pediatric patients must be well equipped to differentiate fracture from the numerous mimics of fracture that exist in this population. Fracture mimics include developmental variations of the growth plates and secondary ossification centers,[6] normal osseous landmarks that simulate fracture lines, and metabolic disorders that affect the pattern and rate of ossification. There are various imaging clues that allow for distinguishing fractures from mimics on plain radiographs, although MR imaging may be useful when there is uncertainty or when expedited diagnosis is required (Table 1).

PHYSEAL INJURIES AND MIMICS

The most common source of pitfalls in diagnosing skeletal trauma in pediatric patients is the growth centers. Physeal injuries represent approximately 20% of pediatric fractures.[7,8] A baseline understanding of the normal appearance of the physis is critical to differentiating fractures from normal growth centers. Although the cartilaginous physis of long bones is flat at birth, over time it develops irregularities in response to increased biomechanical forces.[9] These undulations serve to increase the shear strength of the physis.[1] The physis represents a source of weakness within the skeleton, which accounts for why fractures so often involve this structure.[10,11] The Salter-Harris classification is the most commonly used classification system for physeal injures. The original five Salter-Harris fracture types are the most widely used when describing physeal fractures. Salter-Harris fractures are distinguished from each other based on the pattern of involvement of the metaphysis, epiphysis, or both.[12] In certain locations

Department of Radiology, Boston Children's Hospital, Harvard Medical School, Main 2, 300 Longwood Avenue, Boston, MA 02115, USA
E-mail address: sarah.bixby@childrens.harvard.edu

Magn Reson Imaging Clin N Am 27 (2019) 721–735
https://doi.org/10.1016/j.mric.2019.07.009
1064-9689/19/© 2019 Elsevier Inc. All rights reserved.

Table 1
Fractures and possible mimics

Injury	Mimic
Salter 2 fracture	Developmental physeal variants
Salter 1 fracture/ chronic physeal stress changes: Slipped capital femoral epiphysis Little Leaguer's shoulder Gymnast's wrist	Metabolic conditions: Rickets Shwachman-Diamond syndrome
Salter 3 fracture	Cleft epiphyses
Avulsion fracture	Accessory ossification centers
Greenstick fracture	Nutrient foramina
Stress fracture	Osteoid osteoma
Vertebral compression fracture	Developmental variants Ring apophysis Fish vertebral end plate Cupid's bow Fish vertebra

normal variants may mimic a physeal fracture. Variants are divided into three categories: (1) those that represent chronic chondro-osseous disruption, (2) those that predispose to traumatic and/or degenerative change, and (3) those that predispose to premature degenerative change.[13]

The Salter 2 fracture is the most common Salter-Harris fracture, constituting approximately 75% of Salter-Harris fractures.[12] In a Salter 2 fracture the plane of the fracture propagates transversely through the physeal cartilage before exiting into the metaphysis. The most common sites include the distal radius,[3] phalanges, and distal tibia.[8] The pattern of injury may be difficult to characterize on plain radiographs alone,[6] and MR imaging is useful (**Fig. 1**). Small metaphyseal or epiphyseal fractures may be missed on plain radiographs, whereas they are plainly visible at MR imaging or computed tomography (CT).[6,14] Physeal variants may mimic a Salter 2 fracture, such as within the distal fibula (**Fig. 2**) or proximal radius (**Fig. 3**). In some patients there is a vertical extension of physeal cartilage extending into the fibular metaphysis at the lateral margin of the physis. Diagnosis may be confounded by recent history of trauma. The normal fibular physis is wider laterally than it is medially, often with irregular ossification patterns at the lateral margin of the distal fibular physis,[15] which may raise concern for a physeal fracture. MR imaging may be helpful to detect more detailed information about the pattern of injury, such as subtle fracture lines, bone marrow edema, or fluid signal within the physis.[6,9,14,16]

In a Salter 1 fracture, the fracture propagates through the physis without metaphyseal or epiphyseal extension. If there is no periosteal disruption, the bone remains appropriately aligned[1] and the only manifestation of the acute fracture is widening or irregularity of the physis (**Fig. 4**). This may be difficult to appreciate given expected physeal irregularity. Abnormal widening of the physis is also present in the context of chronic physeal stress changes. In this background, repetitive, forceful loading activities leading to overuse of an extremity can cause shear injury and microtrauma to the cartilaginous physis. This differs from a Salter 1 fracture, because there is no fracture line but rather disorganized enchondral ossification leading to hypertrophic cartilage extending into the metaphysis.[17,18] Although a Salter 1 fracture usually

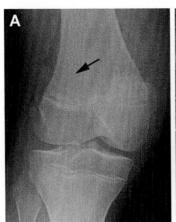
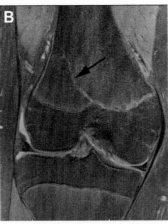

Fig. 1. A 15-year-old boy with knee pain. (*A*) Anteroposterior (AP) radiograph of the knee demonstrates an oblique fracture through the metaphysis (*arrow*). (*B*) Coronal proton density weighted (PDw) fat-suppressed (FS) image through the knee better demonstrates the Salter 2 fracture involving the femoral metaphysis (*arrow*) and medial physis.

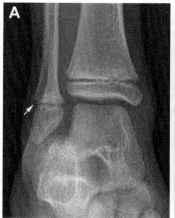
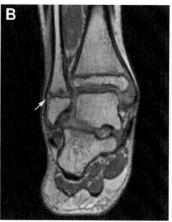

Fig. 2. An 8-year-old girl with ankle pain. (*A*) Mortise view of the ankle demonstrates widening along the lateral aspect of the fibular physis with a tiny bone fragment directed toward the metaphysis (*arrow*). (*B*) Cor T1-weighted image of the ankle confirms a normal physis. The fragment identified on plain radiograph represented irregular ossification of the peripheral physis (*arrow*).

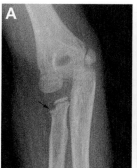
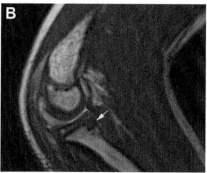

Fig. 3. A 7-year-old girl with elbow pain. (*A*) Oblique elbow radiograph demonstrates focal lucency within the proximal metaphysis in the radial neck (*arrow*). (*B*) Sagittal T1-weighted MR image of the elbow demonstrates a wedge of low signal intensity within the metaphysis extending from the physis (*arrow*) without surrounding edema, consistent with a variant of ossification.

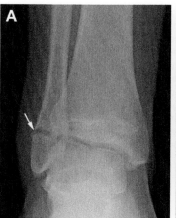
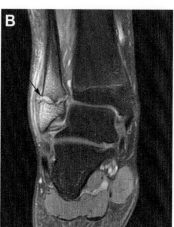

Fig. 4. A 15-year-old boy with ankle pain after trauma. (*A*) AP radiograph of the ankle demonstrates widening and irregularity of the distal fibular physis (*arrow*). (*B*) Coronal PDw FS image of the ankle demonstrates fluid signal within the physis (*arrow*) with surrounding marrow, subperiosteal, and soft tissue edema in keeping with a Salter 1 fracture.

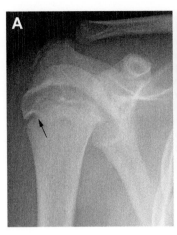
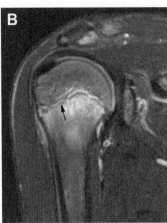

Fig. 5. A 12-year-old baseball pitcher with shoulder pain. (*A*) AP radiograph of the shoulder demonstrates widening and irregularity of the proximal humeral physis (*arrow*). (*B*) Coronal T2-weighted FS MR image better demonstrates fluid within the physis (*arrow*) and surrounding marrow edema in this child with Little Leaguer's shoulder.

involves the entire physis, chronic stress change is focal or diffuse. A classic location includes the proximal humeral physis in overhead throwing athletes, termed Little Leaguer's shoulder. On radiographs this is manifest as a widened proximal humeral physis, which appears asymmetrically irregular when compared with the contralateral side, with associated periphyseal sclerosis (**Fig. 5**). Similar physeal stress changes may occur in the distal radius in patients who engage in sports that involve weightbearing with the upper extremities, such as gymnasts (**Fig. 6**),[19,20] or in the distal femurs or proximal tibiae of children who participate in aggressive physical activity using their lower extremities, such as soccer or running (**Fig. 7**).[17] The physis is wide and irregular and there is periphyseal sclerosis reflecting the healing response. MR imaging is helpful at revealing the presence of marrow edema and fluid within the physis that is present in the setting of trauma. In the hip, slipped capital femoral epiphysis is a condition that is considered a Salter 1 equivalent injury that ultimately results in displacement of the femoral heal, usually in a posteromedial orientation. The diagnosis is most often made with plain radiographs, although when the degree of epiphyseal displacement is subtle or when displacement has not yet occurred the abnormalities are best appreciated at MR imaging (**Fig. 8**).[21]

Certain metabolic conditions that cause disruption of the normal pattern of enchondral ossification at the physis may mimic traumatic or stress-induced injuries, including rickets. Rickets is a group of conditions related to deficiency of (or resistance to) vitamin D or its derivative. This manifests as disordered enchondral ossification with disruption of the normal configuration of the physis. Radiographs demonstrate abnormal widening of the physis associated with decreased density in the zone of provisional calcification (ZPC). MR images demonstrate widening of the physes with increased physeal T2-weighted

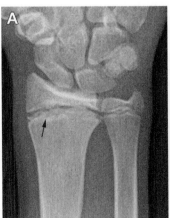
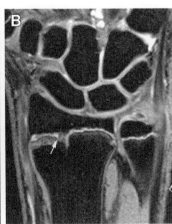

Fig. 6. An 11-year-old gymnast with left wrist pain. (*A*) AP radiograph of the wrist demonstrates widening and irregularity of the distal radial physis (*arrow*). The ulnar physis is normal. (*B*) Coronal gradient echo sequence through the wrist MR image reveals small tongues of physeal cartilage extending into metaphysis (*arrow*) reflecting disorganized enchondral ossification.

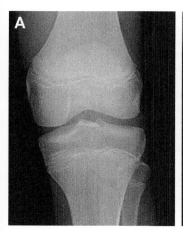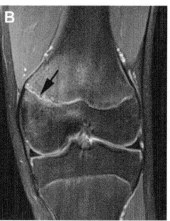

Fig. 7. A 15-year-old boy with knee pain. (A) AP radiograph of the knee demonstrates widening of the medial aspect of the distal femoral physis. (B) Cor PDw FS sequence MR image demonstrates fluid in the physis (arrow) with surrounding marrow edema consistent with stress changes.

signal, with absent ZPC (Fig. 9).[22] Key imaging features that enable differentiating rickets from trauma are the absent ZPC, and lack of metaphyseal marrow edema (or mild edema). The classic radiographic changes may take longer to manifest, and include irregular, cupped, and/or frayed metaphyses.[23] Although these features are easily detected on plain radiographs, they may not be present in the early stages of the disease process. The physes of patients with rickets are at least 50% wider than the physes of normal, age-matched control subjects.[22] In the early stages of rickets, the imaging features mimic stress-related changes. In the appropriate clinical context it should not be necessary to perform MR imaging to distinguish between these two conditions given the subtle radiographic clues that help make the distinction (ie, absent ZPC in rickets) in addition to differing clinical presentations. Stress changes tend to occur in older children known to be involved in activities that would predispose to these types of injuries. Patients with rickets have laboratory abnormalities that coincide with the imaging manifestations of the disease. MR imaging may be useful in confounding cases. Increasingly,

active patients with a history of rickets are developing risk factors for stress-related physeal changes. Plain radiographic imaging may not be well-suited to determine the underlying cause for the physeal change, and treatment choice depends on whether the ZPC is present (in the setting of stress changes) or absent (in the setting or rickets) (Fig. 10).

Patients with other diffuse metabolic conditions may also demonstrate skeletal findings that may mimic physeal microtrauma. Shwachman-Diamond syndrome (SDS) is an autosomal-recessive condition described in patients with pancreatic insufficiency, bone marrow dysfunction, and metaphyseal chondrodysplasia.[24] Skeletal findings are symmetric metaphyseal changes in the hips and knees, such as periphyseal irregularity with mixed lytic and sclerotic areas (Fig. 11).[24,25] In the femoral neck the physis becomes wedge-shaped over time and grows into a cone-shaped defect in the metaphysis.[26] The skeletal manifestations of the disorder are not present in all patients, and the imaging of patients with SDS focuses mainly on the abdominal manifestations of the disease, which includes pancreatic

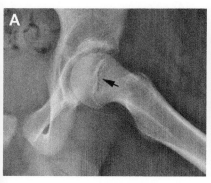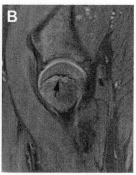

Fig. 8. A 13-year-old boy with left hip pain. (A) Frog-leg lateral radiograph of the left hip demonstrates focal lucency surrounding the central portion of the proximal femoral physis (arrow), which extends into the anterior physis. (B) Sagittal PDw FS MR image better demonstrates the irregularity and widening of the physis in this region (arrow) in keeping with the preslip stage of slipped capital femoral epiphysis.

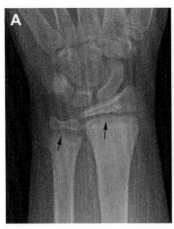 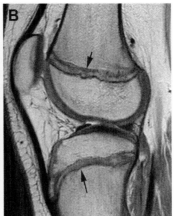

Fig. 9. (*A*) AP radiograph of the wrist in an 11-year-old with rickets demonstrates abnormal widening and irregularity within the physes of the distal radius and ulna (*arrows*) with absence of mineralization noted within the zone of provisional calcification. (*B*) Sagittal PDw knee MR image also reveals widening of the cartilaginous physes of the distal femur and proximal tibia (*arrows*).

lipomatosis.[27] MR imaging is believed to be helpful in the diagnosis of SDS and differentiation from other conditions with exocrine pancreatic insufficiency, such as cystic fibrosis,[28] and the hips may be included in the field of view when evaluating the abdomen. The metaphyseal dysosostosis that affects patients with SDS may mimic an advanced form of physeal stress injury.

In Salter 3 injuries, a physeal fracture extends into the epiphysis as a linear lucency on plain radiographs. These fractures may be confused for variants in normal development including cleft epiphyses. Clefts or defects may be observed in the epiphyses of certain bones usually during adolescence.[29,30] The most common location for such clefts to occur is within the epiphysis of the proximal phalanx of the great toe (**Fig. 12**), although they are also seen within the distal tibia, distal ulna, and calcaneal apophysis.[31] These are variants of normal anatomy not associated with symptoms, and close spontaneously around the time of physeal fusion. These clefts may simulate a Salter 3 fracture, and in some instances there

is little that differentiates these two entities (**Fig. 13**). Imaging features that suggest a fracture over anatomic variant include widening of the physis and displacement of the epiphysis, although displacement of the two halves of the physis has been described in anatomic variants.[31] In most instances, such displacement would raise concern for fracture. Focal pain and tenderness at the site and a history of trauma or injury are helpful clinical clues. Follow-up radiographs within 3 weeks demonstrate healing at sites of fracture, whereas no radiographic change is anticipated at sites of normal variants. MR imaging is useful because the presence of marrow edema and fluid within the physis strongly favors fracture and allows for accurate diagnosis at the time of the acute event, rather than later at follow-up. Stress changes at a physis, as has been previously described, are no less common at a cleft epiphysis than at a normal epiphysis, so it is possible that widening and irregularity of the physis and surrounding marrow edema involving a cleft epiphysis may be present as a chronic feature rather than the

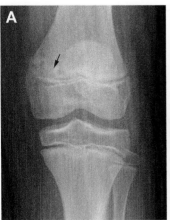 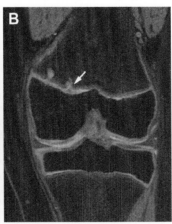

Fig. 10. A 15-year-old with history of treated rickets and knee pain in the setting of rigorous sporting activities. (*A*) AP radiograph of the knee demonstrates widening of the distal femoral physis with periphyseal lucencies along the medial aspect (*arrow*). (*B*) Coronal gradient echo image demonstrates focal extensions of physeal cartilage extending into the metaphysis (*arrow*) with preserved ZPC.

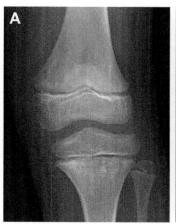
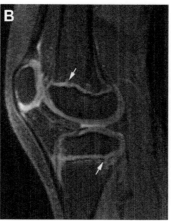

Fig. 11. An 8-year-old girl with Shwachman-Diamond syndrome. (A) AP radiograph of the knee reveals widening of the physes with irregular periphyseal lucencies within the metaphyses. (B) Sagittal gradient echo sequence MR image through the knee also demonstrates irregularity of the physes with small extensions of physeal cartilage projecting into the metaphyses (arrows).

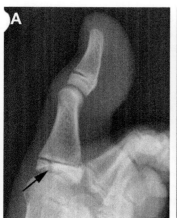
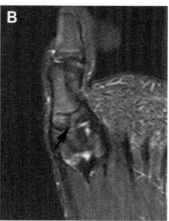

Fig. 12. A 12-year-old boy with toe pain after trauma. (A) Lateral radiograph of the great toe demonstrates a lucency within the epiphysis of the proximal phalanx concerning for a fracture (arrow). (B) T2-weighted MR image reveals the epiphyseal defect (black arrow) with no surrounding marrow edema, consistent with cleft epiphysis.

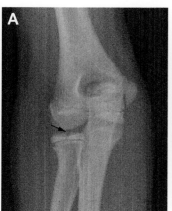
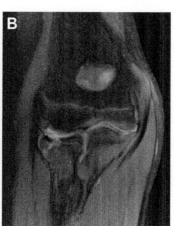

Fig. 13. A 12-year-old girl with elbow pain after fall. (A) AP radiograph of the elbow demonstrates a vertical cleft through the proximal radial epiphysis (arrow). (B) Coronal PDw MR image of the elbow confirms a fracture extending through the epiphysis (arrow).

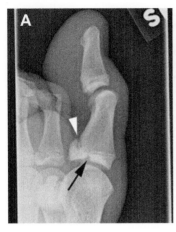
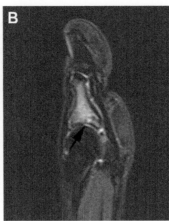

Fig. 14. A 17-year-old boy with toe pain. (*A*) Lateral radiograph of the toe demonstrates displacement of a portion of the proximal epiphysis of the phalanx (*arrowhead*) with a cleft within the epiphysis (*arrow*). (*B*) Sagittal T2-weighted FS MR image demonstrates marrow edema surrounding the cleft (*arrow*) consistent with fracture/stress change superimposed on a normal variant.

result of an acute injury. As Lawson[13] notes, it is possible that traumatic changes may be superimposed on such a variant. In these instances, the radiographic appearance of a normal cleft epiphysis and traumatic or stress changes superimposed on a normal variant are indistinguishable. MR imaging is most helpful in this setting to evaluate for bone marrow edema, and/or fluid signal within the physis or within the surrounding soft tissues, which suggests the presence of superimposed trauma (**Fig. 14**).

Accessory ossification centers are sources of diagnostic error and fracture detection pitfalls. Secondary ossification centers are well described around the patella and may be mistaken for fractures (**Fig. 15**).[32] Another source of confusion

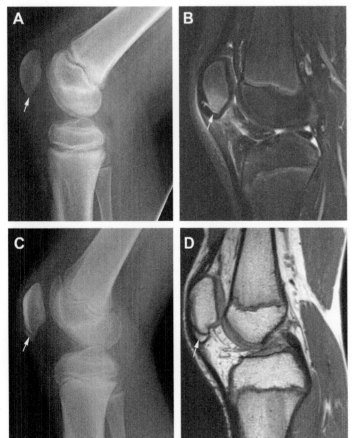

Fig. 15. (*A*) Lateral knee radiograph in a 10-year-old boy with knee pain after trauma demonstrates mild irregularity at the inferior pole of the patella (*arrow*). (*B*) Sagittal T2-weighted FS MR image in same patient reveals a patellar sleeve fracture comprised mainly of unossified cartilage (*arrow*). (*C*) Lateral knee radiograph in a different 10-year-old boy demonstrates a bone fragment projecting along the inferior pole of the patella (*arrow*). (*D*) Sagittal PDw MR image in this patient reveals an unfused secondary ossification center with no surrounding marrow edema (*arrow*).

includes the secondary ossification centers around the ankle, most frequently seen at the tip of the medial malleolus.[15] In the early stages of ossification these may be confused for avulsion fractures. As may also occur around any growth plate, a normal secondary ossification center may become inflamed even without a superimposed fracture, related to abnormal motion at the physis.[33] In such instances, the radiographs reveal a normal, fragmented ossification center, and MR imaging demonstrates abnormal marrow edema. In these situations the identification of a normal-appearing ossification center on plain radiographs does not rule out the possibility of stress changes that requires management. MR imaging is a helpful problem-solving tool in these instances.

In some areas of the body the growth plates are not centered at the ends of long bones, but are located at the site of an apophysis. The pelvis and scapular are bones with several different apophyses, all of which fuse at different points in time. In the scapula, the acromion and the coracoid ossification centers are not fully fused until later in childhood/adolescence. In some patients, the acromial ossification center may not fully fuse until late adolescence/early adulthood.[34] Failure of fusion of the secondary ossification of the acromion by age 18 to 25 results in an os acromiale.[35] An os acromiale may be associated with pain or instability, but in young patients the lack of osseous fusion is considered a normal and expected finding. After physeal fusion, a low signal intensity band may persist at the previous site of the physis, which represents a physeal scar, not to be mistaken for a fracture.[35] MR imaging is helpful for distinguishing between a normal ossification center or a growth plate scar from an acromial fracture, because there should be marrow and soft tissue edema surrounding a fracture.

The appearance of the ossification centers around the shoulder and the variation with age make it challenging to differentiate growth plates from fractures. The glenoid-coracoid interface follows a predictable pattern of skeletal development that aids in the interpretation of imaging studies.[35,36] In the early stages of development the unossified cartilage of the superior glenoid is contiguous with the base of the coracoid, which is also formed of cartilage at this stage. Imaging signs on MR imaging that indicate the presence of a coracoid base growth plate fracture include widening, irregularity, abnormal signal intensity, and adjacent soft tissue edema.[37] Although these are not common injuries, they should be considered in children who have shoulder pain after an injury (Fig. 16).

Before an ossification center has fully ossified, it is challenging to detect a fracture. In a patient with a fracture involving an epiphyseal ossification center, unless there are secondary signs of healing (ie, periosteal new bone formation, periphyseal sclerosis) radiographs are limited in the acute setting. MR imaging is better-suited for detection of nonossified epiphyseal avulsion fractures, such as may occur around the knee (Fig. 17), elbow, or ankle. These displaced injuries represent an important imaging pitfall with plain radiographs that is overcome with MR imaging.

DIAPHYSEAL/METAPHYSEAL FRACTURES AND MIMICS

Pediatric fractures occur with characteristic patterns at the diaphysis or metaphysis of long bones. Typical injury patterns are usually not challenging to detect, but may be mistaken for other normal structures. It is helpful to recognize the imaging features of several classic pediatric-type fractures

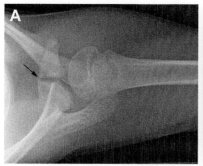
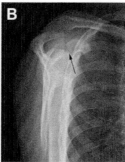
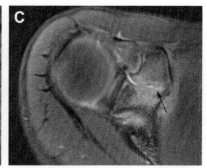

Fig. 16. (*A*) Axillary view of the shoulder demonstrated a normal coracoid physis (*arrow*) in an 8-year-old boy. (*B*) Transcapular Y view in a 14-year-old boy with pain after a fall demonstrates widening of the physis of the coracoid process (*arrow*). (*C*) Axial T2-weighted FS image from a subsequent MR image demonstrates fluid within the coracoid physis (*arrow*) with surrounding bone marrow and soft tissue edema.

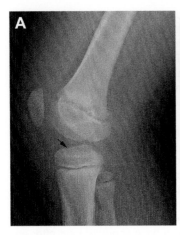
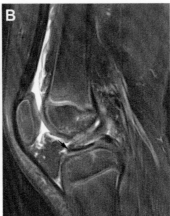

Fig. 17. A 6-year-old boy with knee pain after fall. (*A*) Lateral radiograph of the knee is normal, specifically no abnormality noted in the proximal tibia (*arrow*). (*B*) Sagittal T2-weighted FS MR image of the knee demonstrates avulsion of a bony fragment off the tibial eminence (*arrow*) at the attachment site of the anterior cruciate ligament.

so that these may be easily distinguished from their nontraumatic mimics.

A greenstick fracture is an incomplete fracture that results when the bone producing the fracture fails in tension, dissipating the force of the fracture before the fracture propagates all the way through the bone.[1] The cortex along the compression side of the injury force remains intact. The metaphyses and metadiaphyses of long bones are most susceptible to greenstick fractures, and the radius and ulna are typical sites for these fractures.[38] Plain radiographs are usually sufficient for diagnosis, because the fracture pattern is readily identified especially if a history of trauma is provided at the time of image review.

Stress fractures occur within the long bones when the forces on the bone exceed the ability of the bone's repair mechanism. Stress fractures within the tibia are most often the result of running,[38] although they may occur in any bone in the lower extremity including the metatarsals. Although most stress fractures are oriented transversely with respect to the bone, less frequently they are oriented longitudinally, which makes them less reliably detected on plain radiographs. On plain radiographs, stress fractures manifest as areas of cortical thickening and periosteal new bone formation, often with a central area of bone infraction (**Fig. 18**).[39–41] Stress fractures often manifest at MR imaging with findings of extensive marrow edema, subperiosteal edema, and periosteal new bone formation, which invokes the diagnosis, particularly when a cleft in the cortex of the bone to signify the fracture.[41–44] On other imaging studies, such as plain radiography or CT, the classic marrow edema associated with fractures is not visible, and other entities may be mistaken for a stress fracture.

One particular mimic of a longitudinal stress fracture or a greenstick fracture is nutrient foramina. When the nutrient foramen are imaged at such an angle that the trajectory is elongated they may simulate a fracture line.[45] Additionally, the slight expansion of the cortex and irregularity

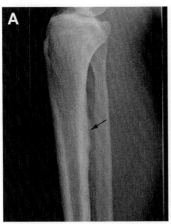
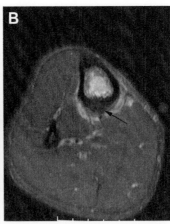

Fig. 18. A 17-year-old with lower leg pain. (*A*) Lateral radiograph of the lower leg demonstrates cortical thickening and periosteal new bone formation posteriorly (*arrow*) concerning for fracture. (*B*) Axial T2-weighted FS MR image of the lower leg demonstrates subperiosteal fluid (*arrow*), surrounding soft issue edema, and intramedullary and intracortical signal abnormality c/w stress fracture.

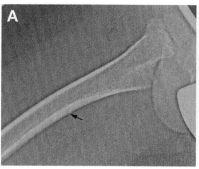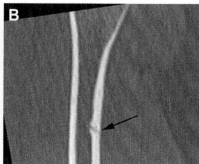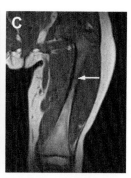

Fig. 19. A 2.5-year-old boy with leg pain and limp. (*A*) Frog-leg lateral radiograph of the femur demonstrates a linear lucency traversing the posterior cortex of the proximal femoral shaft with mild expansion of the cortex (*arrow*). (*B*) Sagittal reformat from a focused CT through this area clearly delineates the cortical lucency (*arrow*). (*C*) Coronal T1-weighted image through the femur confirms normal marrow signal. The lucency corresponds to the entry site of a nutrient vessel (*arrow*) within the proximal diaphysis.

of the periosteum overlying the entry point of the nutrient vessel may raise suspicion for a stress fracture on plain radiographs or CT,[45] particularly for pediatric radiologists who are particularly attuned to attributing subtle bony irregularities to traumatic injuries. Knowledge of the locations of the nutrient foramina on imaging studies is useful so as to not to confuse these for fractures. Cadaveric studies have demonstrated various imaging features of nutrient foramina at CT.[46] In the femur, these vessels may take an upward, downward, or transverse course.[46] In the femur these are located most commonly within the middle segment of the femur. Similarly, nutrient foramina are visible at imaging within the tibia.[47] Unfortunately, in some settings these foramina may be confused for a greenstick or stress fracture when a child presents with pain or injury. If this is not immediately recognized as a normal finding on plan radiographs, additional advanced imaging may be requested to confirm diagnosis.

In most cases MR imaging is the modality of choice in light of the radiation concerns with CT. MR imaging findings are reassuring when there is no associated marrow or cortical edema to confirm fracture. An additional clue to correct diagnosis is location. In the femur, stress fractures most often occur along the inferomedial femoral neck,[48] whereas the nutrient foramen is located within the femoral diaphysis (**Fig. 19**).[46]

Osteoid osteoma (OO) is a benign bone tumor that occurs in patients younger than 20 years of age who present with classic triad of pain most severe at night, and relieved by salicylates. The metaphysis and diaphysis of the femur and tibia are the most common sites of involvement, although OO may occur in other areas including the spine, upper limb, pelvis, and hands/feet.[49,50] Typical radiographic features include an intracortical nidus with variable amounts of mineralization that measures less than 1 cm with a surrounding rim of cortical thickening and reactive sclerosis.[40]

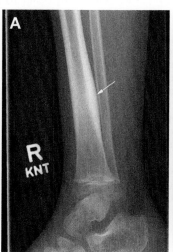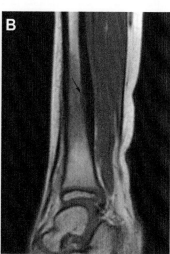

Fig. 20. A 5-year-old boy with lower leg pain. (*A*) Lateral radiograph of the lower leg demonstrates cortical thickening and periosteal new bone formation posteriorly (*arrow*) concerning for fracture. (*B*) Sagittal T1-weighted MR image of the lower leg demonstrates an intracortical nidus of an osteoid osteoma (*arrow*) with surrounding marrow edema.

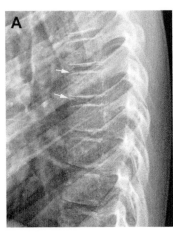 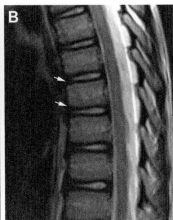

Fig. 21. An 11-year-old girl with back pain. (A) Lateral radiograph of the thoracic spine demonstrates multiple unfused ring apophyses (arrows) along the anterior end plates of the vertebral bodies. (B) Sagittal T2-weighted MR image on this patient demonstrates normal marrow signal surrounding the unfused ring apophyses (arrows).

In some cases the nidus may be so small that it is undetectable or resembles a stress fracture.[40] Cross-sectional imaging is useful to differentiate between stress fracture and OO. In the setting of OO, CT demonstrates a nidus to be low in attenuation with a tiny central focus of high attenuation that represents mineralized osteoid.[51] MR imaging has limited value in depicting the central nidus in an OO.[52] MR imaging reveals edema within the surrounding bone marrow and soft tissues as bright on fluid-sensitive sequences, with a low to intermediate signal nidus on T1-weighted images.[40] Contrast-enhanced MR imaging is more effective at depicting the hypervascular nidus of an OO.[53–55] The imaging features of an OO overlap with the imaging features of a healing stress fracture (Fig. 20).

VERTEBRAL FRACTURES

Fractures in the vertebral bodies are challenging, because these manifest differently from fractures of the long bones. Vertebral bodies collapse in response to compressive forces. Fracture is suggested when there is a diminished height in a vertebral body, or a contour abnormality along the end plate, or both.[56] This may be confusing in younger patients in whom cortical or end plate irregularities pre-exist. The detection of vertebral fracture is compounded by technical factors, such as projection angle, and patient factors, such as patient body mass index and patient positioning. Vertebral body compression fractures are uncommon injuries outside of high-impact trauma given the force required to compress the bony architecture. One should be wary of invoking a compression fracture in a child without a history of antecedent trauma unless there is underlying bone disorder (ie, generalized nutritional deficiency, steroid use).

The vertebral physis is a slow-growing physis compared with physes of the long bones.[57] The end plates consist of ZPCs that first exist as cartilaginous growth plates before they ossify at

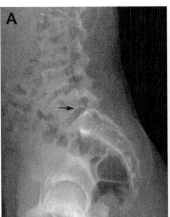 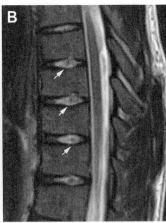

Fig. 22. A 15-year-old boy with back pain. (A) Lateral radiograph of the lumbar spine demonstrates a focal depression in the posterior aspect of the inferior end plate of L5 with loss of height of the vertebral body consistent with a Cupid's bow contour (arrow). (B) Sagittal T2-weighted thoracic spine MR image in same patient demonstrates the balloon-shaped disks (arrows) contributing to the Cupid's bow contour of the vertebral bodies.

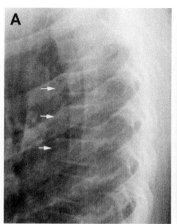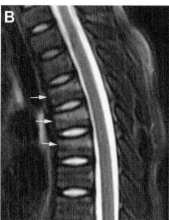

Fig. 23. A 9-year-old boy with pain after trauma. (*A*) Lateral radiograph of the thoracic spine in a 9-year-old boy demonstrates compression deformities of three midthoracic vertebral bodies (*arrows*). (*B*) Sagittal T2-weighted MR image of the thoracic spine demonstrates marrow edema in the compression deformities of three midthoracic vertebral bodies (*arrows*).

skeletal maturity.[56] The "ring apophysis" refers to the peripheral aspect of the vertebral end plates, whose shape is determined by the elliptical contour of the intervertebral disk and the primary vertebral ossification center (**Fig. 21**).[58] Between the ages of 11 and 14 years of age, this small ring ossification center develops at the end plate epiphysis peripherally, and completes ossification by 12 to 15 years of age. Fractures may occur at the cartilage end plate given that the attachment to the osseous end plate represents a point of weakness of the vertebral body.[57,59] Distinguishing between normal ring apophysis and an end plate fracture may be difficult with plain radiographs and better depicted at MR imaging.

In normal patients there may exist undulations within the end plates of the vertebral bodies secondary to the biomechanical stress of everyday living. These undulations should not be mistaken for compression fractures (**Fig. 22**). The cupid's bow deformity is a parasagittal concave curvature of the inferior end plate of the vertebral body at the level of the lumbar spine,[60] which is unrelated to trauma or stress changes (**Fig. 23**). The fish vertebral end plate is defined as a smooth concavity extended throughout the vertebral end plate[60] also considered a normal variant. These variants are present in older children and adults. These variants may be mistaken for compression deformities given that the height of the vertebral body is diminished at the level of the concavity, although vertebral compression fractures tend to have more angular deformities at the end plate rather than smooth, gentle convexities.[60] Following the appearance of the vertebral body over time with serial radiographs is not useful, because fracture and variant may evolve/resolve in a similar manner over time. MR imaging is useful when there is uncertainty in the diagnosis, because MR imaging can detect marrow edema and subtle fracture lines that are missed at plain radiography and CT.[61]

SUMMARY

There are a variety of conditions in the pediatric skeleton that may simulate fractures or other traumatic conditions. The growth plates represent sites where fractures are often suspected based on variations in normal physeal anatomy. Symmetry may be a helpful clue to the correct diagnosis. Follow-up radiographs in the context of equivocal findings may also be helpful. In most cases, regardless of location, MR imaging provides a more definitive diagnosis in the acute setting. As MR imaging technology improves and examination times become faster, MR imaging may be called on more often in children in settings where radiographic imaging findings are indeterminate.

REFERENCES

1. Flynn JM Jr, Skaggs DL, Waters PM. Rockwood and Wilkins' fractures in children. 8th edition. Philadelphia: Wolters Kluwer; 2015.
2. Landin LA. Epidemiology of children's fractures. J Pediatr Orthop B 1997;6(2):79–83.
3. Little JT, Klionsky NB, Chaturvedi A, et al. Pediatric distal forearm and wrist injury: an imaging review. Radiographics 2013;34(2):472–90.
4. Frost HM, Schonau E. The "muscle-bone unit" in children and adolescents: a 2000 overview. J Pediatr Endocrinol Metab 2000;13(6):571–90.
5. Caine D, DiFiori J, Maffulli N. Physeal injuries in children's and youth sports: reasons for concern? Br J Sports Med 2006;40(9):749–60.

6. Lohman M, Kivisaari P, Kallio P, et al. Acute paediatric ankle trauma: MRI versus plain radiography. Skeletal Radiol 2001;30:504–11.

7. Poland J. Traumatic separation of the epiphyses. London: Smith, Elder and Co.; 1898.

8. Mizuta T, Benson WM, Foster BK, et al. Statistical analysis of the incidence of physeal injuries. J Pediatr Orthop 1987;7(5):518–23.

9. Nguyen JC, Markhardt BK, Merrow AC, et al. Imaging of pediatric growth plate disturbances. Radiographics 2017;37:1791–812.

10. Carter SR, Aldridge MJ, Fitzgerald R, et al. Stress changes of the wrist in adolescent gymnasts. Br J Radiol 1988;61(722):109–12.

11. Wu M, Fallon R, Heyworth BE. Overuse injuries in the pediatric population. Sports Med Arthrosc Rev 2016;24(4):150–8.

12. Rogers LF, Poznanski AK. Imaging of epiphyseal injuries. Radiology 1994;191(2):297–308.

13. Lawson JP. Not-so-normal variants. Orthop Clin North Am 1990;3:483–95.

14. Petit P, Panuel M, Faure F, et al. Acute fracture of the distal tibial physis: role of gradient-echo MR imaging versus plain film examination. Am J Roentgenol 1996;166:1203–6.

15. Ogden JA, McCarthy SM. Radiology of postnatal skeletal development. VIII: distal tibia and fibula. Skeletal Radiol 1983;10:209–20.

16. Shi DP, Zhu SC, Li Y, et al. Epiphyseal and physeal injury: comparison of conventional radiography and magnetic resonance imaging. Clin Imaging 2009;33(5):379–83.

17. Laor T, Wall EJ, Vu LP. Physeal widening in the knee due to stress injury in child athletes. Am J Roentgenol 2006;186(5):1260–4.

18. Jaramillo D, Laor T, Zaleske DJ. Indirect trauma to the growth plate: results of MR imaging after epiphyseal and metaphyseal injury in rabbits. Radiology 1993;187(1):171–8.

19. DiFiori JP, Puffer JC, Aish B, et al. Wrist pain, distal radial physeal injury, and ulnar variance in young gymnasts: does a relationship exist? Am J Sports Med 2002;30(6):879–85.

20. Huckaby MC, Kruse D, Gibbs LH. MRI findings of bilateral proximal radial physeal injury in a gymnast. Pediatr Radiol 2012;42:1395–400.

21. Hesper T, Zilkens C, Bittersohl B, et al. Imaging modalities in patients with slipped capital femoral epiphysis. J Child Orthop 2017;11:99–106.

22. Ecklund E, Doria AS, Jaramillo D. Rickets on MR images. Pediatr Radiol 1999;29:673–5.

23. Burnstein MI, Kottamasu SR, Pettifor JM, et al. Metabolic bone disease in pseuodohypoparathyroidism: radiologic features. Radiology 1985;155:351–6.

24. Levin TL, Mäkitie O, Berdon WE, et al. Scwachman-Bodian-Diamond syndrome: metaphyseal chondrodysplasia in children with pancreatic insufficiency and neutropenia. Pediatr Radiol 2015;45:1066–71.

25. Taybi H, Mitchell AD, Friedman GD. Metaphyseal dysostosis and the associated syndrome of pancreatic insufficiency and blood disorders. Radiology 1969;93:563–71.

26. Stanley P, Sutcliffe J. Metaphyseal chondrodysplasia with dwarfism, pancreatic insufficiency and neutropenia. Pediatr Radiol 1973;1:119–26.

27. Bom EP, van der Sande FM, Tham RTOJA, et al. Case report: Shwachman syndrome: CT and MR diagnosis. J Comput Assist Tomogr 1993;17(3):474–6.

28. Lacaille F, Mamou TM, Francis B, et al. Magnetic resonance imaging for diagnosis of Shwachman's syndrome. J Pediatr Gastroenterol Nutr 1996;23(5):599–603.

29. Williams H. Normal anatomical variants and other mimics of skeletal trauma. In: Johnson KJ, editor. Imaging in pediatric skeletal trauma: techniques and applications. Berlin: Springer; 2008. p. 107–9.

30. Berquist TH. Pediatric foot and ankle disorders. Imaging of the foot and ankle. 3rd edition. Philadelphia: Lippincott Williams and Wilkins; 2010. p. 557.

31. Harrison RB, Keats TE. Epiphyseal clefts. Skeletal Radiol 1980;5(1):23–7.

32. Ogden JA. Radiology of postnatal skeletal development. X. Patella and tibial tuberosity. Skeletal Radiol 1984;11:246–57.

33. Stanitski CL, Micheli LJ. Observations on symptomatic medial malleolar ossification centers. J Pediatr Orthop 1993;12:164–8.

34. Winfield M, Rosenberg ZS, Wang A, et al. Differentiating os acromiale from normally developing acromial ossification centers using magnetic resonance imaging. Skeletal Radiol 2015;44(5):667–72.

35. Zember JS, Rosenberg ZS, Kwong S, et al. Normal skeletal maturation and imaging pitfalls in the pediatric shoulder. Radiographics 2015;35:1108–22.

36. Kothary S, Rosenberg ZS, Poncinelli LL, et al. Skeletal development of the glenoid and glenoid-coracoid interface in the pediatric population: MRI features. Skeletal Radiol 2014;43(9):1281–8.

37. Alaia EF, Rosenberg ZS, Rossi I, et al. Growth plate injury at the base of the coracoid: MRI features. Skeletal Radiol 2017;46(11):1507–12.

38. Ho-Fung VM, Zapala MA, Lee EY. Musculoskeletal traumatic injuries in children: characteristic imaging findings and mimickers. Radiol Clin North Am 2017;55:785–802.

39. Levine SM, Lambiase RE, Petchprapa CN. Cortical lesions of the tibia: characteristic appearances at conventional radiography. Radiographics 2003;23(1):157–77.

40. Chai JW, Hong SH, Choi JY, et al. Radiologic diagnosis of osteoid osteoma: from simple to challenging findings. Radiographics 2010;30:737–49.

41. Matcuk GR Jr, Mahanty SR, Skalski MR, et al. Stress fractures: pathophysiology, clinical presentation, imaging features, and treatment options. Emerg Radiol 2016;23(4):365–75.

42. Craig JG, Widman D, van Holsbeek M. Longitudinal stress fracture: patterns of edema and the importance of the nutrient foramen. Skeletal Radiol 2003; 32(1):22–7.

43. Umans HR, Kaye JJ. Longitudinal stress fractures of the tibia: diagnosis by magnetic resonance imaging. Skeletal Radiol 1996;25(4):319–24.

44. Jaimes C, Jimenez M, Shabshin N, et al. Taking the stress out of stress fractures in children. Radiographics 2012;32:537–55.

45. Cha H, Park SB, Kim HJ. Focal increased Tc-99m MDP uptake in the nutrient foramen of the femoral diaphysis on bone SPECT/CT. Nucl Med Mol Imaging 2018;52:162–5.

46. Imre N, Battal B, Acikel CH, et al. The demonstration of the number, course, and the location of nutrient artery canals of the femur by multidetector computed tomography. Surg Radiol Anat 2012;34:427–32.

47. Li J, Zhang H, Yin P, et al. A new measurement technique of the characteristics of nutrient artery canals in tibias using Materialise's Interactive medical image control system software. Biomed Res Int 2015; 2015:17162.

48. Pathria MN, Chung CB, Resnick DL. Acute and stress-related injuries of bone and cartilage: pertinent anatomy, basic biomechanics, and imaging perspective. Radiology 2016;280:21–38.

49. Mirra JM, Picci P, Gold RH. Bone tumors: clinical, radiologic, and pathologic correlations. Philadelphia: Lea & Febiger; 1989.

50. Resnick D, Niwayama G. Diagnosis of bone and joint disorders. 2nd edition. Philadelphia: WB Saunders; 1988.

51. Gamba JL, Martinez S, Apple J, et al. Computed tomography of axial skeleton osteoid osteomas. Am J Roentgenol 1984;142:769–72.

52. Assoun J, Richardi G, Railhac JJ, et al. Osteoid osteoma: MR imaging versus CT. Radiology 1994;191: 217–23.

53. Liu PT, Chivers FS, Roberts CC, et al. Imaging of osteoid osteoma with dynamic gadolinium-enhanced MR imaging. Radiology 2003;227: 691–700.

54. Zampa V, Bargellini I, Ortori S, et al. Osteoid osteoma in atypical locations: the added value of dynamic gadolinium-enhanced MR imaging. Eur J Radiol 2009;71:527–53.

55. Pottecher P, Sibileau E, Aho S, et al. Dynamic contrast-enhanced MR imaging in osteoid osteoma: relationships with clinical and CT characteristics. Skeletal Radiol 2017;46:935–48.

56. Jaremko JL, Siminoski K, Firth GH, et al. Common normal variants of pediatric vertebral development that mimic fractures: a pictorial review from a national longitudinal bone health study. Pediatr Radiol 2015;45:593–605.

57. Labrom RD. Growth and maturation of the spine from birth to adolescence. J Bone Joint Surg Am 2007;89(Suppl 1):3–7.

58. Bick EM, Copel JW. Longitudinal growth of the human vertebra; a contribution to human osteogeny. J Bone Joint Surg Am 1950;32:803–14.

59. Singal A, Mitra A, Cochrane D, et al. Ring apophysis fracture in pediatric lumbar disc herniation: a common entity. Pediatr Neurosurg 2013;49: 16–20.

60. Chan KK, Sartoris DJ, Haghighi P, et al. Cupid's bow contour of the vertebral body: evaluation of pathogenesis with bone densitometry and imaging-histopathologic correlation. Radiology 1997;202: 253–6.

61. Leroux J, Vivier PH, Ould Slimane M, et al. Early diagnosis of thoracolumbar spine fractures in children, a prospective study. Orthop Traumatol Surg Res 2013;99:60–5.

Radiographic/MR Imaging Correlation of the Pediatric Knee Growth

Héloïse Lerisson, MD, Céline Tillaux, MD, Nathalie Boutry, MD, PhD*

KEYWORDS

- Child • Knee joint • Conventional radiography • MR imaging • Normal bone growth
- Ossification variant • Femur • Tibia

KEY POINTS

- This article reviews normal developmental changes in the pediatric knee on imaging (radiography/MR imaging.
- Knowledge of these changes is important to avoid confusing normal growth with disease.
- In distal femur, normal variants are spiculation of epiphyseal ossification centers, subchondral anomalies in posterior femoral condyles, and periosteal desmoid.
- In proximal tibial, fragmentation of the tibial tuberosity during ongoing ossification may be misleading on imaging.
- Dorsal defect, bipartite patella, and lower pole fragmentation are the most common variations in patellar ossification.

With the increasing development of sports activities in children, imaging is more and more often performed in the presence of clinical symptoms and can lead to diagnostic errors. Indeed, some variants of endochondral ossification may mimic pathologic entities, whereas others may be symptomatic. This article discusses the normal aspects and main variants of endochondral knee ossification in children at radiography and MR imaging.

NORMAL BONE GROWTH OF THE KNEE

It mainly involves endochondral ossification and to a lesser degree, membranous ossification. In the process of endochondral ossification, mesenchymal cells condense and differentiate into chondrocytes to form a cartilage model before bone tissue formation, whereas in the process of membranous ossification, mesenchymal cells condense and differentiate directly into osteoforming cells.[1] A long bone such as the femur or tibia has an epiphysis, metaphysis, and diaphysis. In children and adolescents, the physeal cartilage (or growth plate) separates the epiphysis from the metaphysis. Patella is an epiphyseal equivalent.

EPIPHYSIS

Its surface is covered with a layer of articular cartilage. The epiphysis is initially entirely cartilaginous. Epiphyseal cartilage and articular cartilage consist of hyaline cartilage with a different composition: epiphyseal cartilage is rich in chondrocytes and water, with vascular channels,

Disclosure Statement: The authors have nothing to disclose.
Funded by: FRENCH.
Department of Pediatric Imaging, Hôpital Jeanne de Flandre, CHU Lille, Avenue Eugène Avinée, Lille F-59000, France
* Corresponding author.
E-mail addresses: nathalie.boutry@chru-lille.fr; nboutry@gmail.com

Magn Reson Imaging Clin N Am 27 (2019) 737–751
https://doi.org/10.1016/j.mric.2019.07.013
1064-9689/19/© 2019 Elsevier Inc. All rights reserved.

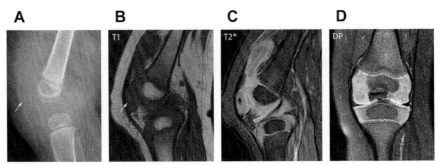

Fig. 1. Normal epiphyses. (*A*) In this 2-year-old child with JIA, the lateral knee radiograph shows ossified epiphyses of the femur and tibia. The primary ossification center of the patella (*arrow* in *A* and *B*) is still punctiform. (*B*) On sagittal T1-W and (*C*) T2-W gradient echo (T2*) and (*D*) frontal T2-W fat-suppressed (FS) MR imaging, the cartilaginous component of the epiphyses shows isointense T1 signal and hyperintense T2 signal. The patellar ossification center shows increased T1 signal. JIA, juvenile idiopathic arthritis. DP, proton density.

whereas articular cartilage is poor in chondrocytes and water, without vessels.[2] On radiographs, the unossified epiphysis is invisible (**Fig. 1**). On MR imaging, it is hypointense to muscle on T1-weighted (T1-W) imaging and mildly hyperintense on T2-W imaging (see **Fig. 1**). As a result of various mechanisms specific to endochondral ossification (chondrocyte hypertrophy, apoptosis, angiogenesis, osteoblast inflow),[1] a secondary ossification center appears within the cartilaginous epiphysis. It is visible on radiographs around 36 weeks' gestation at the distal end of the femur (Beclard's point) and 38 weeks' gestation at the proximal end of the tibia (Todd's point). First spherical in shape, this ossification center becomes hemispherical to adapt to the metaphysis. On MR imaging, the secondary ossification center is visible on T1-W imaging (see **Fig. 1**). At birth and during the first year of life, epiphyseal cartilage is traversed by vascular channels. Initially parallel to each other, these channels then affect a radial arrangement from the secondary ossification center.[3] In toddlers or young children with local hyperemia, these channels can be visualized with MR imaging after administration of gadolinium[4] (**Fig. 2**). Vascular channels tend to disappear over time.[5]

The secondary ossification center is surrounded at its periphery by a secondary physis, also called acrophysis. The part of the ossification center in immediate contact with the

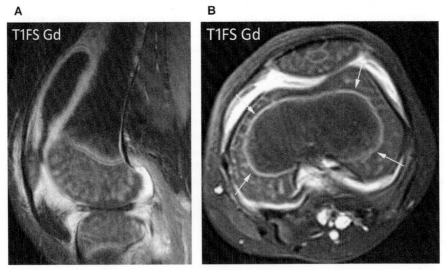

Fig. 2. Epiphyseal vascular channels on MR imaging. Same child as **Fig. 1**. (*A*) Sagittal and (*B*) axial T1-W FS gadolinium-enhanced (Gd) MR imaging show the enhancement of the epiphyseal vascular channels due to hyperemia. Note on the axial image, the enhancement of the primary metaphyseal spongiosa adjacent to the acrophysis (*arrows*) and the radial arrangement of the vascular channels from the secondary ossification center.

acrophysis is equivalent to the metaphyseal primary spongiosa: it is visible on MR imaging in the form of a linear hyperintensity on T2-W and postcontrast T1-W imaging (see **Fig. 2**). Acrophysis (or secondary physis) has the same histologic nature as physeal cartilage (or primary physis) but is thinner. Through acrophysis, endochondral ossification is involved in the hemispheric bone growth of the epiphysis.[3]

The appearance of the secondary ossification center is preceded by the development of preossification centers.[3] The latter are sometimes visible on MR imaging in the form of well-limited, lobulated structures of high signal intensity, within the epiphyseal cartilage[6] (**Fig. 3**). Articular cartilage is also visible on MR imaging: on T1-W images, its signal merges with that of the cartilaginous epiphysis but it becomes visible on T2-W images, in the form of a hypersignal rim around the epiphysis. Homogeneous in young children, the articular cartilage signal becomes more heterogeneous with age and gait acquisition. Along the weight-bearing joint surface, a decrease in T2 signal intensity appears, clearly visible at the middle portion of the femoral condyles (**Fig. 4**).

Physeal Cartilage

Also called growth plate or primary physis, the physeal cartilage is roughly disc-shaped, thick

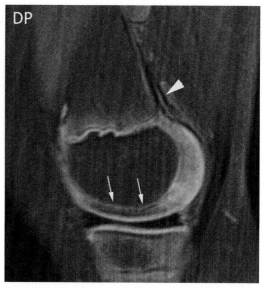

Fig. 4. Changes in the articular cartilage signal on MR imaging. Note the T2 hypointensity of the articular cartilage in the weight-bearing area (*arrows*). The peripheral sleeve surrounding the growth plate is clearly visible (*arrowhead*).

and smooth in young children, whereas thin and wavy in older children. Histologically, the physeal cartilage is formed of 3 successive cellular layers, from the epiphysis to the metaphysis (**Fig. 5**):

- A thin *germinal layer (or reserve zone)* composed of spherical chondrocytes separated by an abundant extracellular matrix, rich in proteoglycans;

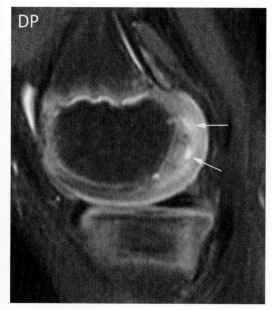

Fig. 3. Preossification centers on MR imaging. They are visible at the posterior medial femoral condyle (*arrows*) as well-demarcated areas exhibiting hyperintensity on T2-W MR imaging.

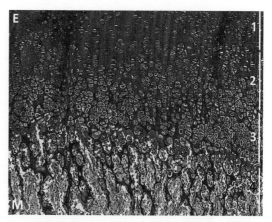

Fig. 5. Histologic section showing the different cellular layers of the physis. (1) Germinal layer; (2) proliferative layer; (3) hypertrophic layer; and (4) endochondral ossification and primary metaphyseal spongiosa. E, epiphysis; M, metaphysis. (*Courtesy of S. Aubert, MD, PhD, Lille Cedex, France.*)

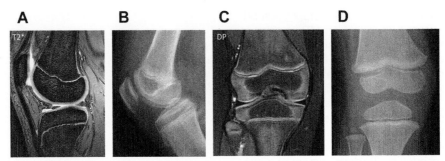

Fig. 6. Normal physes on MR imaging. (*A*) Sagittal T2-W* sequence shows the femoral and tibial physes in hypersignal, contrasting with the hyposignal intensity of the bone. (*B*) Corresponding lateral knee radiograph. (*C*) Coronal T2-W FS MR imaging reveals the trilamellar appearance of the physis with the primary metaphysis spongiosa, the provisional calcification zone, and the other cartilaginous layers, from metaphysis to epiphysis. (*D*) Corresponding anteroposterior (AP) radiograph.

- A thick *proliferative layer (or serial zone)*, where the chondrocytes flatten and arrange themselves in longitudinal columns, parallel to the major axis of the bone, within an extracellular matrix rich in type II collagen;
- A *hypertrophic layer (or hypertrophic zone)* composed of chondrocytes organized in 3 zones: chondrocytic maturation, chondrocytic degeneration, and provisional calcification. The provisional calcification zone, also known as the epiphyseal ossification front, faces the primary metaphyseal spongiosa.

At MR imaging, T2-W gradient-recalled-echo sequences are used to differentiate the hyperintense physeal cartilage from the adjacent hypointense cancellous bone but not to individualize the different cartilage layers of the physis[7] (**Fig. 6**). Conversely, T2-W sequences with fat signal suppression (short T1 inversion-recovery, proton density) distinguish the provisional calcification zone (linear hyposignal) from other cartilage layers (linear hypersignal). Because the primary metaphyseal spongiosa already appears as a linear hypersignal on T2-W sequences, MR imaging shows on T2-W imaging

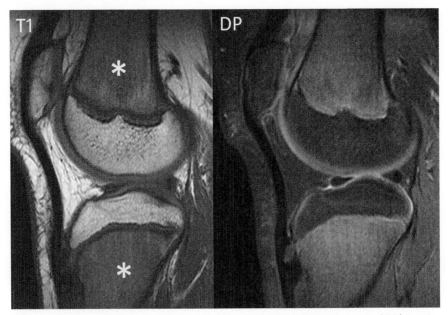

Fig. 7. Normal metaphyses on MR imaging. Sagittal T1-W and T2-W FS MR imaging reveal T1 hyposignal intensity within the femoral and tibial metaphyses (*asterisks*), of linear aspect, due to the presence of red, hematopoietic bone marrow, contrasting with the fatty signal intensity of the epiphyses. On T2-W imaging, this hyposignal intensity is replaced by mild hyperintensity.

a trilamellar aspect, characteristic of the junction between the epiphysis and the metaphysis (see **Fig. 6**).

Physeal cartilage vascularization involves an epiphyseal arterial network and a metaphyseal arterial network. During the first 18 months of life, transphyseal vessels provide anastomoses between these 2 networks but they eventually disappear.[2] Epiphyseal arteries are distributed to the secondary ossification center from which they pass through the epiphyseal cartilage, within the vascular channels and to the epiphyseal side of the physis (germinal layer). Metaphyseal arteries supply the area of provisional calcification (or epiphyseal ossification front). In total, the central part of the physeal cartilage (hypertrophic zone) is not vascularized. Dynamic MR imaging may show the early enhancement of physis and acrophysis and if the spatial resolution is sufficient enough, distinguish between the intense enhancement of the provisional calcification zone (metaphyseal network), the absence of enhancement of the hypertrophic zone, and the moderate enhancement of the germinal zone (epiphyseal network).

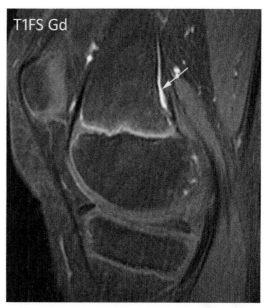

Fig. 8. Normal periosteum on MR imaging. On sagittal T1-W FS Gd MR imaging, a band of fibroconjunctive tissue separating the periosteum from the bone cortex is clearly visible (*arrow*).

Metaphysis and Diaphysis

The metaphysis is richer than the diaphysis in red, hematopoietic bone. At MR imaging, this is reflected by the presence within trabecular bone of poorly limited areas of low signal intensity relative to muscle on T1-W imaging[3] (**Fig. 7**). MR imaging findings are generally symmetric between right and left sides. A similar appearance may be seen at the periphery of the epiphysis, in the form of a linear, subchondral hyposignal intensity. Bone growth in length and width for the metaphysis and diaphysis involves endochondral ossification (via the physeal cartilage) and membranous ossification, respectively. Unlike the epiphysis, the diaphysis and metaphysis are covered by the periosteum formed by a deep cellular layer and a fibrous superficial layer. Periosteum is thicker in children than in adults. It is also less adherent to the bone cortex from which it is separated by fibrovascular tissue that enhances after administration of gadolinium. This aspect is clearly visible on MR imaging at the posterior part of the distal femoral metaphysis[3] (**Fig. 8**). With respect to the physeal cartilage, the fibrous layer of the periosteum is

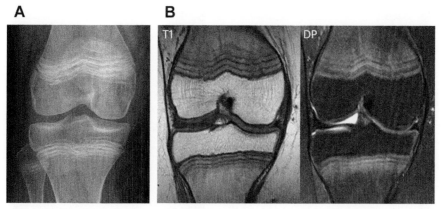

Fig. 9. "Growth arrest lines." (*A*) AP radiograph shows multiple and dense metaphyseal lines in femur, tibia, and fibula related to prior administration of biphosphonates. (*B*) On coronal sequences, these lines are hypointense on both T1-W and T2-W imaging.

in continuity with a fibro-chondro-osseous sleeve encircling the growth plate, consisting of the groove of Ranvier and the perichondrial ring of LaCroix.[4] This peripheral sleeve contributes to the growth and mechanical strength of the growth plate. It appears on MR imaging as a short hypointense band, extending from metaphysis to epiphysis[3] (see **Fig. 4**). The periosteum is essential for circumferential bone growth.

Normal Bone Growth

This is not a continuous but a cyclical phenomenon. In long bones, a physiologic arrest of bone growth results on radiographs in transverse lines of sclerosis, parallel to the growth plate, within the metaphysis (**Fig. 9**). Also called "growth arrest lines," "Harris-Park's lines," or "growth recovery lines," these lines then move toward the diaphysis as bone growth progresses. When numerous, growth arrest lines indicate an intercurrent condition or prior administration of biphosphonates (see **Fig. 9**). When they adopt an oblique path with respect to the growth plate, premature epiphysiodesis should be considered, especially after trauma. In flat bones such as the patella, growth arrest lines produce a "bone within bone"

appearance (**Fig. 10**). On MR imaging, these lines appear hypointense on all sequences (see **Figs. 9** and **10**).

As normal bone growth progresses, the growth plate becomes thinner and then closes partially and finally completely. At the distal end of the femur and the proximal end of the tibia, physiologic closure begins at the central part of the growth plate and then extends to the peripheral part.[8] An onset of physiologic closure is sometimes visible on MR imaging as a focal bridge interrupting the normal hyperintensity of the growth plate on T2-W imaging and may be accompanied by signal abnormalities of the adjacent bone marrow (**Fig. 11**). These MR imaging findings may be associated with knee pain.[8,9] The femur, tibia, and, more rarely, fibula are affected. The acronym "FOPE" is used in the Anglo-Saxon literature to describe these MR imaging abnormalities. They eventually regress with time and the physiologic closure of the growth plate.[9]

OSSIFICATION VARIANTS OF THE FEMUR AND TIBIA
Epiphyseal Irregularities

On both femoral and tibial sides, the contours of the ossification centers may be irregular or even openly spattered[10] (**Fig. 12**). This corresponds to

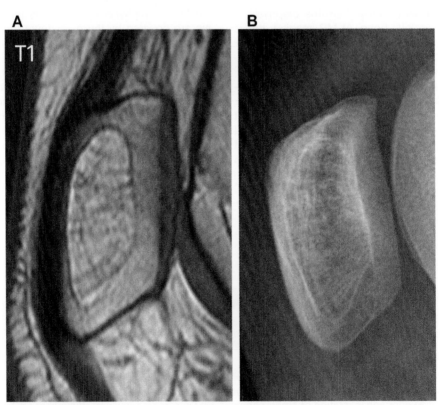

Fig. 10. "Bone within bone" appearance. (*A*) Sagittal T1-W MR imaging reveals a "bone within bone" appearance of the patella. (*B*) Corresponding lateral knee radiograph.

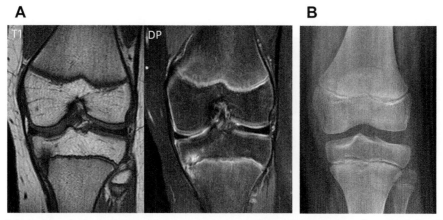

Fig. 11. Periphyseal focal edema (FOPE). (*A*) Coronal T1-W and T2-W FS MR imagings show focal signal anomalies on both sides of the tibial physis at its medial part. (*B*) Corresponding lateral knee radiograph.

variants of endochondral ossification. In the femur, the medial condyle is more often involved than the lateral condyle.

Subchondral Anomalies of the Posterior Part of the Femoral Condyles

They are often encountered incidentally in young children, before the age of 10 years in girls and 13 years in boys.[11] They are reported to be present in just more than 20% of cases.[12] These anomalies typically occur on the posterior third of the femoral condyles and at a distance from the intercondylar fossa, unlike osteochondrosis.[11] The medial femoral condyle is more often affected than the lateral condyle.[11] MR imaging may show irregular contours, a subchondral defect (**Fig. 13**), or a "puzzle" appearance of the subchondral bone plate (ie, an ossified structure more or less

completely filling an arciform subchondral defect).[11,12] There is no associated joint effusion or subchondral bone edema.[11] The articular cartilage overlying these abnormalities is normal. Nodular T2 hyperintensity areas are sometimes visible at the interface between bone and epiphyseal cartilage. They correspond to the preossification centers described earlier (see **Fig. 3**). Subchondral anomalies of the posterior part of the femoral condyles decrease with the progressive closure of the physeal cartilage and eventually disappear at the end of bone growth.[11]

Periosteal Desmoid

Also called "cortical desmoid," it corresponds to a benign subperiosteal lesion, characteristically located at the posteromedial aspect of the distal femoral metaphysis. At radiography, it appears

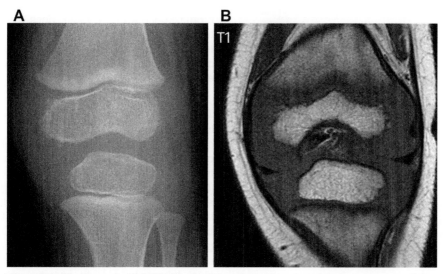

Fig. 12. Epiphyseal contour irregularities. (*A*) On the AP radiograph, a speculated appearance of the medial side of the medial femoral condyle is visible. (*B*) This feature is more visible on MR imaging and involves both the femur and tibia.

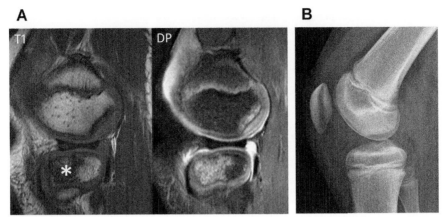

Fig. 13. Defect of the posterior part of the femoral condyles in imaging. (*A*) The posterior third of the lateral femoral condyle is involved in this child who also had a lateral discoid meniscus and a fracture impaction of the anterior tibial epiphysis (*asterisk*) with associated joint effusion on MR imaging. (*B*) Corresponding lateral knee radiograph.

as a bone erosion sometimes associated with a chronic periosteal reaction or small osseous spicules (**Fig. 14**). This variant ossification is reported to be more common in children or adolescents involved in sports activities and results from repeated microtractions at the insertion site of the medial head of the gastrocnemius muscle or the large adductor muscle. At MR imaging, the signal of the lesion is not specific but there is no signal anomaly of the adjacent bone marrow (**Fig. 15**), in the absence of associated trauma.[4,13] In some children, periosteal desmoid is sometimes visible on the anteroposterior (AP) radiograph as a rounded image, finely circled by a reactive sclerotic border that may be confusing with tumor or infectious pathology (**Fig. 16**). At MR imaging, in addition to its evocative location, periosteal desmoid is surrounded by a hypointense rim on all sequences. In case of gadolinium injection, enhancement is generally limited, peripheral, contrasting with a hypointense center (see **Fig. 16**). Unlike fibrous cortical defect/nonossifying fibroma, periosteal desmoid does not migrate toward the diaphysis with bone growth.[4] Periosteal desmoid should not lead to percutaneous biopsy to avoid diagnostic errors on pathology examination.

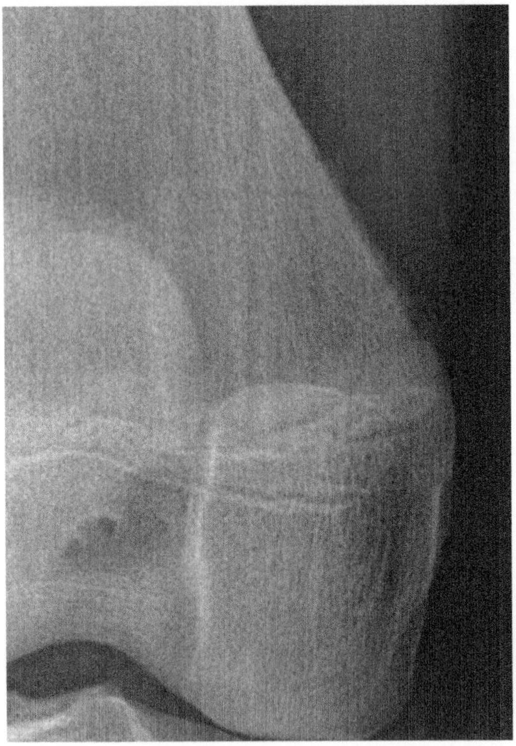

Ossification of the Tibial Tuberosity

In young children, the tibial tuberosity is purely cartilaginous. On a lateral knee radiograph, the proximal tibial metaphysis thus presents a longitudinal depression, with anterior concavity (**Fig. 17**). On MR imaging, sagittal images show a tonguelike structure exhibiting moderate T2 hyperintensity corresponding to the cartilaginous tuberosity (**Fig. 18**). From the age of 10 years in girls and 12 years in boys, one or more secondary ossification centers appear at the distal part of the tibial tuberosity.[4,14,15] In imaging, an isolated, painless fragmentation of the tibial tuberosity can therefore be considered as a normal

Fig. 14. Periosteal desmoid on radiography. Note the presence of small bony spicules at the medial side of the distal femoral metaphysis.

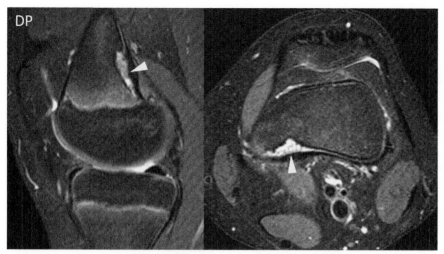

Fig. 15. Periosteal desmoid on MR imaging. Sagittal and axial T2-W FS MR imaging show a bone defect, well limited by a hyposignal rim (*arrowheads*), due to the insertion of the medial gastrocnemius muscle.

variant[4,14–16] (**Fig. 19**). These ossification centers gradually increase in size and eventually coalesce. At the same time, ossification of the proximal tibial epiphysis progresses toward tibial tuberosity to form a single osseous structure, separated from the proximal tibial metaphysis by the physeal cartilage. The latter closes first at its front and central part, then at its back and peripheral part.[17,18] The closure of the proximal tibial physis precedes that of tibial tuberosity, which occurs around the age of 13 to 15 years in girls and 15 to 19 years in boys.[4] In practice, the endochondral ossification of the tibial tuberosity should not be confused with osteochondrosis or Osgood-Schlatter disease. In this case, the child complains of elective pain over tibial tuberosity associated with local MR imaging signal abnormalities. At MR imaging, other rarer diagnoses can be reported: distal patellar enthesitis in juvenile idiopathic arthritis (JIA) (particularly in the form of "arthritis associated with enthesitis") or bone damage in chronic recurrent multifocal osteomyelitis (CRMO). The presence of extensive bone edema, which extends well beyond the tibial tuberosity, as well as edema topography (enthesis in JIA, epiphysometaphyseal area in CRMO) are in favor of an inflammatory pathology (**Fig. 20**).

OSSIFICATION VARIANTS OF THE PATELLA
Normal Development

The patella begins to ossify between the ages of 3 and 7 years.[15,19] Before this age, it is cartilaginous and therefore invisible on radiographs, while it already has its definitive morphology on MR imaging. Most often, patella is ossified from a single primary ossification center (77% of cases).[20] More

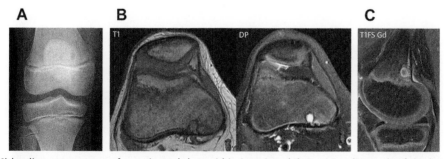

Fig. 16. Misleading appearance of a periosteal desmoid in imaging. (*A*) On AP radiograph of the knee, an oval lacuna with a border of reactive osteosclerosis is seen in projection of the patella. (*B*) Axial T1-W and T2-W FS MR imaging show that the lesion is actually located in the posteromedial cortex of the distal femoral metaphysis. (*C*) Sagittal T1-W FS Gd MR imaging shows limited, peripheral enhancement. There are no adjacent bone marrow signal abnormalities on both T1-W and T2-W sequences.

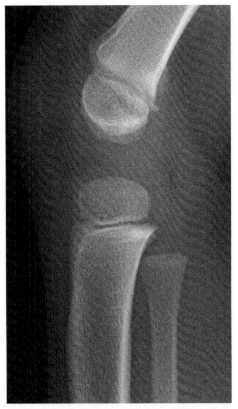

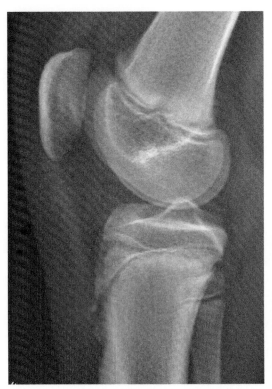

Fig. 17. Normal tibial tuberosity on radiography. In this 3-year-old child, the tibial tuberosity is still entirely cartilaginous. This explains the depression seen at the anterior part of the proximal tibial metaphysis on the lateral knee radiograph.

Fig. 19. Normal appearance of the tibial tuberosity during ossification. Endochondral ossification is responsible for the fragmentation of the tibial tuberosity. The child was asymptomatic.

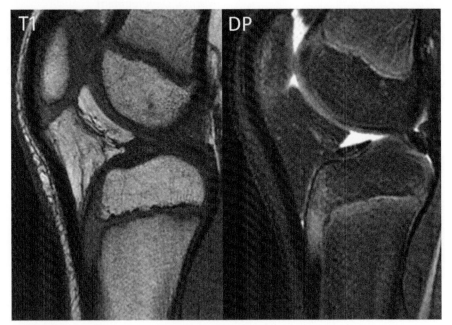

Fig. 18. Normal tibial tuberosity on MR imaging. In this 7-year-old child, the tibial tuberosity is isointense to the muscle on T1-W and mildly hypersignal on T2-W sagittal MR images.

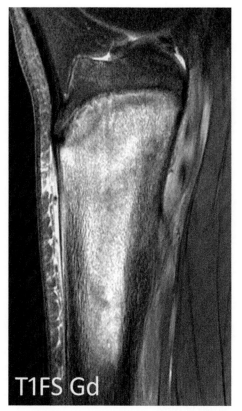

T1FS Gd

Fig. 20. CRMO on MR imaging. Note on this sagittal T1-W FS Gd MR imaging, the hyperintensity of the bone marrow and anterior soft tissues as well as cortical tibial thickening. The tibial tuberosity itself is spared.

rarely, it is ossified from 2 to 3 distinct ossification centers, one of which corresponds to the superior pole of patella.[20,21] These primary ossification centers gradually increase in size and sometimes have irregular contours in radiography (**Fig. 21**). They then merge with each other. Around the age of 12 years, secondary ossification centers may appear, particularly at the upper pole of the

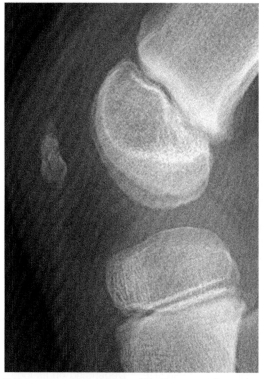

Fig. 21. Normal patellar ossification on radiography. The coalescence of several primary ossification centers explains the irregular contours.

patella. Normally, they also end up merging with the rest of the patella.

Dorsal Defect of Patella

The dorsal defect of the patella (DDP) corresponds to a subchondral lesion, typically located at the upper pole of the patella.[22,23] The DDP can be uni- or bilateral, isolated or associated with a bipartite patella.[22–24] Its origin remains unclear: the commonly accepted theory is that of a disorder of

A **B**

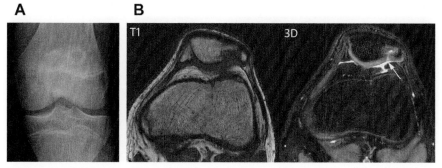

T1 3D

Fig. 22. DDP in imaging. (*A*) The AP radiograph of the knee shows a lytic, round lesion with well-defined sclerotic margins in the superolateral quadrant of the patella. (*B*) Corresponding axial T1-W and T2-W 3-dimensional gradient echo (T2*) MR imaging. The latter shows the perforation of the patellar articular cartilage (*white arrow*).

endochondral ossification secondary to repetitive strain injuries on insertion site of the vastus lateralis muscle.[23,25] The articular cartilage overlying the DDP is intact or perforated,[26] without any link to the symptomatic nature of the lesion.[23] At radiography, DDP appears as a small, well-limited, bone defect, usually surrounded by a reactive rim of osteosclerosis (**Fig. 22**). MR imaging is useful to assess the articular cartilage overlying the DDP[27] (see **Fig. 22**). It can also reveal surrounding bone edema that would be better correlated with the presence of knee pain.[28] DDP may persist or regress, spontaneously or following biopsy or surgical curettage. In practice, the main differential diagnosis of DDP is patellar osteochondrosis, which has a distinct topography from the DDP (ie, distal part of the patella and convex subchondral areas). Other differential diagnoses are bone infection (Brodie's abscess) and patellar tumors (chondroblastoma, osteoid osteoma, aneurysmal bone cyst, etc.).

Bipartite Patella

It corresponds to a fragmented patella. The fragment is of variable size.[29] Depending on its location, there are 3 types of bipartite patella[30]:

- Type I, at the lower pole of the patella (2% of cases),
- Type II, on the lateral side of the patella (20% of cases), and
- Type III, at the superior pole of the patella (75% of cases).

For some investigators,[31] type I would actually correspond to an unknown patellar fracture. In type III, the fragment is sometimes double (tripartite patella) or even multiple (multipartite patella) (**Fig. 23**). Bipartite patella is found in 2% to 6% of the population.[32] It can be uni- or bilateral. It is

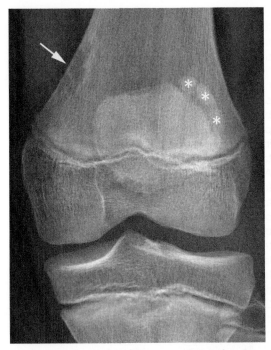

Fig. 23. Patella multipartite on radiography. Bone fragments are visible in the superolateral quadrant of the patella (*asterisks*). There is also a small fibrous cortical defect at the medial side of the distal femoral metaphysis (*arrow*).

more frequent in boys than in girls.[33] Bipartite patella would result from the absence of fusion between the primary ossification center of the upper pole of the patella and the rest of the patella and/or the absence of fusion between one of the secondary ossification centers and the rest of the patella. In radiography, a radiolucent gap separates the bone fragment from the patella; the contours of the bone fragment are regular. On MR imaging, the fragment signal is variable on T1-W and T2-W sequences[29,33] (**Fig. 24**). These signal

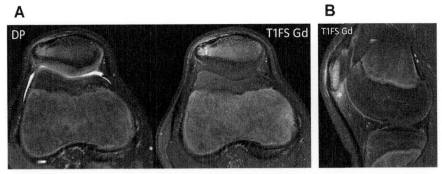

Fig. 24. Patella bipartite on MR imaging. (*A*) Axial T2-W FS and T1-W FS Gd MR imaging show hypersignal intensity within the bone fragment, overflowing on the patella, and contrast enhancement between the fragment and the patella. (*B*) On sagittal T1-W image, the "inflammation" extends to the Hoffa's fat pad. This patient was symptomatic, with no other cause found on MR imaging except bipartite patella.

anomalies may overflow onto the adjacent patella (see **Fig. 24**). The interspace between the bone fragment and the patella may be filled by fibrous tissue (synfibrosis), cartilage (synchondrosis), or fluid (pseudarthrosis).[29,33] The presence of fluid has no pathologic value.[34] On the other hand, signal abnormalities of the bone marrow would be better correlated with the presence of knee pain[33,34] (see **Fig. 24**). MR imaging also provides information on the articular cartilage of the detached bone fragment, especially if it is large.[29] At both radiography and MR imaging, the main differential diagnosis of bipartite patella is patellar avulsion fracture. In general, the bilateral nature of the anomalies; well-defined and corticalized contours for both the bone fragment and the patella; and a meeting of the 2 parts giving a patella larger than a normal patella are all arguments in favor of bipartite patella. Type I bipartite patella poses more diagnostic problems. A Sinding-Larsen-Johansson disease, fragmentation in the context of cerebral palsy, or a true fracture must first be eliminated. The orientation of the continuity solution (concave down in the bipartite patella; transverse in the fracture) also makes a difference.[35]

Fragmentation of the Lower Pole of the Patella

An irregular or even fragmented appearance of the lower pole of the patella is sometimes observed in young children on a lateral knee radiograph (**Fig. 25**) or with MR imaging[16] (**Fig. 26**). This may

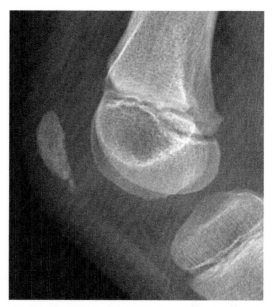

Fig. 25. Physiologic fragmentation of the lower pole of the patella on radiograph.

also occur in case of cerebral palsy with flexion knee contracture.[36] It does not always correspond to a simple normal variant ossification, especially when the child complains of anterior knee pain and/or when MR imaging shows adjacent soft tissue abnormalities on T2-W and contrast-enhanced T1-W images: bone marrow hyperintensity at the lower border of the patella sometimes extending to the Hoffa's fat pad and/or prepatellar

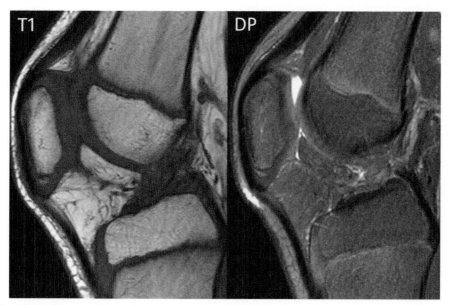

Fig. 26. Physiologic fragmentation of the lower pole of patella on MR imaging. There is no signal anomaly on sagittal T1-W and T2-W FS MR images.

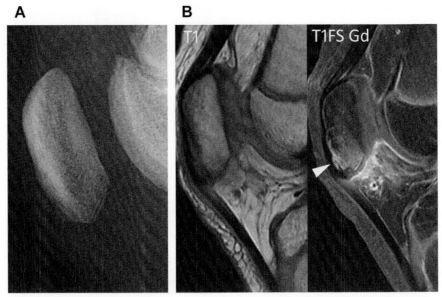

Fig. 27. Fragmentation of the lower pole of the patella on MR imaging. (*A*) An irregular appearance of the patellar apex is seen on a lateral knee radiograph of a young athlete complaining of anterior knee pain. (*B*) Corresponding sagittal T1-W and T1-W FS Gd MR imaging show local "inflammatory" changes and an incipient avulsion of the cartilaginous cover (*arrowhead*).

subcutaneous soft tissues (**Fig. 27**). In this case, other diagnoses should be mentioned: a Sinding-Larsen-Johansson disease; a fracture-avulsion of the patellar apex or proximal patellar enthesitis in the context of JIA (particularly in the form of "arthritis associated with enthesitis").

In conclusion, imaging shows many variants of endochondral ossification of the knee in children. In practice, these variants must be known so as not to lead to confusion with an authentic pathology. On the other hand, not all abnormalities seen on radiographs in children are always simple variants; they can be responsible for knee pain and require additional MR imaging, first and foremost to look for other causes of clinical symptoms.

REFERENCES

1. Kronenberg HM. Developmental regulation of the growth plate. Nature 2003;423:332–6.
2. Jaimes C, Chauvin NA, Delgado J, et al. MR imaging of normal epiphyseal development and common epiphyseal disorders. Radiographics 2014;34:449–71.
3. Laor T, Jaramillo D. MR imaging insights into skeletal maturation: what is normal? Radiology 2009;250:28–38.
4. Stein-Wexler R, Wootton-Gorges SL, Ozonoff MB. Pediatric orthopedic imaging. Berlin (Germany): Springer-Verlag; 2015.
5. Jaramillo D, Villegas-Medina OL, Doty DK, et al. Age-related vascular changes in the epiphysis, physis, and metaphysis : normal findings on gadolinium-enhanced MRI of piglets. AJR Am J Roentgenol 2004;182:353–60.
6. Chapman WM, Nimkin K, Jaramillo D. The preossification center: normal CT and MRI findings in the trochlea. Skeletal Radiol 2004;33:725–7.
7. Yun HH, Kim HJ, Jeong MS, et al. Changes of the growth plate in children: 3-dimensional magnetic resonance imaging analysis. Korean J Pediatr 2018;61:226–30.
8. Zbojniewicz AM, Laor T. Focal periphyseal edema (FOPE) zone on MRI of the adolescent knee: a potentially painful manifestation of physiologic physeal fusion? AJR Am J Roentgenol 2011;197:998–1004.
9. Bochmann T, Forrester R, Smith J. Case report: imaging the clinical course of FOPE-a cause of adolescent knee pain. J Surg Case Rep 2016;11.
10. Ogden JA. Radiology of postnatal skeletal development. IX. Proximal tibia and fibula. Skeletal Radiol 1984;11:169–77.
11. Jans LB, Jaremko JL, Ditchfield M, et al. MRI differentiates femoral condylar ossification evolution from osteochondritis dissecans. A new sign. Eur Radiol 2011;21:1170–9.
12. Jans LB, Jaremko JL, Ditchfield M, et al. Evolution of femoral condylar ossification at MR imaging: frequency and patient age distribution. Radiology 2011;258:880–8.
13. Vieira RL, Bencardino JT, Rosenberg ZS, et al. MRI features of cortical desmoid in acute knee trauma. AJR Am J Roentgenol 2011;196:424–8.

14. Hirano A, Fukubayashi T, Ishii T, et al. Magnetic resonance imaging of Osgood-Schlatter disease: the course of the disease. Skeletal Radiol 2002;31: 334–42.

15. Ogden JA. Radiology of postnatal skeletal development. X. Patella and tibial tuberosity. Skeletal Radiol 1984;11:246–57.

16. Keats T, Anderson M. Atlas of normal variants that may simulate disease. 7th edition. St Louis (MO): Mosby; 2001.

17. Dvonch VM, Bunch WH. Pattern of closure of the proximal femoral and tibial epiphyses in man. J Pediatr Orthop 1983;3:498–501.

18. Sasaki T, Ishibashi Y, Okamura Y, et al. MRI evaluation of growth plate closure rate and pattern in the normal knee joint. J Knee Surg 2002;15:72–6.

19. Kan JH, Vogelius ES, Orth RC, et al. Inferior patellar pole fragmentation in children: just a normal variant? Pediatr Radiol 2015;45:882–7.

20. Green WT Jr. Painful bipartite patellae. A report of three cases. Clin Orthop Relat Res 1975;110:197–200.

21. Dwek JR, Chung CB. The patellar extensor apparatus of the knee. Pediatr Radiol 2008;38:925–35.

22. Goergen TG, Resnick D, Greenway G, et al. Dorsal defect of the patella (DDP): a characteristic radiographic lesion. Radiology 1979;130:333–6.

23. van Holsbeeck M, Vandamme B, Marchal G, et al. Dorsal defect of the patella: concept of its origin and relationship with bipartite and multipartite patella. Skeletal Radiol 1987;16:304–11.

24. Johnson JF, Brogdon BG. Dorsal defect of the patella: incidence and distribution. AJR Am J Roentgenol 1982;139:339–40.

25. Ogden JA, McCarthy SM, Jokl P. The painful bipartite patella. J Pediatr Orthop 1982;2:263–9.

26. Sueyoshi Y, Shimozaki E, Matsumoto T, et al. Two cases of dorsal defect of the patella with arthroscopically visible cartilage surface perforations. Arthroscopy 1993;9:164–9.

27. Ho VB, Kransdorf MJ, Jelinek JS, et al. Dorsal defect of the patella: MR features. J Comput Assist Tomogr 1991;15:474–6.

28. Kwee TC, Sonneveld H, Nix M. Successful conservative management of symptomatic bilateral dorsal patellar defects presenting with cartilage involvement and bone marrow edema: MRI findings. Skeletal Radiol 2016;45:723–7.

29. Vaishya R, Chopra S, Vijay V, et al. Bipartite patella causing knee pain in young adults: a report of 5 cases. J Orthop Surg 2015;23:127–30.

30. Oohashi Y, Noriki S, Koshino T, et al. Histopathological abnormalities in painful bipartite patellae in adolescents. Knee 2006;13:189–93.

31. Oohashi Y, Oohashi Y. A concern regarding the diagnosis of injury of a bipartite patella at the lower part of the patella. Arch Orthop Trauma Surg 2011; 131:1467.

32. Collings CL. Scintigraphic findings on examination of the multipartite patella. Clin Nucl Med 1994;19: 865–6.

33. Kavanagh EC, Zoga A, Omar I, et al. MRI findings in bipartite patella. Skeletal Radiol 2007;36:209–14.

34. O'Brien J, Murphy C, Halpenny D, et al. Magnetic resonance imaging features of asymptomatic bipartite patella. Eur J Radiol 2011;78:425–9.

35. Mason RW, Moore TE, Walker CW, et al. Patellar fatigue fractures. Skeletal Radiol 1996;25:329–32.

36. Senaran H, Holden C, Dabney KW, et al. Anterior knee pain in children with cerebral palsy. J Pediatr Orthop 2007;27:12–6.

Imaging Features of Bone Tumors

Conventional Radiographs and MR Imaging Correlation

Ioan N. Gemescu, MD[a],*, Kolja M. Thierfelder, MD, MSc[b],
Christoph Rehnitz, MD[c], Marc-André Weber, MD, MSc[b]

KEYWORDS

- Bone tumors • Bone tumor semiology • Tumor matrix • X-rays • Radiographs • MR imaging

KEY POINTS

- The imaging of bone tumors often causes uncertainty, especially outside dedicated sarcoma treatment centers.
- To make the correct diagnosis, a systematic approach that addresses all semiological aspects is necessary.
- Conventional radiography is still the backbone of bone tumor diagnostics, but MR imaging also has its role.
- Although radiographs are crucial for assessing the tumor matrix and aggressiveness, MR imaging is the best modality for local staging.

Bone tumors represent a pathologic entity that can cause debates and uncertainty when considering correct diagnosis and treatment, especially outside dedicated sarcoma treatment centers. Although primary malignant bone tumors are relatively rare in Europe and the United States,[1] it is important to correctly raise the suspicion if necessary and to refer to a dedicated sarcoma treatment center, if not diagnose them accurately. Therefore, the European Society of Musculoskeletal Radiology has recently published a consensus to better guide radiologists and clinicians in evaluating bone[2] as well as soft tissue tumors.[3]

During the last decades, the role of Computed tomography (CT) and MR imaging in making the correct diagnosis has become much more important, being now the core of residency training.

Furthermore, new advanced imaging methods such as diffusion-weighted imaging, dynamic contrast enhanced MR imaging, and Dixon-type techniques have become important elements in the systemic approach to bone tumors.[4] This led to a decrease in teaching about conventional radiographs in the training of radiology residents. However, the conventional bone radiograph remains the key method in diagnosing bone tumors,[2,5] especially because it provides critical information on the aggressiveness and matrix formation of the tumor. Of note, not all semiological aspects can be observed on MR imaging in every case, often owing to marrow and soft tissue edema caused by the high aggressiveness of the tumor,[6–8] further strengthening the idea that both MR imaging and radiographs (or CT)

[a] Department of Radiology and Medical Imaging, University Emergency Hospital Bucharest, Splaiul Independentei, 169, 050098, Bucharest, Romania; [b] Institute of Diagnostic and Interventional Radiology, Pediatric Radiology and Neuroradiology, Rostock University Medical Centre, Ernst-Heydemann-Str. 6, 18057, Rostock, Germany; [c] Department of Diagnostic and Interventional Radiology, Heidelberg University Hospital, Im Neuenheimer Feld 672, 69120, Heidelberg, Germany
* Corresponding author.
E-mail address: dr.gemescu.ioan@gmail.com

Magn Reson Imaging Clin N Am 27 (2019) 753–767
https://doi.org/10.1016/j.mric.2019.07.008
1064-9689/19/© 2019 Elsevier Inc. All rights reserved.

are required for an accurate diagnosis.[9] Residents should learn to never make a diagnosis of a bone tumor solely on MR imaging without having a conventional radiograph available and MR imaging alone can cause confusion.[2,5] However, MR imaging is required for local staging as well as for detecting vessel, nerve and joint infiltration and for extracompartimental spread,[10] features that cannot be detected accurately by radiographs.

This article reviews basic bone tumor semiology, highlighting their aspects on both standard radiographs and MR imaging, pointing out each technique's advantages and disadvantages. It will help the radiologist to better recognize and understand the semiology of bone tumors. Particularly, the following aspects of bone tumors will be discussed: patient age, tumor localization, pattern of bone destruction/margins, matrix, periosteal reaction (PR), cortical involvement, size, and number.

PATIENT AGE, TUMOR LOCALIZATION, AND LESION SIZE AND NUMBER

Before characterizing a lesion, a few basic elements that should be taken into consideration to shorten the differential diagnosis list. First, patient age is extremely important. With a few exceptions, most bone tumors have a predilection for a specific age group.[5] For example, Ewing's sarcoma is most frequent in 10- to 20-year -old patients; a patient older than 40 years with a similar lesion is more likely to have a metastatic lesion or multiple myeloma.[5,11] Another rule of thumb is that a spinal lesion in patients under 30 is more likely to be benign, with the rare exceptions of Ewing's sarcoma and osteosarcoma.[12] **Table 1** depicts the general distribution of aggressive versus nonaggressive bone tumors.[2,5,13]

Tumor localization is also crucial. Most lesions have a higher incidence in the long bones of the limbs, although some are located more frequently the spine or pelvis (osteoid osteoma, lymphoma, chondrosarcoma, Ewing's sarcoma, myeloma).[13] Within the long bones, most tumors have predilection for the either diaphysis, metaphysis, or epiphysis (**Table 2**). The size of a tumor cannot reliably predict the malignancy, although lesions with a size over 6 cm are most likely malignant.[13] The criterion on size also differentiates between osteoid osteoma and osteoblastoma: there are several thresholds suggested, with 1.5 cm being the most common.[13] Furthermore, when differentiating between an enchondroma and chondrosarcoma, a lesion smaller than 2 cm is likely to be an enchondroma and a lesion of more than 5 to 6 cm is more often a chondrosarcoma.[13] In osteochondromas, the size of the cartilage cap is suggestive of malignant degeneration, with a suggested threshold of greater than 1.5 cm (**Fig. 1**).[13] Furthermore, lesions that grow over time and lesions located next to the spine and pelvis require special focus owing to the risk of malignancy and/or complications. Regarding the number of lesions, it is well-known that most bone tumors are solitary lesions. In children, multifocal lesions are associated with leukemia, eosinophilic granuloma (circumscribed form of Langerhans cell histiocytosis), or metastases. In adults, multifocal osteolytic disease usually means metastases or multiple myeloma.

Table 1
Predilection of bone tumors depending on patient age (in alphabetical order)

Age (y)	Aggressive	Nonaggressive
0–10	Eosinophilic granuloma, Ewing's sarcoma, hematologic malignancies, neuroblastoma	Aneurysmal bone cyst, eosinophilic granuloma, simple bone cyst
10–20	Adamantinoma, Ewing's sarcoma, giant cell tumor, osteosarcoma	Adamantinoma, aneurysmal bone cyst, chondroblastoma, chondromyxoid fibroma, fibrous dysplasia, nonossifying fibroma, osteochondroma, simple bone cyst
20–40	Chondrosarcoma, periosteal osteosarcoma, pleomorphic sarcoma	Enchondroma, giant cell tumor
>40	Chondrosarcoma, chordoma, lymphoma, metastases, multiple myeloma, osteosarcoma (Paget's associated), plasmacytoma, pleomorphic sarcoma	Geode or subchondral cyst, intraosseous ganglion

Adapted from Lalam R, Bloem JL, Noebauer-Huhmann IM, et al. ESSR Consensus Document for Detection, Characterization, and Referral Pathway for Tumors and Tumorlike Lesions of Bone. Semin Musculoskelet Radiol 2017;21(5):630–47.

Table 2
Differential diagnosis of bone tumors based on patient age and location (in alphabetical order)

Age (y)	Diaphysis	Metaphysis	Epiphysis
<20	Adamantinoma, eosinophilic granuloma, Ewing's sarcoma, fibrous dysplasia, lymphoma, osteoid osteoma	Aneurysmal bone cyst, chondromyxoid fibroma, enchondroma, nonossifying fibroma, osteochondroma, osteosarcoma, simple bone cyst	Chondroblastoma, infection
20–40	Adamantinoma, eosinophilic granuloma, Ewing's sarcoma, fibrous dysplasia, lymphoma, osteoid osteoma	Enchondroma, giant cell tumor, nonossifying fibroma, osteochondroma, osteosarcoma,	Giant cell tumor, osteosarcoma
>40	Fibrous dysplasia, metastases, myeloma	Lymphoma, metastases, myeloma, osteochondroma	Clear cell chondrosarcoma, Paget's disease, subchondral cyst

Adapted from Lalam R, Bloem JL, Noebauer-Huhmann IM, et al. ESSR Consensus Document for Detection, Characterization, and Referral Pathway for Tumors and Tumorlike Lesions of Bone. Semin Musculoskelet Radiol 2017;21(5):630-647; with permission.

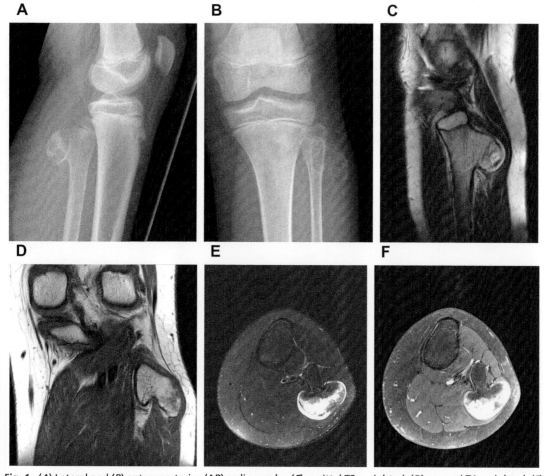

Fig. 1. (*A*) Lateral and (*B*) anteroposterior (AP) radiographs, (*C*) sagittal T2-weighted, (*D*) coronal T1-weighted, (*E*) axial T2-weighted fat-saturated, and (*F*) axial T1-weighted fat-saturated postgadolinium depicting an osteochondroma in the proximal fibula of the left lower limb. Note the continuation of cancellous bone from the fibula into the tumor and the thin sclerotic margin extending from the bone cortex, surrounding a predominantly cartilaginous matrix.

Important exceptions are enchondromatosis and fibrous dysplasia.[11]

MARGINS AND PATTERN OF BONE DESTRUCTION

The Lodwick-Madewell classification remains very useful to determine the biologic activity of a tumor by assessing the bone response on a radiograph.[14–17] Because bone response is slow, a slow-growing lesion will give the bone enough time to create solid osseous tissue around the lesion. In contrast, a fast-growing lesion will cause a more disorganized response.[14] The Lodwick-Madewell classification refers to lytic lesions and divides them into 5 subtypes: type IA (geographic with sclerotic margins), type IB (geographic without sclerotic margins), type IC (geographic with poorly defined margins), moth-eaten (type II), and permeative (type III) (**Fig. 2**).

In other words, a nonaggressive lesion presents a narrow zone of transition leaves the cortex intact and has a nonaggressive or absent PR. In contrast, an aggressive lesion results in a wide zone of transition with cortical destruction and aggressive PR.[18] Furthermore, a nonaggressive lesion usually has a geographic pattern with sclerotic rim and no soft tissue extension, whereas an aggressive lesion can have ill-defined margins, permeative destruction, and soft tissue masses.[12] Exceptions in which benign lesions can present aggressively are aneurysmal bone cysts (ABC), aggressive hemangiomas and Langerhans cell histiocytosis (eosinophilic granuloma).[12]

Type IA is assigned to geographic well-defined lesions with sclerotic margins. It is typical for a slowly or nongrowing lesion such as nonossifying fibroma, simple bone cyst, fibrous dysplasia, intraosseous ganglion, or lipoma (**Fig. 3**).[11,13,19] The sclerotic margin appears as a rim of signal void on both T1- and T2-weighted sequences. In contrast, clear cell chondrosarcomas, malignant fibrous histiocytomas, or Ewing's sarcomas may have sclerotic margins.[20] A statement should be made about the inner and outer margins of the sclerotic rim: clear-cut inner and ill-defined outer margins are usually found in osteomyelitis, eosinophilic granuloma, and avascular necrosis, whereas clear-cut inner and outer sclerotic rim borders are observed in osteomyelitis, benign tumors and occasionally in slow-growing malignant tumors, and tumor-like lesions. Furthermore, mottled sclerosis can be seen in both malignant and benign lesions.[11]

A type IB lesion is geographic and well-defined, but without a sclerotic margin. On a radiograph, type IB lesions are better detected in areas with cancellous bone. In the diaphysis, sometimes endosteal scalloping is the only sign of the existence of a type IB lesion. Usually, type IB lesions are cartilaginous or fibrous. Common benign examples are giant cell tumor (GCT), enchondroma, eosinophilic granuloma, and fibrous dysplasia,

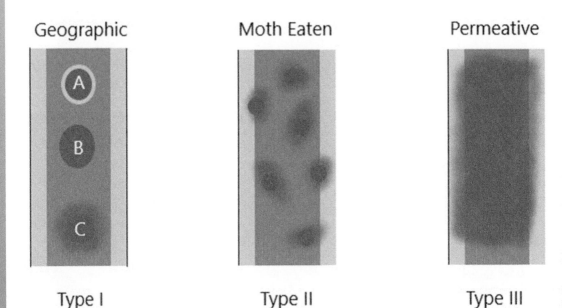

Fig. 2. Patterns of bone destruction according to the Lodwick-Madewell classification. (*Adapted from* Lalam R, Bloem JL, Noebauer-Huhmann IM, et al. ESSR Consensus Document for Detection, Characterization, and Referral Pathway for Tumors and Tumorlike Lesions of Bone. Semin Musculoskelet Radiol 2017;21(5):630-647; with permission.)

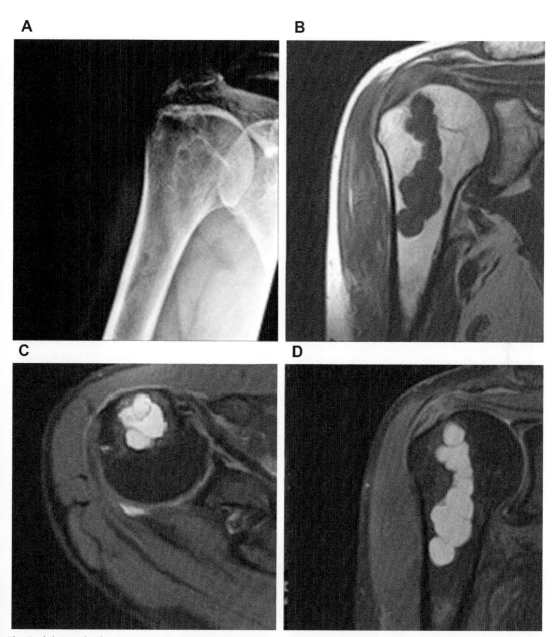

Fig. 3. (*A*) Standard anteroposterior radiograph, (*B*) coronal T1-weighted, (*C*) axial proton density-weighted fat-saturated, and (*D*) coronal proton density-weighted fat-saturated of a large ganglion cyst in the right proximal humerus of a 54-year-old man. The lesion is well-defined, homogenous, hypointense on T1-weighted imaging, and hyperintense on fluid-sensitive sequences.

although multiple myeloma and some low-grade sarcomas are included in this category.[13]

A type IC lesion is still geographic, but with indistinct margins which suggest infiltration and increased activity. Examples include GCT, enchondroma, metastasis, and sarcoma.[13]

A type II lesion has a moth-eaten pattern and represents an increased aggressiveness. It is defined by multiple ovoid areas parallel to the long axis of the bone, with a diameter of 2 to 5 mm. Type II lesions usually infiltrate rapidly and lead to an indistinct endosteal scalloping. Typical examples of this category include metastasis, multiple myeloma, osteosarcoma, chondrosarcoma, and lymphoma.[13,21]

The type III pattern, also called permeative, is the most aggressive subtype. It is represented by multiple ill-defined oval lesions, with a wide zone of transition, cortical destruction, and a soft tissue mass. It is frequently seen in malignant conditions such as metastasis, multiple myeloma, lymphoma, Ewing's sarcoma, osteosarcoma, and high-grade chondrosarcoma.[11,13]

The shape of the margin can also provide additional information, thereby shortening the differential diagnosis list. For example, a lobulated contour can be seen in malignant conditions, such as chondrosarcoma, chordoma, or adamantinoma, as well as benign lesions such as large enchondromas, chondroblastomas, and chondromyxoid fibromas (**Figs. 4** and **5**).[19,20,22,23]

Regarding the MR sequences to use when evaluating tumor margins within the bone and fatty bone marrow replacement, most authors agree that unenhanced T1-weighted sequences are most suitable, with no clinically significant underestimation or overestimation (like in the case of short-tau inversion recovery and T1-weighted fat-saturated images).[24] Within the muscles, contrast-enhanced T1-weighted fat-saturated or fluid-sensitive fat-saturated sequences are to be preferred to assess tumor margins. Furthermore, some investigators suggest to use postgadolinium sequences to assess joint involvement and T1-weighted and short-tau inversion recovery imaging for examining epiphyseal involvement.[24] It has also been shown that intraoperative MR imaging is adequate for guiding resection and can provide rapid information regarding tumor resection margins before the end of the surgery or help the pathologist focus on uncertain areas.[25]

TUMOR MATRIX

Traditionally, on a conventional radiograph, a tumor can be described as lytic or sclerotic, with lytic lesions to become only evident on radiographs when there is a minimum of about 30% lysis. MR imaging can also provide useful information when characterizing a lesion. In some cases, it can directly diagnose certain lesions such as ABC or intraosseous lipoma.[18,26] Furthermore, MR imaging is useful in detecting medullary lesions and soft tissue extension.[18,27] It is important to note that an MR imaging protocol for sarcomas must include sequences with a large field of view to evaluate the entire bone longitudinally to detect skip lesions. Postgadolinium sequences are useful for evaluating the soft tissue mass and for differentiating necrosis and hemorrhage.[18] CT is preferred over MR imaging for characterizing subtle mineralization or cortical involvement.[18,26]

With a few exceptions, bone tumors have an osteoid, a chondroid, or a fibrous matrix, which refers to the acellular material produced by the tumor cells.[12,13,20,28,29] However, there is a significant overlap and therefore more semiological aspects need to be taken into consideration when making a diagnosis.

Most musculoskeletal tumors are hyperintense on T2-weighted sequences, but there are exceptions.[30] Dense osteoblastic lesions appear hypointense on T1- and T2-weighted sequences. They include osteoid osteoma, osteoblastoma, osteoblastic metastasis, lymphoma. and osteosarcoma.[12,13,31] On a radiograph, an osseous matrix appears dense and cloud-like.[32] It is important to

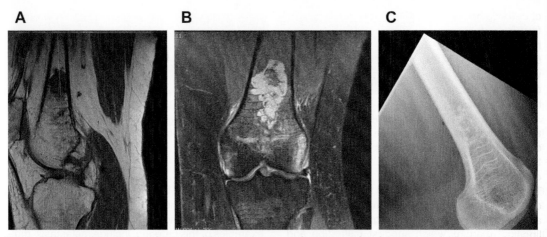

Fig. 4. (*A*) Sagittal T1-weighted image, (*B*) coronal proton density-weighted image, and (*C*) standard lateral radiograph, depicting an enchondroma in the distal femur of a 23-year-old woman. The lesion has a mixed matrix: the cartilaginous part is lytic on the radiograph, hypointense on T1-weighted image, and hyperintense on fluid-sensitive sequences; the calcified part is dense on the radiograph and hypointense on all MR imaging pulse sequences. Also note the zebra stripe sign caused by osteogenesis imperfecta in this patient. (*From* Holl N, Weber MA. [Incidental findings in recurrent patella dislocation]. Radiologe 2019;59(1):43-45; with permission.)

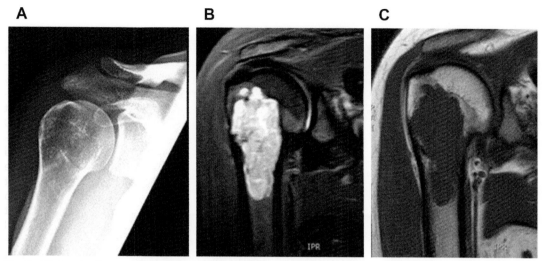

Fig. 5. (*A*) Standard anteroposterior radiograph, (*B*) coronal proton density-weighted fat-saturated image, and (*C*) coronal T1-weighted image depicting an enchondroma in the proximal humerus of a 38-year-old woman. The matrix is cartilaginous (lytic on the radiograph and hyperintense on fluid sensitive MR sequences). Note the lobulated contour and the endosteal scalloping.

note that, in the case of a mixed lesion such as osteosarcoma, the mineralized part is hypointense on T1- and T2-weighted MR imaging, while the lytic part is hypointense on T1-weighted sequences and hyperintense on T2-weighted sequences.[20] A chondroid matrix is usually hypointense in T1-weighted and hyperintense in T2-weighted sequences owing to an increased amount of water in the tumor (see **Figs. 4** and **5**).[23] Postcontrast images depict a pattern of enhancing rings and arcs.[33] Cartilage-forming tumors include both malignant and benign lesions, such as osteochondroma, chondroblastoma, chondrosarcoma, and chordoma.[12,33] Finally, a fibrous matrix is not specific on MR imaging; it has an intermediate T1 signal and a variable T2 signal. It is, however, easily observed on CT, where it typically has a ground-glass appearance owing to a mixture of collagen fibers and bone.[12,13]

Examining the calcification pattern, which appear as foci of signal void on MR imaging, can also provide clues. Chondrogenic calcifications appear as punctate comma-like, ring-like, or annular foci of signal void (see **Fig. 4**).[12,23] They are seen in enchondromas and chondrosarcomas, but can also be seen in chondromas with an amorphous and unspecific aspect.[20,34] A lipoma, however, may have central dystrophic calcifications owing to fat necrosis.[13,19] Punctate or linear calcifications can also be seen in focal osteonecrosis, at the interface between healthy and necrotic bone, but with a serpiginous pattern.[13]

Similar to calcifications, trabeculations may also help. They are either the formation of new bone or residual trabeculae. A thick and coarse pattern may be seen in chondromyxoid fibroma or desmoplastic fibroma, thin/delicate in GCT, lobulated in nonossifying fibroma, striated/radiating in hemangioma, and horizontal in ABC (**Fig. 6**).[35]

Finally, MR imaging is by far the best method to detect fluid–fluid levels (see **Fig. 6**),[36] being most evident on T2-weighted imaging. They are seen in primary and secondary ABC, but are not pathognomonic because they are sometimes encountered also in fibrous dysplasia, osteoblastoma, chondroblastoma, telangiectatic osteosarcoma, Brown tumor, GCT, and simple cysts.[36] Multiple fluid–fluid levels that occupy more than one-half of the lesion's volume can be seen in ABC, osteoblastoma, teleangiectatic osteosarcoma, Brown tumor, and GCT.[36] Frequently, fluid–fluid levels are related to a history of intralesional hemorrhage or necrosis.[36] The fluid nature can be demonstrated by the persistence of a horizontal level after the repositioning of the patient.[36,37] To summarize, fluid–fluid levels are most frequent in ABC, but can also occur as an associated lesion[36,38]; thus, it is important to look for solid areas in a cystic lesion with fluid–fluid levels and this area should be biopsied.

Furthermore, the association with aggressive aspects such as cortical destruction or Codman's triangle may suggest a malignant condition, because they are very rare in ABCs. It was also stated that fluid–fluid characteristics might vary between benign and malignant: serous fluid and

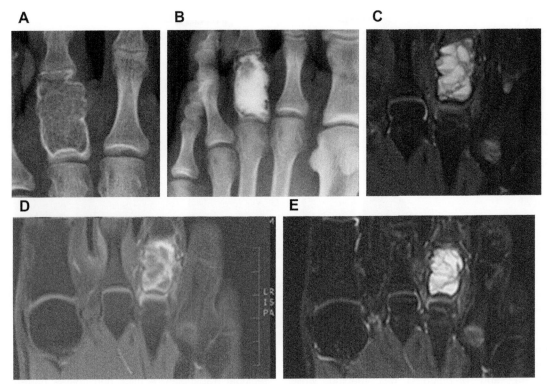

Fig. 6. (*A*) Standard preoperative radiograph, (*B*) postoperative radiograph, (*C*) coronal PD fat-saturated image, (*D*) coronal T1-weighted fat-saturated image, and (*E*) coronal short-tau inversion recovery image of an 18-year-old man with an ABC in the proximal phalanx of third digit of the foot.

old hemorrhage is found in benign lesions, while recent hemorrhage and liquefaction necrosis are more often present in malignant lesions.[36,39]

PERIOSTEAL REACTION

The periosteum is a tissue that covers almost the entire part of the bone, except those covered by cartilage. It consists of 2 layers: an outer fibrous layer and an inner cellular layer. The periosteum is attached to the bone cortex through collagen fibers that run perpendicular to the bone and are also named Sharpey fibers.[13,40] Under stimulating mechanical factors, the periosteum can produce new bone tissue.[40] Therefore, the PR results from an insult to the cortical bone, such as tumors, infections, or trauma, being also an attempt to heal the bone.[41,42] A PR may be positive (the adding of new bone, which will be discussed) or negative (the removal of bone; ie, hyperparathyroidism) and its aspect reflects the aggressiveness of the lesion.[11,13]

When assessing PRs, it is important to note that the radiologist should describe it as aggressive or nonaggressive. Although there is some overlap, an aggressive lesion is fast growing, and a nonaggressive one is slow growing.[40,41,43] As stated,

the terms aggressive or nonaggressive are to be preferred, because some benign conditions such as osteomyelitis may cause an aggressive PR and some malignant lesions can appear nonaggressive. A bilateral localization of PR indicates a systemic cause.[44] Also, it is important to note that PR is not specific to a lesion; it reflects the biological activity, intensity, duration, and aggressiveness of the trigger: usually, processes that are highly active and have a fast evolution lead to an aggressive type of PR.[11,43,45,46] It needs to be associated with other semiological aspects to make the correct diagnosis or to limit the list of differential diagnoses to a minimum.[13,43] As stated, PR should be classified into nonaggressive and aggressive, with each being made of several subtypes.

Regarding imaging, the elevated periosteum is only visible after mineralization, which happens between 10 and 21 days after injury of the periosteum.[13,43,46] Usually, MR imaging is used for local staging of a bone tumor and CT scanning is the best modality for body staging, taking into account the fact that CT scans can also detect subtle bony changes faster than conventional radiographs.[43,45,46] Although normal periosteum may not be visible on MR imaging, PR is viewed as low signal lines on pulse sequences, such as T2-weighted fat-saturated and short-tau inversion recovery.[43,45–48] It was also demonstrated that detecting and characterizing PR with MR imaging has a high specificity, a high negative predictive value, and a moderate sensitivity. In addition, there was almost perfect interobserver agreement for detecting the changes on MR imaging and on radiographs.[45] Although 1 study observed no difference between MR imaging and conventional radiographs regarding their ability to classify PR,[45] another study found that MR imaging is superior to radiographs for the detection of PR in osteomyelitis.[49]

The first category of PR is represented by thin, solid, thick irregular, and septated forms with the solid form being the most frequent. Besides some tumors, these can be associated with osteogenesis imperfecta, Caffey disease (infantile cortical hyperostosis), hypervitaminosis A, fluorosis, psoriatic arthritis, hypertrophic osteoarthropathy, and thyroid acropathy.[41,44,50] The aggressive forms are the laminated, spiculated (hair-on-end and sunburst), disorganized, and interrupted (Codman's triangle).[40,41,44,51] Interruptions appear as the result of tumor extension that prevents the formation of new bone, or through osteoclastic activity caused by pressure and hyperemia.[13,46]

The recent bone tumor consensus published by the European Society of Musculoskeletal Radiology divides PR into aggressive (smooth, solid) and nonaggressive (irregular, interrupted, complex).[2] In **Fig. 7**, the different types of PR are illustrated.

The *solid* reaction can be thick or thin; it is stable over time and reflects the ossification of multiple layers of periosteal bone in response to a slowly growing benign process (such as osteoid osteoma, or a healing fracture) and is rarely malignant[11,13,41,46] (**Figs. 8** and **9**).

The laminated PR can be further subdivided into single layered and multilayered. The single layered laminated PR appears as a result of hyperemia, which causes the inactive fibroblasts to become osteoclasts. This hyperemia results in a single layer of bone at 1 to 2 mm from the cortex, separated by edema, vessels, blood, pus, or tumor, and appearing as a line of signal void near the cortex.[13,46] Between the cortex and the periosteum, the tissue is usually T1-weighted isointense, T2-weighted hyperintense, and enhances after gadolinium administration.[46] The single layer laminated PR is frequently seen in benign processes such as osteomyelitis, healing or stress fracture and eosinophilic granuloma, although it was also reported in malignant cases such as Ewing's sarcoma.[13,16,52]

The multilayered laminated PR, also known as onion skin, is defined as the existence of numerous layers of parallel and concentric bone, separated by dilated vessels and connective tissue.[43,46] Although the underlying mechanism is not entirely known, it has been suggested that it either forms as a result of repeated injury to the underlying bone or as a result from hyperemia that extends beyond the first layer of PR, thereby stimulating new osteoblastic formation.[13,46] It can be present in benign lesions, such as osteomyelitis, chondroblastoma, ABC, or stress fractures, but also malignant conditions such as Ewing's sarcoma and osteosarcoma, making it an intermediate PR in terms of aggressiveness[40,41,43,52–54] (**Fig. 10**).

The spiculated PR can be subdivided into perpendicular (or hair-on-end) and divergent (sunburst). They develop along vascular channels and Sharpey fibers, which become stretched by cellular infiltration.[13,43,46] The direction of the spiculae indicate the direction of tumor growth, although this type of PR is not exclusive to neoplasms.[46]

In the hair-on-end PR, the spicules are parallel to each other and perpendicular to the cortex. They are long and thin, forming along blood vessels oriented radially. The spicules themselves are not neoplastic, but merely originate from the ossifications along Sharpey fibers or vascular channels. They are longer at the center and decrease in height as they progress toward the periphery. The space between them may later contain tumor tissue.[13,43,46,52] This form of PR can be seen in cases of thalassemia and other chronic anemias in the calvarium, in cases of osteomyelitis or rarely in healing fractures where the spicules are short and thick. However, they are more common in osteosarcoma, Ewing's sarcoma, hematologic malignancies such as leukemia (**Fig. 11**) and rarely in metastasis, having a thick and irregular aspect.[11,13,46,52]

The sunburst pattern is considered the most aggressive type of PR. It consists of a combination of radial bands of PR and osteoid matrix caused by the tumor.[13,51] It is usually present around malignant lesions and suggestive for osteosarcoma, although not pathognomonic.[40,51] It can also be encountered in aggressive blastic metastases (eg, in prostate cancer, breast cancer, children's retinoblastoma and leukemia) and occasionally in aggressive forms of osteoblastoma.[13,43,46,55]

The interrupted PR pattern reflects an infiltrating aggressive process. It can be single or multilamellated or spiculated. The Codman's

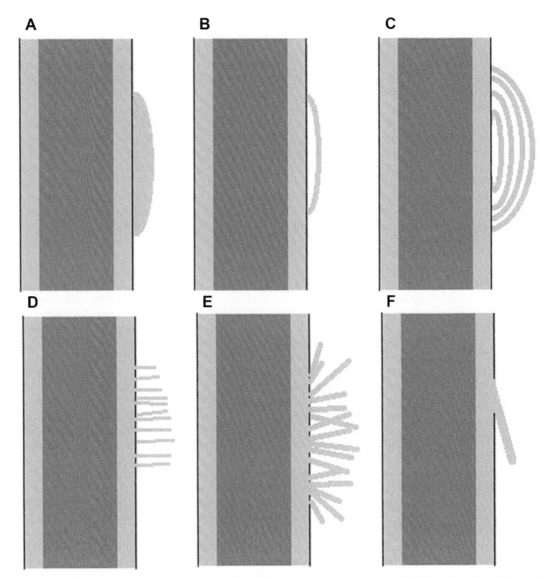

Fig. 7. Illustration of the different types of PR: (*A*) solid, (*B*) laminated single layered, (*C*) laminated multilayered, (*D*) hair-on-end, (*E*) sunburst and (*F*) Codman's triangle. (*From* Lalam R, Bloem JL, Noebauer-Huhmann IM, et al. ESSR Consensus Document for Detection, Characterization, and Referral Pathway for Tumors and Tumorlike Lesions of Bone. Semin Musculoskelet Radiol 2017;21(5):630-647; with permission.)

triangle is the classical pattern of interrupted PR, being a form of infiltrating lamellar PR.[43] The periosteum is elevated by pus, hemorrhage, or the tip of the tumor.[5,46] It usually indicates a malignant process such as osteosarcoma, Ewing's sarcoma or metastasis, or rarely benign lesions such as ABC, osteomyelitis, trauma, and subperiosteal hematoma.[13,43,46]

These forms of PR can also have a disorganized appearance. It is usually associated with very aggressive cases of osteosarcoma or the complication of a benign or malignant lesion by infection or fracture.[46]

CORTICAL INVOLVEMENT

Cortical bone is made out of osseous tissue around a Haversian canal. It is surrounded by an inner and an outer fibrovascular layer: the endosteum and the periosteum. The cortical appearance on MR imaging is a low signal on pulse sequences.[35] When involved, the cortex may appear gray and mottled on both spin echo and inversion recovery sequences, called dirty cortical bone[7] (**Fig. 12**).

There are several aspects to be taken into consideration when discussing cortical involvement,

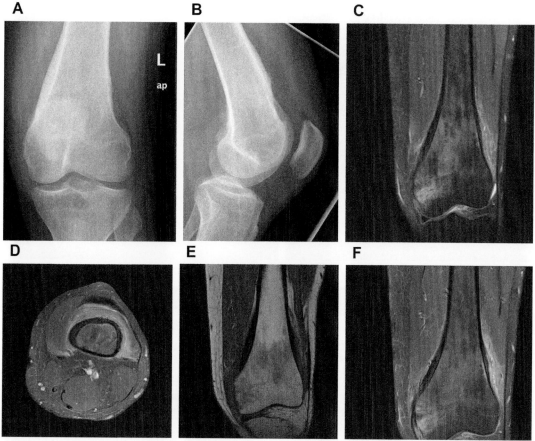

Fig. 8. (*A*) Anteroposterior and (*B*) lateral radiographs, (*C*) coronal proton density-weighted fat-saturated image, (*D*) axial T1-weighted fat-saturated postgadolinium image, (*E*) coronal T1-weighted image, and (*F*) T1-weighted fat-saturated image depicting a solid PR at the medial side of the femur in a patient with osteomyelitis.

namely, scalloping, thickening, and destruction/penetration.

Scalloping represents the erosion of the bone as a result of a lesion.[56] Most commonly, it is an endosteal scalloping owing to a medullary lesion. It is seen in both malignant and benign conditions such as enchondroma, chondrosarcoma, and fibrous dysplasia as typical examples (see

Fig. 5).[5,19,20,56,57] However, outer scalloping has also been described as a result of a periosteal osteosarcoma or juxtacortical chondrosarcoma.[20] The degree of endosteal scalloping can, however, indicate if a lesion is more likely to be benign or malignant.[34] When uncertain between an enchondroma and a low-grade chondrosarcoma, an erosion of more than two-thirds of the cortical

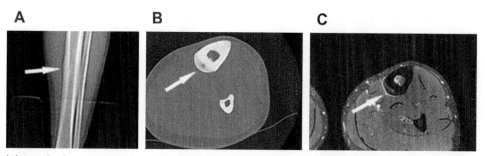

Fig. 9. (*A*) Standard anteroposterior radiograph, (*B*) axial CT scan, and (*C*) axial proton density-weighted fat-saturated image of an osteoid osteoma in the left tibia of a 17-year-old man. Note the lucent nidus (*arrows*) surrounded by solid PR.

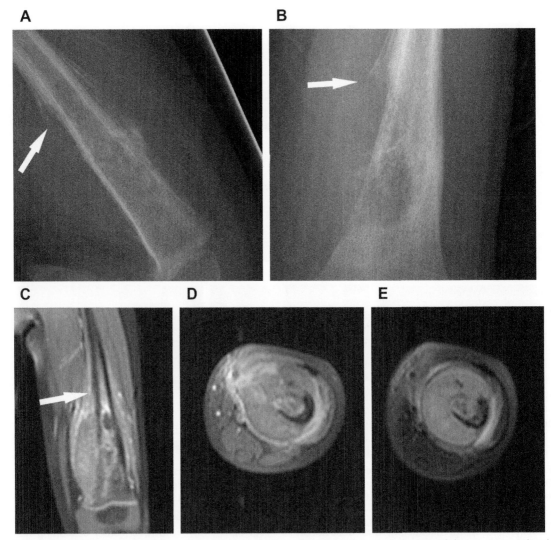

Fig. 10. (*A*, *B*) Conventional lateral and anteroposterior radiographs, (*C*) coronal postgadolinium T1-weighted fat-saturated image, (*D*) axial postgadolinium T1-weighted fat-saturated image, and (*E*) axial T2-weighted fat-saturated image of an Ewing's sarcoma in the left femur of a 3-year-old boy. Note the multilayered (onion skin) PR being interrupted by the tumor that extends into the soft tissues; this process also leads to the appearance of a Codman's triangle (*arrows*) at the upper border of the tumor.

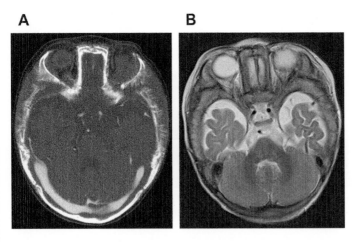

Fig. 11. (*A*) Axial contrast-enhanced CT scan and (*B*) axial T2-weighted MR imaging in a 6-month-old boy with acute undifferentiated leukemia. Note the spiculated, thin PR of the skull.

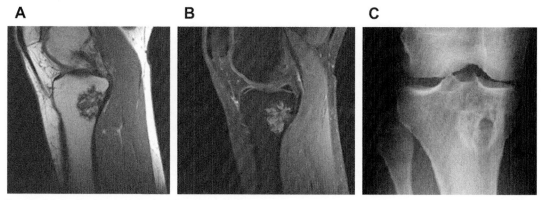

Fig. 12. (*A*) Sagittal T1-weighted, (*B*) sagittal proton density-weighted fat-saturated, and (*C*) anteroposterior radiographs of a nonossifying fibroma in the proximal tibia of a 23-year-old woman. The lesion has a mixed matrix, thin trabeculations, and sclerotic margins. There is a partial destruction of the adjacent cortex, which appears slightly more hyperintense (dirty cortex sign).

thickness is more likely to be the cause of the latter.[22,58]

Cortical thickening can be seen in various types of osteosarcoma, central chondrosarcoma, Ewing's sarcoma, osteochondroma, and osteoid osteoma.[20,59,60] It is a sign that favors chondrosarcoma versus an enchondroma, being a sign of malignancy in long bones.[61] Furthermore, the cortex can also be thinned, as in the case of a clear cell chondrosarcoma or a hemangioendothelioma.[20]

Cortical destruction is a sign of malignancy in both short and long bones.[61] In Lodwick's classification, a partial or no cortical penetration would fall into grades IA or IB, while a total penetration would be type IC or higher.[15,16] It can be seen in numerous types of lesions, the most notable ones being nonossifying fibroma (see **Fig. 12**), fibrous dysplasia, ABC, GCT, Ewing's sarcoma, and osteoblastoma.[20,52,53,57,58,60,62] Regarding the differentiation between an enchondroma or a chondosarcoma or atypical cartilaginous tumor; cortical destruction is more likely to be seen in the second category.[34,57,58] It should also be stated that cortical destruction in association with a soft tissue mass is a sign of a sarcoma until proven otherwise.[20]

SUMMARY

Bone tumors continue to represent a challenging field of musculoskeletal radiology. To make a successful diagnosis, one must approach the case systematically, assessing each semiological aspect. Conventional radiography is the backbone of bone tumor diagnostics, but MR imaging also has its defined role. Essentially, radiographs are important for assessing the tumor matrix and aggressiveness, whereas MR imaging is the best modality for local staging.

REFERENCES

1. Stiller CA, Trama A, Serraino D, et al. Descriptive epidemiology of sarcomas in Europe: report from the RARECARE project. Eur J Cancer 2013;49(3):684–95.
2. Lalam R, Bloem JL, Noebauer-Huhmann IM, et al. ESSR consensus document for detection, characterization, and referral pathway for tumors and Tumorlike lesions of bone. Semin Musculoskelet Radiol 2017;21(5):630–47.
3. Noebauer-Huhmann IM, Weber MA, Lalam R, et al. Soft tissue tumors in adults: ESSR-approved guidelines for diagnostic imaging. Semin Musculoskelet Radiol 2015;19(5):e1.
4. Weber MA, Lalam R. Bone and soft tissue tumors. Semin Musculoskelet Radiol 2019;23(1):1–2.
5. Miller TT. Bone tumors and tumorlike conditions: analysis with conventional radiography. Radiology 2008;246(3):662–74.
6. Seeger LL, Dungan DH, Eckardt JJ, et al. Nonspecific findings on MR imaging. The importance of correlative studies and clinical information. Clin Orthop Relat Res 1991;(270):306–12.
7. Hayes CW, Conway WF, Sundaram M. Misleading aggressive MR imaging appearance of some benign musculoskeletal lesions. Radiographics 1992;12(6):1119–34 [discussion: 1135–6].
8. Ma LD, Frassica FJ, Scott WW Jr, et al. Differentiation of benign and malignant musculoskeletal tumors: potential pitfalls with MR imaging. Radiographics 1995;15(2):349–66.
9. Brown KT, Kattapuram SV, Rosenthal DI. Computed tomography analysis of bone tumors: patterns of cortical destruction and soft tissue extension. Skeletal Radiol 1986;15(6):448–51.
10. Holzapfel K, Regler J, Baum T, et al. Local staging of soft-tissue sarcoma: emphasis on assessment of neurovascular encasement-value of MR imaging in 174 confirmed cases. Radiology 2015;275(2):501–9.

11. Priolo F, Cerase A. The current role of radiography in the assessment of skeletal tumors and tumor-like lesions. Eur J Radiol 1998;27(Suppl 1):S77–85.

12. Rodallec MH, Feydy A, Larousserie F, et al. Diagnostic imaging of solitary tumors of the spine: what to do and say. Radiographics 2008;28(4): 1019–41.

13. Nichols RE, Dixon LB. Radiographic analysis of solitary bone lesions. Radiol Clin North Am 2011;49(6): 1095–114, v.

14. Madewell JE, Ragsdale BD, Sweet DE. Radiologic and pathologic analysis of solitary bone lesions. Part I: internal margins. Radiol Clin North Am 1981; 19(4):715–48.

15. Lodwick GS, Wilson AJ, Farrell C, et al. Determining growth rates of focal lesions of bone from radiographs. Radiology 1980;134(3):577–83.

16. Lodwick GS, Wilson AJ, Farrell C, et al. Estimating rate of growth in bone lesions: observer performance and error. Radiology 1980;134(3):585–90.

17. Caracciolo JT, Temple HT, Letson GD, et al. A modified Lodwick-Madewell grading system for the evaluation of Lytic bone lesions. AJR Am J Roentgenol 2016;207(1):150–6.

18. Stacy GS, Mahal RS, Peabody TD. Staging of bone tumors: a review with illustrative examples. AJR Am J Roentgenol 2006;186(4):967–76.

19. Motamedi K, Seeger LL. Benign bone tumors. Radiol Clin North Am 2011;49(6):1115–34, v.

20. Rajiah P, Ilaslan H, Sundaram M. Imaging of primary malignant bone tumors (nonhematological). Radiol Clin North Am 2011;49(6):1135–61, v.

21. Weber MA, Papakonstantinou O, Nikodinovska VV, et al. Ewing's sarcoma and primary osseous lymphoma: spectrum of imaging appearances. Semin Musculoskelet Radiol 2019;23(1):36–57.

22. Bierry G, Kerr DA, Nielsen GP, et al. Enchondromas in children: imaging appearance with pathological correlation. Skeletal Radiol 2012;41(10):1223–9.

23. Afonso PD, Isaac A, Villagran JM. Chondroid tumors as incidental findings and differential diagnosis between enchondromas and low-grade chondrosarcomas. Semin Musculoskelet Radiol 2019;23(1):3–18.

24. Putta T, Gibikote S, Madhuri V, et al. Accuracy of various MRI sequences in determining the tumour margin in musculoskeletal tumours. Pol J Radiol 2016;81:540–8.

25. Vandergugten S, Traore SY, Cartiaux O, et al. MRI evaluation of resection margins in bone tumour surgery. Sarcoma 2014;2014:967848.

26. Balach T, Stacy GS, Peabody TD. The clinical evaluation of bone tumors. Radiol Clin North Am 2011; 49(6):1079–93, v.

27. Pettersson H, Gillespy T 3rd, Hamlin DJ, et al. Primary musculoskeletal tumors: examination with MR imaging compared with conventional modalities. Radiology 1987;164(1):237–41.

28. Flanagan AM, Lindsay D. A diagnostic approach to bone tumours. Pathology 2017;49(7):675–87.

29. Perera JR, Saifuddin A, Pollock R. Management of benign bone tumours. Orthopaedics and Trauma 2017;31(3):151–60.

30. Papakonstantinou O, Isaac A, Dalili D, et al. T2-weighted hypointense tumors and tumor-like lesions. Semin Musculoskelet Radiol 2019;23(1):58–75.

31. Cerase A, Priolo F. Skeletal benign bone-forming lesions. Eur J Radiol 1998;27(Suppl 1):S91–7.

32. Sweet DE, Madewell JE, Ragsdale BD. Radiologic and pathologic analysis of solitary bone lesions. Part III: matrix patterns. Radiol Clin North Am 1981;19(4):785–814.

33. Fayad LM, Ahlawat S, Khan MS, et al. Chondrosarcomas of the hands and feet: a case series and systematic review of the literature. Eur J Radiol 2015; 84(10):2004–12.

34. Jamshidi K, Mirzaei A. Long bone enchondroma vs. low-grade chondrosarcoma: current concepts review. Shafa Orthooedic Journal 2016;4(1):e9155.

35. Resnick DL. Bone and joint imaging. Philadelphia: Elsevier; 2005.

36. Van Dyck P, Vanhoenacker FM, Vogel J, et al. Prevalence, extension and characteristics of fluid-fluid levels in bone and soft tissue tumors. Eur Radiol 2006;16(12):2644–51.

37. Ehara S, Sone M, Tamakawa Y, et al. Fluid-fluid levels in cavernous hemangioma of soft tissue. Skeletal Radiol 1994;23(2):107–9.

38. O'Donnell P, Saifuddin A. The prevalence and diagnostic significance of fluid-fluid levels in focal lesions of bone. Skeletal Radiol 2004;33(6):330–6.

39. Tsai JC, Dalinka MK, Fallon MD, et al. Fluid-fluid level: a nonspecific finding in tumors of bone and soft tissue. Radiology 1990;175(3):779–82.

40. Ragsdale BD, Madewell JE, Sweet DE. Radiologic and pathologic analysis of solitary bone lesions. Part II: periosteal reactions. Radiol Clin North Am 1981;19(4):749–83.

41. Rana RS, Wu JS, Eisenberg RL. Periosteal reaction. AJR Am J Roentgenol 2009;193(4):W259–72.

42. Kriss VM, Kindle JJ. Periosteal reaction in children. Contemp Diagn Radiol 1999;22(11).

43. Nogueira-Barbosa MH, de Sá JL, Trad CS, et al. Magnetic resonance imaging in the evaluation of periosteal reactions. Radiol Bras 2010;43(4): 266–71.

44. Chen EM, Masih S, Chow K, et al. Periosteal reaction: review of various patterns associated with specific pathology. Contemp Diagn Radiol 2012; 35(17):1–5.

45. de Sa Neto JL, Simão MN, Crema MD, et al. Diagnostic performance of magnetic resonance imaging in the assessment of periosteal reactions in bone sarcomas using conventional radiography as the reference. Radiol Bras 2017;50(3):176–81.

46. Wenaden AE, Szyszko TA, Saifuddin A. Imaging of periosteal reactions associated with focal lesions of bone. Clin Radiol 2005;60(4):439–56.

47. Fayad LM, Jacobs MA, Wang X, et al. Musculoskeletal tumors: how to use anatomic, functional, and metabolic MR techniques. Radiology 2012;265(2): 340–56.

48. Steiner GC, Schweitzer ME, Kenan S, et al. Chondrosarcoma of the femur with histology-imaging correlation of tumor growth–preliminary observations concerning periosteal new bone formation and soft tissue extension. Bull NYU Hosp Jt Dis 2011;69(2): 158–67.

49. Spaeth HJ, Chandnani VP, Beltran J, et al. Magnetic resonance imaging detection of early experimental periostitis. Comparison of magnetic resonance imaging, computed tomography, and plain radiography with histopathologic correlation. Invest Radiol 1991;26(4):304–8.

50. Taneja S, Jain R, Nadri G, et al. Tibial periosteal reaction. Pediatric Oncall Journal 2014;12(3):92.

51. Gross M, Stevens K. Sunburst periosteal reaction in osteogenic sarcoma. Pediatr Radiol 2005;35: 647–8.

52. McCarville MB, Chen JY, Coleman JL, et al. Distinguishing osteomyelitis from Ewing sarcoma on radiography and MRI. AJR Am J Roentgenol 2015; 205(3):640–50 [quiz: 651].

53. Gongidi P, Jasti S, Rafferty W, et al. Adult intramedullary ewing sarcoma of the proximal hip. Case Rep Radiol 2014;2014:916935.

54. Freeman AK, Sumathi VP, Jeys L. Primary malignant tumours of the bone. Surgery 2017;36(1):27–34.

55. Lehrer HZ, Maxfield WS, Nice CM. The periosteal "sunburst" pattern in metastatic bone tumors. Am J Roentgenol Radium Ther Nucl Med 1970;108(1): 154–61.

56. Ridley WE, Xiang H, Han J, et al. Endosteal scalloping: pattern of bone erosion. J Med Imaging Radiat Oncol 2018;62(Suppl 1):131–2.

57. Errani C, Tsukamoto S, Ciani G, et al. Risk factors for local recurrence from atypical cartilaginous tumour and enchondroma of the long bones. Eur J Orthop Surg Traumatol 2017;27(6):805–11.

58. Douis H, Parry M, Vaiyapuri S, et al. What are the differentiating clinical and MRI-features of enchondromas from low-grade chondrosarcomas? Eur Radiol 2018;28(1):398–409.

59. Okada K, Hasegawa T, Tateishi U, et al. Dedifferentiated chondrosarcoma with telangiectatic osteosarcoma-like features. J Clin Pathol 2006;59(11): 1200–2.

60. Levine SM, Lambiase RE, Petchprapa CN. Cortical lesions of the tibia: characteristic appearances at conventional radiography. Radiographics 2003; 23(1):157–77.

61. Kendell SD, Collins MS, Adkins MC, et al. Radiographic differentiation of enchondroma from low-grade chondrosarcoma in the fibula. Skeletal Radiol 2004;33(8):458–66.

62. Cui J, Chen H, Hao D, et al. Imaging features of primary leiomyosarcoma of bone. Int J Clin Exp Med 2017;10(7):10846–51.

Radiographic/MR Imaging Correlation of Soft Tissues

Filip M. Vanhoenacker, MD, PhD[a],*, Frederik Bosmans, MD[b]

KEYWORDS

- Radiography • MR imaging • Soft tissue musculoskeletal disease

KEY POINTS

- Plain films have a low sensitivity in the diagnosis of soft tissue tumors or tumor-like conditions, but the presence of intralesional soft tissue calcification may be useful for tissue specific diagnosis.
- Mineralization in myositis ossificans follows a time-dependent centripetal pattern from the periphery toward the center. The mineralization pattern in extraskeletal osteosarcoma (ESO) is more amorphous and occurs from the center to the periphery.
- MR imaging and histology may simulate ESO in the early stage of myositis ossificans. Biopsy should be avoided in the early stage of myositis ossificans.
- The use of fat suppression may decrease conspicuity of accessory muscles.
- The presence of intralesional air may enhance the specificity of gas-forming infection and of necrotizing soft tissue infections.

INTRODUCTION

Because of its high soft tissue contrast and exquisite anatomic resolution, MR imaging is regarded as the imaging modality of choice for evaluation of musculoskeletal soft tissue lesions.

However, most of these abnormalities may be suspected on conventional radiography (CR) by analysis of subtle or indirect signs. These signs are well recognized by experienced radiologists, but are less known and often forgotten by young colleagues who are currently well trained in interpretation of MR imaging. As CR remains often the initial imaging tool in the evaluation of many musculoskeletal disorders, it is important to remember these signs as potential markers of relevant soft tissue pathology. Correct identification and interpretation of soft tissue signs on CR may be helpful to select patients who

need to be referred for further MR imaging. On the other hand, in certain scenarios, meticulous analysis of plain film findings may even lead to a more specific tissue diagnosis of soft tissue abnormalities, such as demonstration of phleboliths in slow-flow vascular malformation or the presence of peripheral calcifications in myositis ossificans.

Therefore, correlation of MR imaging findings and radiographic findings is highly recommended, as the information derived from both imaging techniques is often complementary.

The aim of this article is to remind readers of the most valuable signs that may suggest the presence of soft tissue pathology on CR and to discuss their diagnostic strength compared with MR imaging findings.

Discussion of musculoskeletal soft tissue diseases on plain films will be done along with the

Disclosure Statement: The authors have nothing to disclose.
a Department of Radiology, AZ Sint-Maarten Mechelen, University Hospital Antwerp, Ghent University, Liersesteenweg 435, Mechelen 2800, Belgium; b Department of Radiology, AZ Sint-Maarten Mechelen, University Hospital Antwerp, Liersesteenweg 435, Mechelen 2800, Belgium
* Corresponding author.
E-mail address: Filip.vanhoenacker@telenet.be

Magn Reson Imaging Clin N Am 27 (2019) 769–789
https://doi.org/10.1016/j.mric.2019.07.007

radiographic density of its major macroscopic components (**Table 1**).

LESIONS CONTAINING SOFT TISSUE MINERALIZATION

Mineralization in the soft tissues may occur in a large spectrum of disorders including congenital, metabolic, endocrine, traumatic, and parasitic infections. Mineralization is often far better identified on plain films or computed tomography (CT) than on MR imaging. In addition, meticulous analysis of the pattern of intralesional calcification or ossification may be helpful for a more tissue-specific diagnosis of a soft tissue lesion.[1,2]

Basic Calcium Phosphate Crystal Deposition Disease

Basic calcium phosphate (BCP) crystal deposition disease consists of BCP crystal deposition in either periarticular soft tissues or less frequently the joints. It is also designated as hydroxyapatite deposition disease (HADD), as the deposits are predominantly composed of hydroxyapatite and less commonly of tricalcium phosphate and octacalcium phosphate.[3,4]

Calcific tendinopathy of the shoulder tendons is the most common manifestation, accounting for 60% of cases, followed by involvement of the tendons of the hip, knee, elbow, wrist, and hand.[4] Virtually any tendon can be involved. Other periarticular tissues such as bursae (**Fig. 1**), capsule, and ligaments may be also involved. The disease can be divided in a precalcific, calcific, and postcalcific stages, of which the calcific stage is further subdivided into formative, resting, and resorptive phases.[5]

In the formative and resting phases, dense, homogeneous and well-defined calcium deposits are seen on plain radiographs. Calcifications in the formative and resting stages are often more difficult to characterize on MR imaging, because of the low contrast with surrounding tendons.

Patients are often asymptomatic at these stages or may present with only a mild discomfort. On the contrary, acute pain typically accompanies the resorptive phase, in which deposits migrate in surrounding tissues, bursae, joints, or even bones. On radiographs, the calcification becomes fluffy, ill-defined, and less dense, or may even become invisible.[3] Associated bone erosions, bone marrow edema on MR imaging, intraosseous migration, or increased uptake on nuclear medicine studies may mimic a tumor or infection.[6,7] The clue to the correct diagnosis is the location of the lesion at its specific tendon insertion at the bone and correlation of MR imaging with the presence of calcification on plain radiographs. A targeted CT scan may be useful to demonstrate minute calcifications and bone erosions in complex anatomic areas such as the pelvis (**Fig. 2**).

Symptomatic BCP in the capsule and ligaments may be associated with adjacent bone marrow and soft tissue edema on MR imaging, whereas the underlying calcification is better seen on corresponding radiographs (**Fig. 3**).

Calcific tendinopathy of the longus colli is a specific spinal manifestation of BCP disease and may clinically and on MR imaging mimic a retropharyngeal abscess. The identification of calcifications in the longus colli underneath the anterior arc of C1 is the clue to the correct diagnosis (**Fig. 4**).[8–10]

Calcium Pyrophosphate Dihydrate Crystal Deposition

Calcium pyrophosphate dihydrate (CPPD) crystal deposition disease refers to deposition of CPPD in hyaline cartilages and fibrocartilage of the joints (menisci, acetabular labrum, pubic symphysis, and intervertebral discs), but also in other soft tissue such as ligaments, capsules, and tendons. Both articular and periarticular deposition may be complicated by subsequent inflammation and may result in CPPD arthropathy or painful tophaceous pseudogout of the soft tissues, respectively. In the soft tissues, radiographs show a more linear and/or stratified appearance compared with BCP (HADD), and it should be noted that CPPD crystal deposition occurs in an older population.[3] Overall, the use of MR imaging for evaluation of CPPD of the soft tissues is disappointing or may mimic other soft tissue lesions.[11] On MR imaging, CPPD deposits are of low signal on all pulse sequences. Like other calcifications, they are often difficult to detect and characterize on MR imaging. Gradient-echo

Table 1	
Radiographic grayscale of macroscopic components occurring in soft tissue lesions	
Grayscale	**Soft Tissue Component**
Black	Air
Dark gray	Fat
Light gray	Water and most other soft tissue
White (moderate)	Calcification, ossification
White (marked)	Metal, iron

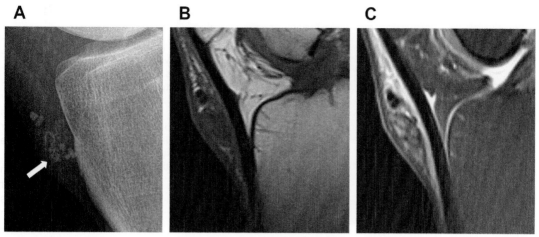

Fig. 1. Chronic calcified infrapatellar bursitis. (*A*) Lateral radiograph of the right knee shows multiple amorphous calcifications in a prepatellar soft tissue mass (*white arrow*). (*B*) Sagittal T1-weighted imaging and (*C*) sagittal fat-suppressed T2-weight imaging. The calcifications are hypointense on both pulse sequences, but the number and extent of the calcifications are less conspicuous on MR imaging than on plain films.

sequences may enhance their conspicuity.[12] As meniscal chondrocalcinosis can mimic a meniscal tear, correlation of radiographs with all MR imaging is important to avoid overdiagnosis[3] (**Fig. 5**).

Calcifications involving the transverse ligament and adjacent to the odontoid process, designated as the crowned dens syndrome, comprise a spinal manifestation of CPPD. Calcifications are often an incidental finding on imaging, but they may be associated with fever, neck pain, and stiffness, and may even mimic meningitis clinically.[3,13]

Traction Fibro-Osteosis at the Insertion of Tendons at the Bones

Bone production at the insertion of tendons at the bones is common at different locations, and is generally found incidentally on imaging. It is readily detected on plain films but is often more difficult to detect on corresponding MR imaging unless it is

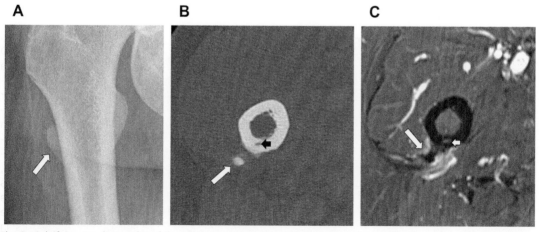

Fig. 2. Calcifying tendinopathy of the gluteus maximus in a patient presenting with pain at the right upper leg. A metastasis at the right femur was suspected on bone scintigraphy. (*A*) AP radiograph of the right upper leg showing calcification adjacent to the posterolateral cortex of the right femoral diaphysis (*white arrow*). (*B*) Axial CT image of the right femur confirms calcifications (*long white arrow*) with heterogeneous density at the distal insertion of the gluteus maximus at the linea aspera. Note a small intracortical lucency (*short black arrow*). (*C*) Axial fat-suppressed T1-weighted imaging after administration of gadolinium contrast. There is thickening and heterogenous enhancement of the tendon (*long white arrow*) and a subtle intracortical focus of enhancement in the posterior femoral cortex (*short white arrow*).

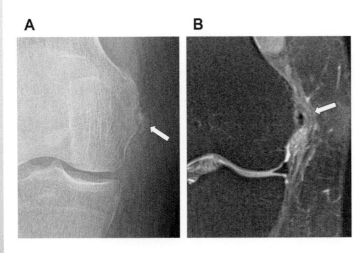

Fig. 3. BCP deposition in the medial collateral ligament of the knee with surrounding inflammation. (*A*) AP radiograph of the left knee showing irregular delineated calcifications adjacent to the medial femoral condyle (*white arrow*). (*B*) Coronal fat-suppressed T2-weighted imaging. Foci of low signal anterior to the femoral insertion of the medial collateral ligament with surrounding strands of high signal indicating inflammatory reaction (*white arrow*).

accompanied by surrounding inflammation or if contains fatty bone marrow (**Fig. 6**).

Collagen Vascular Disease

Soft tissue calcifications are also a typical manifestation in collagen vascular disorders such as progressive systemic sclerosis, systemic lupus erythematosus, dermatomyositis, and polymyositis. Calcifications associated with progressive systemic sclerosis involve the hands and wrists. In systemic lupus erythematosus (SLE), they are preferentially located in the lower extremity, whereas calcifications in polymyositis and dermatomyositis typically affect the fasciae and subcutaneous tissues.[14,15]

Scleroderma-associated calcinosis is usually seen in the finger tips and around the synovial joints of the hands, knees, and elbows.[16]

Patients with scleroderma may present with 1 or more components of the CREST (calcinosis- Raynaud - esophageal dysfunction - sclerodactyly-teleangiectases) syndrome.[16]

Mixed connective tissue disease consists of a combination of SLE, scleroderma, and polymyositis. On MR imaging, calcified lesions are of low signal intensity, both on T1- as on T2-weighted images, and show no contrast uptake after administration of gadolinium contrast[15] (**Fig. 7**). Active inflammation may be of high signal intensity on fluid-sensitive sequences.

Osteochondromatosis

Synovial osteochondromatosis (SC) is characterized by the formation of numerous metaplastic cartilaginous or osteocartilaginous nodules of

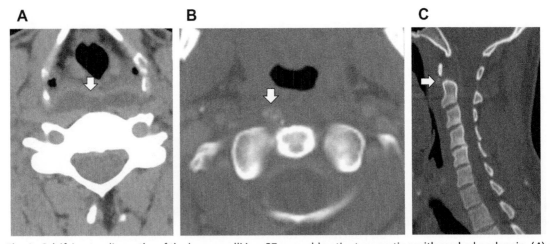

Fig. 4. Calcifying tendinopathy of the longus colli in a 37-year-old patient presenting with marked neck pain. (*A*) Axial CT (soft tissue window) image showing a retropharyngeal collection (*white arrow*). (*B*) Axial and (*C*) sagittal reformatted CT (bone window) shows amorphous calcifications underneath the anterior arc of C1 at the attachment of the right m. longus colli. The calcification is ill-defined, which indicates an acute inflammatory reaction (*white arrows*).

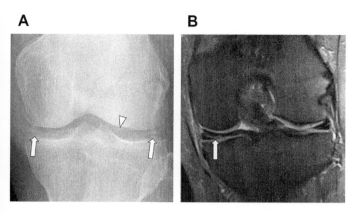

Fig. 5. Chondrocalcinosis mimicking a meniscus tear. (A) AP radiograph of the left knee showing chondrocalcinosis in the medial and lateral meniscus (*white arrows*) and the articular cartilage of the lateral femoral condyle (*white arrowhead*). (B) Coronal fat-suppressed T2-weighted imaging. High signal intensity band extending to the inferior border of the medial meniscus simulating a meniscus tear (*white arrow*).

small size, within the joint, tendon sheath,[17–19] or bursa.[20] Synovial osteochondromatosis commonly occurs in large joints,[17] but virtually any joint may be involved.[17,21]

Primary SC (**Fig. 8**) is defined by cartilaginous metaplasia, synovial hyperplasia, and production of round cartilaginous nodules of similar size. The joint space is spared or may be even enlarged because of pressure erosion. This occurs preferentially in joints with a tense capsule, such as the hip joint.[17]

Secondary SC (**Fig. 9**) is part of degenerative joint disease, arthritis, or trauma, resulting in dislodgement of bony or cartilaginous tissue undergoing concentric layering. The nodules are more irregular, often larger and of heterogeneous size compared with nodules of the primary form.[17] The joint space is narrowed. Milgram proposed the following staging system.[20] In the

initial stage, there is active synovial disease without loose bodies. The transitional stage is characterized by persistent synovial disease and formation of loose bodies, whereas in the third stage, detached intra-articular nodules are present, with burned-out intrasynovial disease. Approximately two-thirds of nodules calcify or ossify.

Plain radiographs are normal in the initial stage, whereas MR imaging shows increased amount of joint fluid and nonspecific synovitis (see **Fig. 9**). Uncalcified nodules are also invisible on plain radiographs in the transitional stage, and are isointense to muscle on T1-weighted images and hypointense to synovial fluid on T2-weighted images (see **Fig. 9**). Calcified lesions are seen as small, round signal voids. Finally, ossified nodules may demonstrate signal intensities of fatty bone marrow. Plain

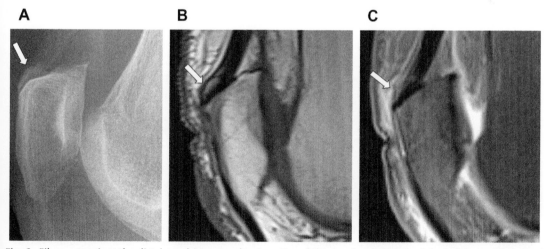

Fig. 6. Fibro-osteosis at the distal quadriceps tendon insertion. (A) Lateral radiograph of the left knee. (B) Sagittal T1-weighted imaging. (C) Sagittal fat-suppressed T2-weighted imaging. Note a focal bony excrescence best seen on plain films (*white arrow*). On T1-weighted imaging, the lesion contains yellow bone marrow (*white arrow*), whereas on FS T2-weighted imaging, the lesion is barely visible because of the lack of contrast of the fibro-osteosis with the fibers of the quadriceps tendon (*white arrow*).

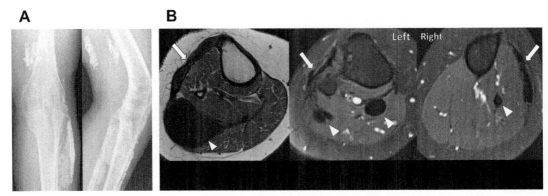

Fig. 7. Mixed connective tissue disease. (*A*) Plain radiograph of the right lower leg. Extensive soft tissue calcification in the anterior and posterior compartment. Note also postsurgical arthrodesis of the right knee. (*B*) Axial T1-weighted imaging of the right lower leg shows hypointense areas adjacent to the fascia cruris anteriorly (*long white arrow*) and at the intermuscular fascia between the soleus and lateral gastrocnemius muscle (*white arrowheads*). Axial FS T2-weighted imaging of both lower legs shows bilateral hypointense areas adjacent to the fascia cruris (*long white arrow*) and in the calf muscles (*white arrowheads*).

radiography and CT demonstrate calcified or ossified nodules (**Fig. 10, Table 2**).

Myositis Ossificans

Myositis ossificans is a benign, solitary, frequently self-limiting, ossifying soft-tissue mass encountered often in young patients and related to trauma in more than half of the cases.[22]

The lesion has a typical zonal organization on histology and imaging.

Three time-dependent stages have been described: early, intermediate, and mature. There may be some overlap between these stages.[23] In the early stage (up to 4 weeks), faint peripheral calcifications may appear at earliest 2 weeks of presentation on ultrasound or CT and soon after on plain radiographs. The signal intensity on

MR imaging is nonspecific, and the lesion may enhance, simulating a soft tissue sarcoma. Biopsy should be avoided in this stage, as histologic findings may show a high mitotic activity, hyperchromatic myofibroblastic cells, and osteoid matrix, simulating an extraskeletal osteosarcoma (ESO). After 4 weeks to 8 weeks (intermediate stage), a well-defined peripheral calcification with central lucency or hypodensity becomes more apparent on plain radiographs and CT, respectively. MR imaging shows a rim of low SI on all pulse sequences, corresponding to calcifications, but generally calcifications are less conspicuous on MR imaging. There is perilesional edema that gradually disappears after 4 weeks. In the mature stage starting at 8 weeks until 6 to 12 months, calcifications are gradually replaced by ossification,

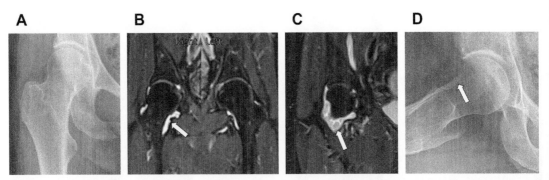

Fig. 8. Primary osteochondromatosis of the right hip in a 51-year-old patient presenting with a decreased range of motion of the right hip. (*A*) Initial plain radiograph shows no abnormalities. (*B*) Coronal fat-suppressed T2-weighted imaging 5 weeks later shows a subtle increase of fluid in the right hip (*long white arrow*) compared with the left hip. (*C*) Coronal fat-suppressed T2-weighted imaging 4 years later showing persisting joint effusion at the right hip and multiple intra-articular nodules (*long white arrow*). Note also an erosion at the lateral femoral neck. (*D*) Plain radiograph at that moment shows sclerotic delineated erosions at the anterolateral aspect of the femoral neck (*long white arrow*), although the intra-articular nodules are not calcified.

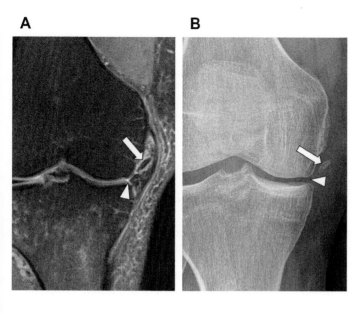

Fig. 9. Secondary osteochondroma mimicking a displaced meniscus fragment on MR imaging. (*A*) Coronal fat-suppressed T2-weighted imaging shows a hypointense fragment underneath the medial collateral ligament mimicking a displaced meniscus fragment (*long white arrow*). The medial meniscus is shortened because of previous partial meniscectomy (*white arrowhead*). (*B*) Correlation with plain radiographs shows an ossified fragment adjacent to the medial femoral condyle (*long white arrow*). Note also narrowing of the joint space caused by cartilage loss (*white arrowhead*).

with no residual central lucency on plain radiographs. The calcification-ossification front further develops following a centripetal pattern, with lamellar bone at the periphery proceeding toward the center (**Figs. 11** and **12**).[24,25] This centripetal pattern is important in the differential diagnosis with ESO, in which the lesion calcifies from the center to the periphery. MR imaging demonstrates low signal intensity on all sequences in mature lamellar bone with hyperintense areas on T1-weighted images, corresponding to fatty bone marrow formation between the bone trabeculae. The perilesional edema is absent in this stage.[23–25] Between months 6 and 12, the lesion may spontaneously regress slightly or completely and appear smaller on repeated radiographs (see **Fig. 11**).[23]

Florid reactive periostitis and soft tissue aneurysmal bone cysts are lesions that are closely related to myositis ossificans.[2] Florid reactive periostitis is attached to the underlying cortex,

whereas myositis is usually separated from the cortex. Soft tissue ABC contains fluid-fluid levels on MR imaging.[2]

Calcific Myonecrosis

Calcific myonecrosis is an uncommon late sequela of trauma, with a reported delay ranging from 10 to 64 years after an initial traumatic event.[26–28] It typically affects the lower extremities in the anterior and lateral compartments of the leg.[29] More rarely, the foot[26,30] and upper extremities are involved.[31]

Plain radiographs show a fusiform mass along with the long axis of the muscles with peripheral calcifications, with a typical linear plate- or plaque-like configuration.

On MR imaging, the periphery of the lesion is of low intensity on T1-weighted images, corresponding to abundant calcification (**Fig. 13**). T1- and T2-weighted images may demonstrate lesion

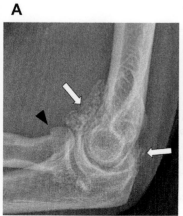
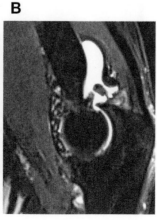

Fig. 10. Secondary synovial osteochondromatosis of the elbow. (*A*) Plain radiographs show multiple intra-articular ossified nodules (*long white arrows*). There is osteophyte formation at the radial neck (*black arrowhead*). (*B*) On sagittal fat-suppressed T2-weighted imaging, these nodules have a mixed signal consisting of central high signal and a peripheral rim of low signal. The central core of high signal correlates with cartilage, whereas the peripheral rim consists of ossification. Note also increased joint fluid.

Table 2
Radiographic-magnetic resonance correlation of synovial chondromatosis

Stage	Radiographs	T1-Weighted Imaging	T2-Weighted Imaging
Early	Normal	Hypointense joint fluid	Hyperintense increased joint fluid
Intermediate	Normal	Nodules isointense with muscle	Nodules of high signal
Late-stage calcified nodules	Calcified nodules	Low signal nodules	Low signal nodules
Late-stage ossified nodules	Ossified nodules with concentric rings	Ringlike nodules containing central fat	Ringlike nodules containing alternating fat and cartilage

heterogeneity caused by repeated intralesional hemorrhage with accumulation of blood products, liquefaction necrosis, and calcified areas. The lesion does not enhance, unless there is superimposed inflammation, often caused by mobilization of plaque and penetration through the muscle fascia.[29,32]

Vascular Calcifications

Arterial and venous calcifications are frequently seen in older patients and readily detected on plain radiographs, but they are usually not visible on MR imaging. Extensive venous calcifications may sometimes cause areas of low signal on both pulse sequences (**Fig. 14**).

Tumoral Calcinosis

Idiopathic tumoral calcinosis is characterized by the presence of progressively enlarging juxta-articular calcified soft tissue masses. These deposits contain a mixture of amorphous calcium carbonate, calcium phosphate, and hydroxyapatite crystals.[33,34] The exact pathogenesis is not known. An inborn error of phosphorus and vitamin D metabolism is suggested. Hyperphosphatemia is observed in only one-third of cases,[35–38] the hip joint being the most common site.[39] The disease may be multifocal.[36] A secondary form may be caused by chronic renal failure.[40] On radiographs, the characteristic appearance of tumoral calcinosis is a well-demarcated lobulated calcified mass located in the periarticular soft tissue, commonly at the extensor side. The lobules are separated by radiolucent lines, histologically corresponding to fibrous septa. This may cause a chicken wire appearance of plain radiographs. Fluid-calcium levels may be seen on upright radiographs.[39–42] Cortical destruction and intramedullary extension may occur because of chronic pressure erosion (**Fig. 15**).[40] On MR imaging, tumoral calcinosis has a well-circumscribed

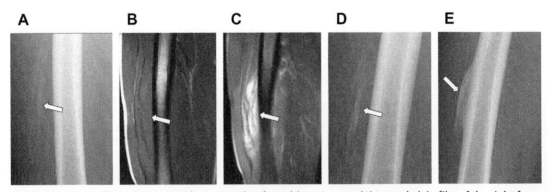

A **B** **C** **D** **E**

Fig. 11. Myositis ossificans in a soccer player 4 weeks after a blunt trauma. (*A*) Lateral plain film of the right femur shows a preferomal shell-like calcification perpendicular to the femoral diaphysis (*long white arrow*). (*B*) Sagittal T1-weighted imaging and (*C*) sagittal fat-suppressed T2-weighted imaging 1 week later. The lesion is heterogeneous on both pulse sequences and has a nonspecific signal intensity (*long white arrows*). Intralesional calcifications are difficult to appreciate. The lesion is surrounded by edema. (*D*) Lateral plain film of the right femur 6 weeks after the first radiograph show further maturation and ossification (*long white arrow*). (*E*) Lateral plain films of the right femur 12 months later show marked decrease of the ossification and fusion with the underlying cortex of the femur (*long white arrow*).

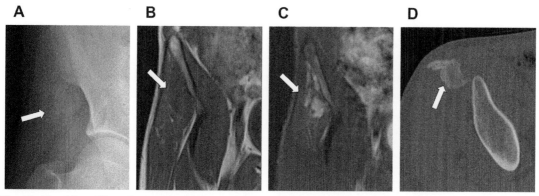

Fig. 12. Myositis ossificans in 27-year-old man. (*A*) Radiograph of the pelvis 2 months after a blunt trauma at the right gluteus region shows a subtle radiodensity with faint calcifications (*long white arrow*). (*B*) Coronal T1-weighted imaging and (*C*) coronal fat-suppressed T2-weighted imaging 5 weeks later. The lesion is heterogeneous on both sequences and contains foci of low signal in keeping with calcifications (*long white arrows*). There is some perilesional edema on (*D*) T2-weighted imaging. Axial CT at the same moment shows mature ossification in the right gluteus minimus (*long white arrow*).

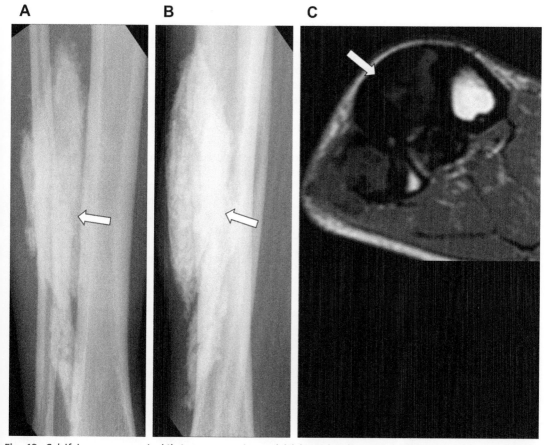

Fig. 13. Calcifying myonecrosis. (*A*) Anteroposterior and (*B*) lateral radiograph of the right lower leg showing typical plate-like calcifications along with longitudinal axis of the muscle in the anterior compartment of the right lower leg (*white arrows*). (*C*) FS T2-weighted imaging of another patient shows a low signal in the anterior and lateral compartment of the right lower leg (*white arrow*). The central part is of intermediate signal, which is more pronounced in the lateral compared with the anterior compartment.

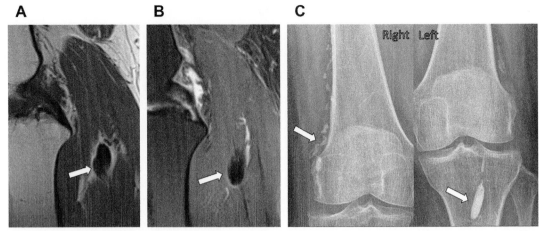

A **B** **C**

Fig. 14. Venous calcifications caused by previous venous thrombosis. (*A*) Sagittal T1-weighted imaging and (*B*) fat-suppressed T2-weighted imaging show a focus of low signal on both pulse sequences within the gastrocnemius muscles (*white arrows*), which is difficult to characterize on MR imaging. Correlation with (*C*) plain radiographs shows bilateral serpiginous calcification in keeping with old calcified thrombi (*white arrows*).

multicystic mass. On T1-weighted images, the mass appears inhomogeneous and is of intermediate to low signal. The lesion is heterogeneous and may contain areas of low[43] and relatively high signal on T2-weighted images. This hyperintense T2 signal may be attributed to the granulomatous foreign body reaction,[44] the hypervascularity of the lesion,[33] or to the partial fluid nature of the calcium material (milk of calcium).[45] Multiple fluid-fluid or fluid-calcium levels may be seen.[42] The calcified areas are of low intensity on T1- and T2-weighted images.[46] The septa separating the cysts are of low signal on T1-weighted images and variable signal on T2-weighted images and enhance after gadolinium contrast injection.[45]

Soft Tissue Tumors Containing Intralesional Mineralization

MR imaging is the preferred modality for evaluation of soft tissue tumors. Various benign and malignant soft tissue tumors may contain intralesional calcifications or ossifications. **Box 1** summarizes the most common soft tissue lesions. Based on the analysis of the distribution and pattern of mineralized foci, tissue specific diagnosis may be suggested.

Phleboliths are circular foci with a lucent center and are characteristic for soft tissue hemangioma (slow flow vascular malformation) (**Fig. 16**).

Ring-and-arc calcification in soft tissue lesions reveals the chondroid nature of the lesions and may be seen in several benign or malignant cartilage tumors or other soft tissue lesions containing chondroid foci.[2]

Soft tissue chondroma most commonly involves the hands (**Fig. 17**) and feet.[2,47,48] In addition to intralesional curvilinear calcifications, the lesion may cause pressure erosion of the underlying bone. MR imaging is useful to demonstrate the cartilaginous matrix, which is hyperintense

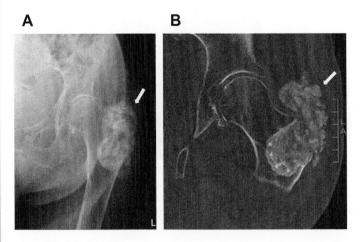

A **B**

Fig. 15. Secondary tumoral calcinosis caused by chronic renal failure. (*A*) Plain radiograph of the left hip shows a large lobulated calcified mass adjacent to the greater trochanter (*white arrow*). (*B*) Coronal reformatted CT shows cortical destruction of the greater trochanter with extension of calcifications within the adjacent medullary cavity (*white arrow*). (*Adapted from* Van Muylder L, Declercq H, Vanhoenacker FM. Secondary tumoral calcinosis with intraosseous extension. JBR-BTR 2013;96(1):50; with permission.)

on T2-weighted images and has a lobular appearance.[49]

Poorly defined, amorphous calcifications are seen in up to 30% of synovial sarcomas[50]

and approximately 50% of extraskeletal osteosarcomas.[1,2]

Metal and Other Foreign Bodies

Foreign bodies such as plastic, wood, glass, and silica may penetrate the soft tissues. Most foreign bodies are of slightly higher density than the surrounding soft tissue except for metal or a postoperative textiloma which appear radiopaque.

Although ultrasound is the modality of choice for further evaluation of foreign bodies, MR imaging may sometimes inadvertently detect foreign bodies.[51]

Foreign bodies are usually low on all MR pulse sequences, because of the presence of few mobile protons.[52–55] Adjacent edema may be seen because of inflammatory reaction. Even small metal fragments (**Fig. 18**) (eg, in metal workers) may cause marked magnetic susceptibility artifacts, which are most pronounced on gradient echo imaging.[56] As intraocular metal fragments, bullets, and shrapnel are risk factors for retinal detachment in MR imaging, patients who have worked with sheet metal or ammunition should have intraocular metal fragments ruled out by radiographs prior to the MR examination. Plain radiography may, however, fail to detect tiny intraocular metallic foreign bodies.[57] Based on a report

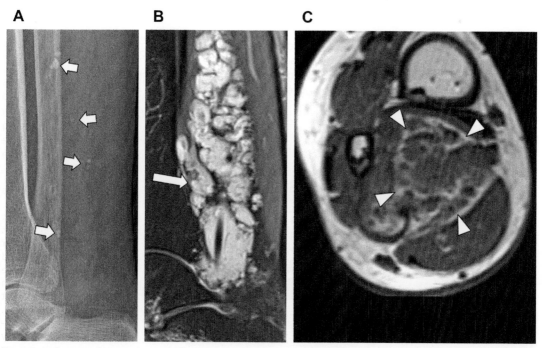

Fig. 16. Soft tissue hemangioma. (*A*) Lateral radiograph of the right lower leg showing multiple phleboliths within the posterior compartment of the lower leg (*white arrows*). The lesion contains also some interspersed fat. (*B*) Sagittal fat-suppressed T2-weighted imaging and (*C*) axial T1-weighted imaging. The mass has a multilobular appearance (*white arrow*), has a high signal on T2-weighted imaging, and is interspersed with fat (*white arrowheads*). Phleboliths are more conspicuous on CR.

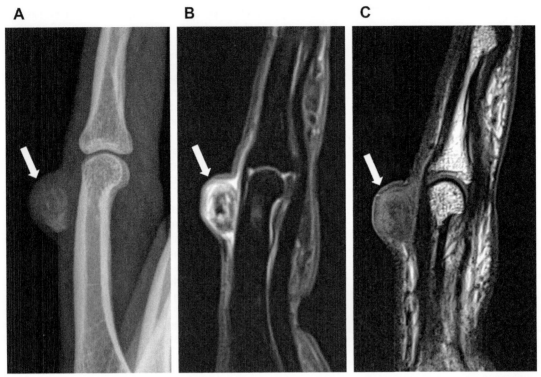

Fig. 17. Soft tissue chondroma. (*A*) Lateral radiograph of the right third finger showing a nodular soft tissue lesion at the extensor side of first phalanx with intralesional ring-and-arc calcifications (*arrow*). (*B*) Sagittal fat-suppressed T2-weighted imaging. The lesion is of low signal at its central part, whereas it is of high signal at the periphery (*arrow*). (*C*) Sagittal T1-weighted imaging. The central part of the lesion is of low signal, whereas the periphery is isointense to muscle (*arrow*).

of 2 cases, Zhang and colleagues[57] suggested that tiny ferromagnetic fragments with a diameter less than 0.5 mm are too small to be visualized by radiographs or CT, but are not likely to cause MR-induced damage of magnetic field strengths less than 1.0 T. Platt and colleagues[51] reported a 3.5-mm intraocular metallic foreign body that was detected by MR imaging in a 10-year-old

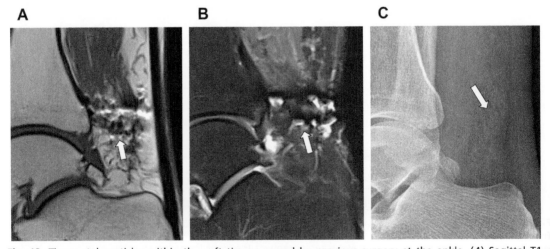

Fig. 18. Tiny metal particles within the soft tissues caused by previous surgery at the ankle. (*A*) Sagittal T1-weighted imaging and (*B*) fat-suppressed T2-weighted imaging show metal artifacts within Kager fat pad (*white arrows*). Correlation with (*C*) plain radiographs of the right ankle shows multiple tiny metal particles (*white arrow*).

patient without causing any damage to the ocular tissues. Further evaluation in in vitro and in vivo animal studies to evaluate the movement and MR safety of tiny intraocular ferromagnetic particles at 1.5 and 3.0T MR is warranted.[57]

Injection granulomas arising from injection of oil-based corticosteroids in bodybuilders contain foci of high signal on T1-weighted images.[58] An intralesional fat-fluid level may be seen at the interface of fatty and necrotic components. The combination of the clinical history and location at typical injection sites (eg, shoulder and gluteus muscles) provides clues to the correct diagnosis of these pseudotumoral soft tissue masses.[59,60]

LESIONS WITH A SLIGHTLY INCREASED DENSITY THAN SURROUNDING SOFT TISSUE
Gout

Gout is a metabolic disorder characterized by hyperuricemia and deposits of uric acid crystals in joints and periarticular soft tissues. The first metatarsophalangeal joint is most commonly involved, followed by the ankle, knee, wrist, fingers, and elbow. Clinical and radiographic findings of articular manifestations are usually diagnostic.[4]

Soft tissue deposition of uric acid crystals is designated as tophaceous gout.[61] Uric acid crystals deposits are slightly denser than the surrounding soft tissues. They are currently often characterized dual-energy CT,[62] whereas ultrasound is useful to identify crystals on the surface of the articular cartilage,[63] rather than within cartilage, as observed with CPPD.[3]

The MR imaging features of gouty arthritis include synovial thickening and joint effusion. Tophaceous gout is of low to intermediate signal intensity on T1-weighted images.[64] T2-weighted image characteristics vary from a heterogeneously hypointense to hyperintense mass on T2-weighted images (**Fig. 19**),[61] depending on the degree of inflammation.[62] Enhancement may be seen.[65]

Pigmented Villonodular Synovitis and Tenosynovial Giant Cell Tumor

Pigmented villonodular synovitis (PVNS) represents a diffuse benign fibrohistiocytic tumor arising from the synovium of joints, characterized by the formation of nodular synovial masses consisting of hemosiderin deposits. The predominantly affected joint of diffuse PVNS is the knee, followed by the ankle, and in rare cases the wrist, hip, shoulder, and elbow. Localized intra-articular forms are designated as localized nodular synovitis (LNS), which most commonly affects Hoffa fat pad. It may also involve

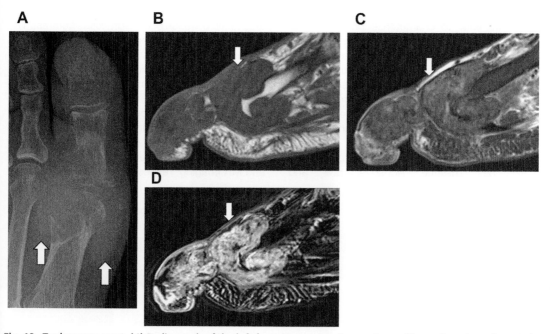

Fig. 19. Tophaceous gout. (*A*) Radiograph of the left foot. Note extensive erosions with overhanging edges at the first metatarsophalangeal joint. The adjacent soft tissue swelling has an increased density compared with the surrounding soft tissues (*white arrows*). (*B*) Sagittal T1-weighted imaging. (*C*) Sagittal fat-suppressed T2-weighted imaging. (*D*) Subtraction image of sagittal fat-suppressed T1-weighted imaging before and after administration of gadolinium contrast. Tophi are of heterogeneous signal intensity on both pulse sequences (*white arrows*), and there is heterogenous contrast enhancement (*white arrows*).

the tendon sheath (tenosynovial giant cell tumors) and bursae (pigmented villonodular bursitis).[66]

Standard radiographs may be normal in an early stage, or may demonstrate well-defined dense soft tissue masses caused by hemosiderin deposition. Calcifications are typically not seen. Later, proliferation of the synovium may cause erosions and marginal sclerosis in the adjacent bone. Erosions occur in a more early stage in joints with a limited capacity to expand, such as the wrist and hip joints.

For early detection and for imaging characterization, MR imaging is the preferred imaging technique and is currently referred as the gold standard.[67]

Both T1- and T2-weighted images reveal hypointense intra-articular masses, indicative of hemosiderin deposition. Fat-suppressed T2-weighted images may show areas of interspersed fluid entrapped within the thickened and hemosiderin-laden synovium.

Gradient echo imaging is useful to demonstrate characteristic blooming artifacts caused by hemosiderin deposits. The lesion usually enhances vividly (**Fig. 20**).[66]

Ganglion Cysts and Enlarged Bursae

Ganglion cysts, synovial cysts, and enlarged bursae are easy to characterize on ultrasound and MR imaging because of their fluid contents and to define the exact location and their relationship to the joint and surrounding structures.[68] The lesions are hyperintense on T2-weighted images, and there is subtle peripheral enhancement.

If large enough, they may be suspected on plain films if a nonspecific soft tissue swelling is seen adjacent to the joint (**Fig. 21**).

Peritrochanteric, subacromial-subdeltoid, ischiogluteal, pes anserine, iliopsoas, pre- and infrapatellar, and retrocalcaneal and olecranon bursae are most commonly involved.[69–75]

An adventitious bursa results from inflammation and fibrinoid necrosis of connective tissue in areas subject to chronic frictional irritation. It is most commonly located at the first metatarsophalangeal joint because of chronic friction over a hallux valgus, but it may be seen in other locations (**Fig. 22**).[68]

Lesions Causing Displacement of Surrounding Fat Pads

A variety of soft tissue lesions of different etiology may cause displacement and distortion of surrounding fat pads. Most lesions cannot be further characterized on radiographs alone. This paragraph will be restricted to accessory muscles. Accessory muscles are variations in muscular anatomy differing from the musculature described in anatomy textbooks.[76] Most accessory muscles are incidental findings on imaging. They may become symptomatic, because they present as a soft tissue mass or may cause compression or displacement of adjacent neurovascular structures and tendons. They also may cause exercise-related pain because of a focal compartment syndrome or inadequate blood supply.[76,77]

On plain radiography, accessory muscles may cause displacement of fat planes, but CR is rarely diagnostic because of low soft tissue contrast. The prototype is an accessory soleus muscle, causing obliteration of Kager fat pad.[78]

Ultrasound and MR imaging are the preferred imaging modalities for direct identification of accessory muscles. The clues to differentiate accessory muscles from true soft tissue neoplasms are the knowledge of the variant anatomy, their specific location, and their similar echotexture and signal to other muscles on ultrasound and MR imaging, respectively.

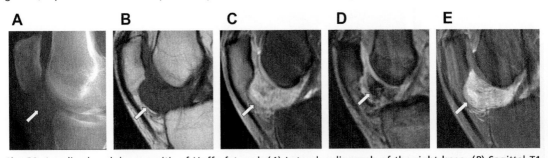

A   B   C   D   E

Fig. 20. Localized nodular synovitis of Hoffa fat pad. (*A*) Lateral radiograph of the right knee. (*B*) Sagittal T1-weighted imaging. (*C*) Sagittal fat-suppressed T2-weighted imaging. (*D*) Sagittal gradient echo imaging. (*E*) Sagittal FS T1-weighted imaging after gadolinium contrast. Nodular mass within Hoffa fat pad (*white arrows*). The lesion is isointense to muscle on T1-weighted imaging and heterogeneous on T2-weighted imaging, and there is marked blooming artifact on gradient echo imaging. Note marked enhancement after gadolinium contrast.

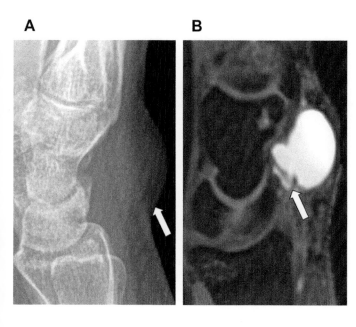

Fig. 21. Arthrosynovial cyst of left wrist. (*A*) Lateral radiograph of the left wrist showing a nonspecific soft tissue swelling at the dorsal aspect of the wrist (*white arrow*). (*B*) Sagittal T2-weighted imaging. The lesion is of high signal, and there is a connecting stalk to the radiocarpal compartment (*white arrow*).

When fat suppression (FS) is used, accessory muscles are barely distinguishable from the surrounding structures. Therefore, because of their intrinsic contrast with the adjacent intermuscular fat, accessory muscles are best identified on T1-weighted images without FS (**Fig. 23**).[78]

Fat-Containing Lesions

MR imaging is the imaging technique of choice for characterization of adipocytic tumors. CR is rarely diagnostic but may occasionally demonstrate a radiolucent soft tissue mass and/or osseous deformity caused by mass effect (**Fig. 24**).

Air-Containing Lesions

Degenerative disc and joint disease
An intervertebral vacuum phenomenon is defined as the presence of gas in the intervertebral disk spaces.[79] It is a common manifestation of degenerative disc disease.[80] The gas may be located either at the nucleus pulposus or at the peripheral part of the disc, resulting from focal rupture of the annulus fibrosus.

MR imaging is less sensitive than CR or CT to detect vacuum phenomenon.[81] Although gas within the disc is usually of low signal intensity on T2-weighted images because of the lack of water protons, a hyperintense signal less than fluid or even fluid-like signal may be seen in patients with a clear intradiscal vacuum phenomenon on plain films or CT.[80] The presence of fluid or hyperintense signal is correlated to the presence and amount of bone marrow edema and degenerative endplate abnormalities Modic I.[80] It has been postulated that on MR imaging in supine position, fluid transudate flows slowly from adjacent edematous

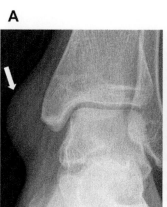
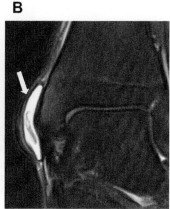

Fig. 22. Adventitious bursa resulting from chronic friction in a skater. (*A*) Anteroposterior radiograph of the left ankle showing a nonspecific soft tissue mass at the medial malleolus (*white arrow*). (*B*) Coronal fat-suppressed T2-weighted imaging reveals a fluid-filled bursa (*white arrow*).

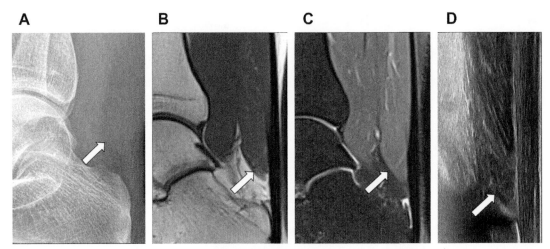

Fig. 23. Accessory soleus. (*A*) Lateral radiograph of the right ankle shows partial obliteration of Kager fat pad (*white arrow*). (*B*) Sagittal T1-weighted imaging and (*C*) FS T2-weighted imaging reveal an accessory soleus (*white arrows*). The lesion is most conspicuous on nonfat-suppressed images. The lesion has a similar signal intensity to muscle on MR imaging and has a muscular architecture on (*D*) ultrasound (*white arrow*).

endplate into the vacuum cleft. On CT, which takes only a few minutes, the time spent in the supine position is too short for migration of fluid into the vacuum cleft.[80]

This hyperintense signal within the disc in patients with a degenerative vacuum phenomenon should not be confused with early spondylodiscitis.

In a similar way, a subtle peripheral vacuum phenomenon in spondylosis deformans may be seen as a hyperintense annular tear on corresponding T2-weighted MR imaging, especially when fluid-sensitive sequences are used.

A vacuum phenomenon may also occur in other joints, including the shoulder, wrist, hip, sacroiliac joint, ankle, subtalar joint, and knee.[82] Its clinical significance is still debated.[83]

Trauma
Soft tissue air may occur in injuries causing leakage of air from a damaged lung or other penetrating (such as open fractures or shotgun wounds), lacerating, or crushing injuries in which the skin is disrupted.[84] The latter are always limited to the region of the injury, never extend into uninjured tissue, and usually rapidly decrease in size and disappear.[84]

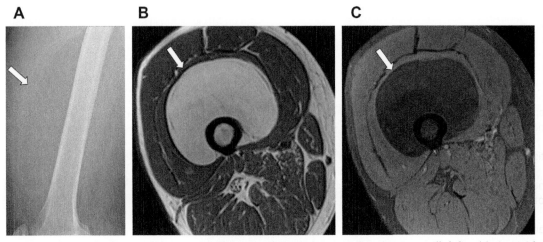

Fig. 24. Intramuscular lipoma. (*A*) Lateral radiograph of the right upper leg shows a well-defined lesion with similar density of the subcutaneous fat (*white arrow*). (*B*) Axial T1-weighted imaging and (*C*) axial FS T1-weighted imaging confirm the lipomatous nature of the lesion with a signal intensity similar to subcutaneous fat (*white arrows*).

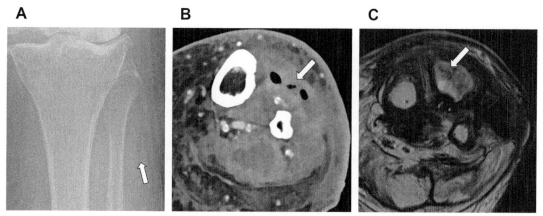

Fig. 25. Intramuscular abscess. (*A*) Anteroposterior radiograph of the left lower leg shows soft tissue gas lateral to the fibula (*white arrow*). (*B*) Axial contrast-enhanced CT showing intramuscular collections with peripheral rim enhancement in the anterior, lateral, and posterior compartments with intralesional gas (*white arrow*). (*C*) Corresponding axial T2-weighted imaging. The intralesional gas bubbles are of low signal (*white arrow*), but their identification and correct interpretation are less straightforward on MR imaging compared with CT.

The combination of the clinical history and plain films is sufficient for the diagnosis, and MR imaging is not mandatory for this indication.

Abscess and necrotizing soft tissue infections

A soft tissue abscess is a fluid collection surrounded by a well-vascularized fibrous pseudocapsule.[85]

On conventional radiography, a soft tissue abscess may cause potential distortion of normal muscle anatomy and fascial planes. This nonspecific sign is of little value, unless there is intralesional gas development in the case of gas-forming infection. Therefore, the diagnosis is usually made on ultrasound, CT, or MR imaging.

On MR imaging, an abscess is hypointense to isointense relative to muscle tissue on T1-weighted imaging. On T2-weighted imaging, the central portion of the abscess is usually hyperintense. Central pus collection may cause diffusion restriction. The inflammatory pseudocapsule can have a variable signal intensity compared with skeletal muscle on T1-weighted imaging. A thick and irregular enhancing peripheral rim corresponds to the inflammatory and cellular component of the abscess.

Peripheral edema in muscle and subcutaneous tissue is hyperintense on T2-weighted imaging.[86]

Intralesional gas bubbles may cause inhomogeneity on T2-weighted images with intralesional foci of signal void[86] (**Fig. 25**).

Pedal abscesses in the diabetic foot are nearly always caused by contiguous spread from an adjacent skin ulcer or sinus tract. The sinus tract and necrotic center of the abscess may show gas and air-fluid levels on plain radiographs. Ulcerations are seen on MR imaging as defects of skin and/or subcutaneous tissue and may be surrounded by heaped-up edges.

Sinus tracts appear as thin bands of high signal on T2-weighted images with a tram track appearance on contrast-enhanced fat-suppressed T1-weighted imaging because of enhancement of the margins of the sinus tract. Associated osteomyelitis is frequently seen.[87] Necrotizing soft tissue infections (NSTIs) are rapidly progressive and lead to sepsis, multisystem organ failure, and sometimes death.[88]

Air tracking on plain films or CT along the soft tissue can also indicate aggressive NSTIs that need urgent surgical debridement.[89] Identifying gas on radiographs or CT images has a high specificity but low sensitivity for NSTI (2).[86]

The overall role of MR imaging in the diagnosis of NSTI is limited.[88]

SUMMARY

Although MR imaging is the preferred imaging modality for evaluation of soft tissue lesions, knowledge and meticulous analysis of often subtle soft tissue signs on conventional radiography may be helpful to select patients who need to be referred for subsequent MR imaging. In addition, certain plain film findings, such as intralesional calcification or gas may allow one to make to a more specific tissue diagnosis and may obviate the need for invasive diagnostic procedures and potential harmful treatment.

KEY POINTS, PEARLS, PITFALLS, VARIANTS

Plain films have a low sensitivity is the diagnosis of soft tissue tumors or tumor-like conditions, but the presence of intralesional soft tissue calcification may be useful for tissue specific diagnosis (eg, in case of myositis ossificans or slow-flow vascular malformations [hemangiomas]).

Mineralization in myositis ossificans follows a time-dependent centripetal pattern from the periphery toward the center. The mineralization pattern in extraskeletal osteosarcoma (ESO) is more amorphous and occurs from the center to the periphery.

The clinical history of trauma is not always present in myositis ossificans. Calcific myonecrosis may present several years after trauma.

MR imaging and histology may simulate ESO in the early stage of myositis ossificans. Biopsy should be avoided in the early stage of myositis ossificans.

The use of fat suppression may decrease conspicuity of accessory muscles. Although plain films have a low sensitivity in the diagnosis of soft tissue infections, the presence of intralesional air may enhance the specificity of gas-forming infection and of necrotizing soft tissue infections.

WHAT THE REFERRING PHYSICIAN NEEDS TO KNOW

MR imaging is the preferred imaging modality for evaluation of most soft tissue lesions because of its high soft tissue contrast.

Although plain radiography is not very sensitive, identification of certain macroscopic components within the lesion may allow a more specific diagnosis. The presence of intralesional calcifications and air yields the greatest diagnostic value. In this regard, plain radiographs may be complementary to MR imaging for characterization of certain soft tissue lesions such as myositis ossificans, calcifying myonecrosis, calcified soft tissue tumors, and gas-forming infection.

MR imaging and histology may simulate ESO in early myositis. In any case of suspected myositis ossificans, biopsy should be avoided, and repeated evaluation by serial radiography or ultrasound is mandatory.

As intraocular metal fragments, bullets, and shrapnel may cause the risk of retinal detachment in MR imaging, patients who have worked with sheet metal or ammunition or intraocular metal fragments should be ruled out by radiographs prior to the MR examination.

REFERENCES

1. Botchu R, James SL, Davies AM. Radiography and computed tomography. In: Vanhoenacker FM, Parizel PM, Gielen JL, editors. Imaging of soft tissue tumors. 4th edition. Cham (Switzerland): Springer International Publishing; 2017. p. 41–57. https://doi.org/10.1007/978-3-319-46679-8_2.
2. Cho S-J, Horvai A. Chondro-osseous lesions of soft tissue. Surg Pathol Clin 2015;8(3):419–44.
3. Freire V, Moser TP, Lepage-Saucier M. Radiological identification and analysis of soft tissue musculoskeletal calcifications. Insights Imaging 2018;9(4):477–92.
4. Jacques T, Michelin P, Badr S, et al. Conventional radiology in crystal arthritis: gout, calcium pyrophosphate deposition, and basic calcium phosphate crystals. Radiol Clin North Am 2017;55(5):967–84.
5. Uhthoff L. Calcific tendinopathy of the rotator cuff: pathogenesis, diagnosis, and management. J Am Acad Orthop Surg 1997;5(4):183–91.
6. Malghem J, Omoumi P, Lecouvet F, et al. Intraosseous migration of tendinous calcifications: cortical erosions, subcortical migration and extensive intramedullary diffusion, a SIMS series. Skeletal Radiol 2015;44(10):1403–12.
7. El-Essawy MT, Vanhoenacker FM. Calcific tendinopathy of the pectoralis major insertion with intracortical protrusion of calcification. JBR-BTR 2012;95(6):374.
8. Alamoudi U, Al-Sayed AA, AlSallumi Y, et al. Acute calcific tendinitis of the longus colli muscle masquerading as a retropharyngeal abscess: a case report and review of the literature. Int J Surg Case Rep 2017;41:343–6.
9. Uchida T, Kanzaki M, Kakumoto T, et al. Longus colli tendinitis in a patient presenting with neck pain and acute systemic inflammation. Intern Med 2018;57(18):2759–61.
10. Razon RVB, Nasir A, Wu GS, et al. Retropharyngeal calcific tendonitis: report of two cases. J Am Board Fam Med 2009;22(1):84–8.
11. Miksanek J, Rosenthal AK. Imaging of calcium pyrophosphate deposition disease. Curr Rheumatol Rep 2015;17(3):20.
12. Steinbach LS. Calcium pyrophosphate dihydrate and calcium hydroxyapatite crystal deposition diseases: imaging perspectives. Radiol Clin North Am 2004;42(1):185–205, vii.
13. Zünkeler B, Schelper R, Menezes AH. Periodontoid calcium pyrophosphate dihydrate deposition disease: "pseudogout" mass lesions of the craniocervical junction. J Neurosurg 1996;85(5):803–9.
14. Schweitzer ME, Cervilla V, Manaster BJ, et al. Cervical paraspinal calcification in collagen vascular diseases. AJR Am J Roentgenol 1991;157(3):523–5.
15. Van de Perre S, Vanhoenacker FM, Op De Beeck B, et al. Paraspinal cervical calcifications associated with scleroderma. JBR-BTR 2003;86(2):80–2.
16. Arginteanu MS, Perin NI. Paraspinal calcinosis associated with progressive systemic sclerosis. Case report. J Neurosurg 1997;87(5):761–3.

17. Murphey MD, Vidal JA, Fanburg-Smith JC, et al. Imaging of synovial chondromatosis with radiologic-pathologic correlation. Radiographics 2007;27(5): 1465–88.

18. Walker EA, Murphey MD, Fetsch JF. Imaging characteristics of tenosynovial and bursal chondromatosis. Skeletal Radiol 2011;40(3):317–25.

19. Christoforou D, Strauss EJ, Abramovici L, et al. Benign extraosseous cartilage tumours of the hand and wrist. J Hand Surg Eur Vol 2012;37(1):8–13.

20. Milgram JW, Hadesman WM. Synovial osteochondromatosis in the subacromial bursa. Clin Orthop Relat Res 1988;236:154–9.

21. Guffens F, Dom M, Vanhoenacker F. Case report: primary osteochondromatosis of the right TMJ. Vienna: European Society of Radiology; 2015. https://doi.org/10.1594/EURORAD/CASE.13176.

22. Devilbiss Z, Hess M, Ho GWK. Myositis ossificans in sport. Curr Sports Med Rep 2018;17(9):290–5.

23. Walczak BE, Johnson CN, Howe BM. Myositis ossificans. J Am Acad Orthop Surg 2015;23(10):612–22.

24. Tyler P, Saifuddin A. The imaging of myositis ossificans. Semin Musculoskelet Radiol 2010;14(02): 201–16.

25. Wang XL, Malghem J, Parizel PM, et al. Myositis ossificans circumscripta. J Belge Radiol 2003;86(5): 278–85.

26. Holobinko JN, Damron TA, Scerpella PR, et al. Calcific myonecrosis: keys to early recognition. Skeletal Radiol 2003;32(1):35–40.

27. Tuncay IC, Demirörs H, Isiklar ZU, et al. Calcific myonecrosis. Int Orthop 1999;23(1):68–70.

28. Peeters J, Vanhoenacker FM, Camerlinck M, et al. Calcific myonecrosis. JBR-BTR 2010;93(2):111.

29. Eyselbergs M, Catry F, Scharpé P, et al. Case 9086 calcific myonecrosis. Vienna: European Society of Radiology; 2011.

30. Papanna MC, Monga P, Wilkes RA. Post-traumatic calcific myonecrosis of flexor hallucis longus. A case report and literature review. Acta Orthop Belg 2010;76(1):137–41.

31. Larson RC, Sierra RJ, Sundaram M, et al. Calcific myonecrosis: a unique presentation in the upper extremity. Skeletal Radiol 2004;33(5):306–9.

32. Gielen JL, Blom RM, Vanhoenacker FM, et al. An elderly man with a slowly growing painless mass in the soft tissues of the lower leg: presentation. Skeletal Radiol 2008;37(4):335, 337-338.

33. Neeman Z, Wood BJ. Angiographic findings in tumoral calcinosis. Clin Imaging 2003;27(3):184–6.

34. Polykandriotis EP, Beutel FK, Horch RE, et al. A case of familial tumoral calcinosis in a neonate and review of the literature. Arch Orthop Trauma Surg 2004; 124(8):563–7.

35. Adams WM, Laitt RD, Davies M, et al. Familial tumoral calcinosis: association with cerebral and peripheral aneurysm formation. Neuroradiology 1999;41(5):351–5.

36. Fujii T, Matsui N, Yamamoto T, et al. Solitary intra-articular tumoral calcinosis of the knee. Arthroscopy 2003;19(1):E1.

37. Geirnaerdt MJ, Kroon HM, van der Heul RO, et al. Tumoral calcinosis. Skeletal Radiol 1995;24(2): 148–51.

38. Yamaguchi T, Sugimoto T, Imai Y, et al. Successful treatment of hyperphosphatemic tumoral calcinosis with long-term acetazolamide. Bone 1995;16(4 Suppl):247S–50S.

39. Noyez JF, Murphree SM, Chen K. Tumoral calcinosis, a clinical report of eleven cases. Acta Orthop Belg 1993;59(3):249–54.

40. Van Muylder L, Declercq H, Vanhoenacker FM. Secondary tumoral calcinosis with intra-osseous extension. JBR-BTR 2013;96(1):50.

41. Bittmann S, Günther MW, Ulus H. Tumoral calcinosis of the gluteal region in a child: case report with overview of different soft-tissue calcifications. J Pediatr Surg 2003;38(8):E4–7.

42. Steinbach LS, Johnston JO, Tepper EF, et al. Tumoral calcinosis: radiologic-pathologic correlation. Skeletal Radiol 1995;24(8):573–8.

43. Ohashi K, Yamada T, Ishikawa T, et al. Idiopathic tumoral calcinosis involving the cervical spine. Skeletal Radiol 1996;25(4):388–90.

44. Martinez S, Vogler JB, Harrelson JM, et al. Imaging of tumoral calcinosis: new observations. Radiology 1990;174(1):215–22.

45. Chaabane S, Chelli-Bouaziz M, Jelassi H, et al. Idiopathic tumoral calcinosis. Acta Orthop Belg 2008; 74(6):837–45.

46. Ovali GY, Tarhan S, Serter S, et al. A rare disorder: idiopathic tumoral calcinosis. Clin Rheumatol 2007; 26(7):1142–4.

47. Khedhaier A, Maalla R, Ennouri K, et al. Soft tissues chondromas of the hand: a report of five cases. Acta Orthop Belg 2007;73(4):458–61.

48. Fetsch JF, Vinh TN, Remotti F, et al. Tenosynovial (extraarticular) chondromatosis: an analysis of 37 cases of an underrecognized clinicopathologic entity with a strong predilection for the hands and feet and a high local recurrence rate. Am J Surg Pathol 2003;27(9):1260–8.

49. Kosaka H, Nishio J, Matsunaga T, et al. Imaging features of periosteal chondroma manifesting as a subcutaneous mass in the index finger. Case Rep Orthop 2014;2014:763480.

50. Horowitz AL, Resnick D, Watson RC. The roentgen features of synovial sarcomas. Clin Radiol 1973; 24(4):481–4.

51. Platt AS, Wajda BG, Ingram AD, et al. Metallic intraocular foreign body as detected by magnetic resonance imaging without complications– a

case report. Am J Ophthalmol Case Rep 2017;7:76–9.

52. Jelinek J, Kransdorf MJ. MR imaging of soft-tissue masses. Mass-like lesions that simulate neoplasms. Magn Reson Imaging Clin N Am 1995;3(4):727–41.

53. Laor T, Barnewolt CE. Nonradiopaque penetrating foreign body: "a sticky situation." Pediatr Radiol 1999;29(9):702–4.

54. Monu JU, McManus CM, Ward WG, et al. Soft-tissue masses caused by long-standing foreign bodies in the extremities: MR imaging findings. AJR Am J Roentgenol 1995;165(2):395–7.

55. Vanhoenacker FM, Eyselbergs M, Van Hul E, et al. Pseudotumoural soft tissue lesions of the hand and wrist: a pictorial review. Insights Imaging 2011;2(3):319–33.

56. Senol S, Gumus K. A rare incidence of metal artifact on MRI. Quant Imaging Med Surg 2017;7(1):142–3.

57. Momoniat HT, England A. An investigation into the accuracy of orbital X-rays, when using CR, in detecting ferromagnetic intraocular foreign bodies. Radiography 2017;23(1):55–9.

58. Lee SY, Lee NH, Chung MJ, et al. Foreign-body granuloma caused by dispersed oil droplets simulating subcutaneous fat tissue on MR images. AJR Am J Roentgenol 2004;182(4):1090–1.

59. Ardies L, De Beule T, Degroote T, et al. Bilateral intramuscular pseudotumor in a bodybuilder. JBR-BTR 2012;95(2):108.

60. Vanhoenacker FM, Verstraete KL. Soft tissue tumors about the shoulder. Semin Musculoskelet Radiol 2015;19(3):284–99.

61. Chaoui A, Garcia J, Kurt AM. Gouty tophus simulating soft tissue tumor in a heart transplant recipient. Skeletal Radiol 1997;26(10):626–8.

62. Bayat S, Baraf HSB, Rech J. Update on imaging in gout: contrasting and comparing the role of dual-energy computed tomography to traditional diagnostic and monitoring techniques. Clin Exp Rheumatol 2018;36. Suppl 1(5):53–60.

63. Wang Y, Deng X, Xu Y, et al. Detection of uric acid crystal deposition by ultrasonography and dual-energy computed tomography: a cross-sectional study in patients with clinically diagnosed gout. Medicine (Baltimore) 2018;97(42):e12834.

64. Van Slyke MA, Moser RP, Madewell JE. MR imaging of periarticular soft-tissue lesions. Magn Reson Imaging Clin N Am 1995;3(4):651–67.

65. Chen CK, Yeh LR, Pan HB, et al. Intra-articular gouty tophi of the knee: CT and MR imaging in 12 patients. Skeletal Radiol 1999;28(2):75–80.

66. Shah A, Botchu R, Davies AM, et al. So-called fibrohistiocytic tumours. In: Vanhoenacker FM, Parizel PM, Gielen JL, editors. Imaging of soft tissue tumors. 4th edition. Cham (Switzerland): Springer International Publishing; 2017. p. 311–37. https://doi.org/10.1007/978-3-319-46679-8_14.

67. Verlinden C, Vanhoenacker FM, Boone P. Pigmented villonodular synovitis of the ankle presenting as a persisting ankle effusion. JBR-BTR 2012;95(2):101.

68. Nikodinovska VV, Vanhoenacker FM. Synovial lesions. In: Vanhoenacker FM, Parizel PM, Gielen JL, editors. Imaging of soft tissue tumors. 4th edition. Cham (Switzerland): Springer; 2017. p. 495–522.

69. Chatra PS. Bursae around the knee joints. Indian J Radiol Imaging 2012;22(1):27–30.

70. Steinbach LS, Stevens KJ. Imaging of cysts and bursae about the knee. Radiol Clin North Am 2013;51(3):433–54.

71. Beaman FD, Peterson JJ. MR imaging of cysts, ganglia, and bursae about the knee. Radiol Clin North Am 2007;45(6):969–82, vi.

72. McCarthy CL, McNally EG. The MRI appearance of cystic lesions around the knee. Skeletal Radiol 2004;33(4):187–209.

73. Draghi F, Scudeller L, Draghi AG, et al. Prevalence of subacromial-subdeltoid bursitis in shoulder pain: an ultrasonographic study. J Ultrasound 2015;18(2):151–8.

74. Yukata K, Nakai S, Goto T, et al. Cystic lesion around the hip joint. World J Orthop 2015;6(9):688.

75. Khodaee M. Common superficial bursitis. Am Fam Physician 2017;95(4):224–31.

76. Martinoli C, Perez MM, Padua L, et al. Muscle variants of the upper and lower limb (with anatomical correlation). Semin Musculoskelet Radiol 2010;14(2):106–21.

77. Sookur PA, Naraghi AM, Bleakney RR, et al. Accessory muscles: anatomy, symptoms, and radiologic evaluation. Radiographics 2008;28(2):481–99.

78. Vanhoenacker FM, Desimpel J, Mespreuve M, et al. Accessory muscles of the extremities. Semin Musculoskelet Radiol 2018;22(3):275–85.

79. Resnick D, Niwayama G, Guerra J, et al. Spinal vacuum phenomena: anatomical study and review. Radiology 1981;139(2):341–8.

80. D'Anastasi M, Birkenmaier C, Schmidt GP, et al. Correlation between vacuum phenomenon on CT and fluid on MRI in degenerative disks. AJR Am J Roentgenol 2011;197(5):1182–9.

81. Coulier B. The spectrum of vacuum phenomenon and gas in spine. JBR-BTR 2004;87(1):9–16.

82. Liu Z, Yan W, Zhang L. Analysis of the vacuum phenomenon in plain hip radiographs in children. Int J Clin Exp Med 2015;8(3):3325–31.

83. Gohil I, Vilensky JA, Weber EC. Vacuum phenomenon: clinical relevance. Clin Anat 2014;27(3):455–62.

84. Rhinehart DA. Air and gas in the soft tissues: a radiologic study. Radiology 1931;17(6):1158–70.

85. Vanhoenacker FM, Mechri Rekik M, Salgado R. Pseudotumoral lesions. In: Vanhoenacker FM, Parizel PM, Gielen JL, editors. Imaging of soft tissue tumors. 4th edition. Cham (Switzerland): Springer International Publishing; 2017. p. 523–75.

86. Wall SD, Fisher MR, Amparo EG, et al. Magnetic resonance imaging in the evaluation of abscesses. AJR Am J Roentgenol 1985;144(6):1217–21.

87. Naidoo P, Liu VJ, Mautone M, et al. Lower limb complications of diabetes mellitus: a comprehensive review with clinicopathological insights from a dedicated high-risk diabetic foot multidisciplinary team. Br J Radiol 2015;88(1053):20150135.

88. Garcia NM, Cai J. Aggressive soft tissue infections. Surg Clin North Am 2018;98(5):1097–108.

89. Gomes DC, Quaresma L. Plain x-ray films in soft tissue infections. Pan Afr Med J 2017;26:149.

UNITED STATES POSTAL SERVICE® Statement of Ownership, Management, and Circulation
(All Periodicals Publications Except Requester Publications)

1. Publication Title	2. Publication Number	3. Filing Date
MAGNETIC RESONANCE IMAGING CLINICS OF NORTH AMERICA	011 – 909	9/18/2019

4. Issue Frequency	5. Number of Issues Published Annually	6. Annual Subscription Price
FEB, MAY, AUG, NOV	4	$404.00

7. Complete Mailing Address of Known Office of Publication *(Not printer)* *(Street, city, county, state, and ZIP+4®)*

ELSEVIER INC.
230 Park Avenue, Suite 800
New York, NY 10169

Contact Person
STEPHEN R. BUSHING

Telephone *(Include area code)*
215-239-3688

8. Complete Mailing Address of Headquarters or General Business Office of Publisher *(Not printer)*

ELSEVIER INC.
230 Park Avenue, Suite 800
New York, NY 10169

9. Full Names and Complete Mailing Addresses of Publisher, Editor, and Managing Editor *(Do not leave blank)*

Publisher *(Name and complete mailing address)*

TAYLOR BALL, ELSEVIER INC.
1600 JOHN F KENNEDY BLVD. SUITE 1800
PHILADELPHIA, PA 19103-2899

Editor *(Name and complete mailing address)*

JOHN VASSALLO, ELSEVIER INC.
1600 JOHN F KENNEDY BLVD. SUITE 1800
PHILADELPHIA, PA 19103-2899

Managing Editor *(Name and complete mailing address)*

PATRICK MANLEY, ELSEVIER INC.
1600 JOHN F KENNEDY BLVD. SUITE 1800
PHILADELPHIA, PA 19103-2899

10. Owner *(Do not leave blank. If the publication is owned by a corporation, give the name and address of the corporation immediately followed by the names and addresses of all stockholders owning or holding 1 percent or more of the total amount of stock. If not owned by a corporation, give the names and addresses of the individual owners. If owned by a partnership or other unincorporated firm, give its name and address as well as those of each individual owner. If the publication is published by a nonprofit organization, give its name and address.)*

Full Name	Complete Mailing Address
WHOLLY OWNED SUBSIDIARY OF REED/ELSEVIER, US HOLDINGS	1600 JOHN F KENNEDY BLVD. SUITE 1800 PHILADELPHIA, PA 19103-2899

11. Known Bondholders, Mortgagees, and Other Security Holders Owning or Holding 1 Percent or More of Total Amount of Bonds, Mortgages, or Other Securities. If none, check box ▸ ☐ None

Full Name	Complete Mailing Address
N/A	

12. Tax Status *(For completion by nonprofit organizations authorized to mail at nonprofit rates)* *(Check one)*
The purpose, function, and nonprofit status of this organization and the exempt status for federal income tax purposes:
☒ Has Not Changed During Preceding 12 Months
☐ Has Changed During Preceding 12 Months *(Publisher must submit explanation of change with this statement)*

PS Form 3526, July 2014 *[Page 1 of 4 (see instructions page 4)]* PSN 7530-01-000-9931 PRIVACY NOTICE: See our privacy policy on www.usps.com.

---

13. Publication Title	14. Issue Date for Circulation Data Below
MAGNETIC RESONANCE IMAGING CLINICS OF NORTH AMERICA	MAY 2019

15. Extent and Nature of Circulation			Average No. Copies Each Issue During Preceding 12 Months	No. Copies of Single Issue Published Nearest to Filing Date
a. Total Number of Copies *(Net press run)*			301	381
b. Paid Circulation *(By Mail and Outside the Mail)*	(1)	Mailed Outside-County Paid Subscriptions Stated on PS Form 3541 (Include paid distribution above nominal rate, advertiser's proof copies, and exchange copies)	202	295
	(2)	Mailed In-County Paid Subscriptions Stated on PS Form 3541 (Include paid distribution above nominal rate, advertiser's proof copies, and exchange copies)	0	0
	(3)	Paid Distribution Outside the Mails Including Sales Through Dealers and Carriers, Street Vendors, Counter Sales, and Other Paid Distribution Outside USPS®	56	69
	(4)	Paid Distribution by Other Classes of Mail Through the USPS (e.g. First-Class Mail®)	0	0
c. Total Paid Distribution *[Sum of 15b (1), (2), (3), and (4)]*			258	364
d. Free or Nominal Rate Distribution *(By Mail and Outside the Mail)*	(1)	Free or Nominal Rate Outside-County Copies Included on PS Form 3541	38	17
	(2)	Free or Nominal Rate In-County Copies Included on PS Form 3541	0	0
	(3)	Free or Nominal Rate Copies Mailed at Other Classes Through the USPS (e.g. First-Class Mail)	0	0
	(4)	Free or Nominal Rate Distribution Outside the Mail (Carriers or other means)	0	0
e. Total Free or Nominal Rate Distribution *(Sum of 15d (1), (2), (3) and (4))*			38	17
f. Total Distribution *(Sum of 15c and 15e)*			296	381
g. Copies not Distributed *(See Instructions to Publishers #4 (page #3))*			6	0
h. Total *(Sum of 15f and g)*			302	381
i. Percent Paid *(15c divided by 15f times 100)*			87.16%	95.54%

* If you are claiming electronic copies, go to line 16 on page 3. If you are not claiming electronic copies, skip to line 17 on page 3.

16. Electronic Copy Circulation		Average No. Copies Each Issue During Preceding 12 Months	No. Copies of Single Issue Published Nearest to Filing Date
a. Paid Electronic Copies	▸		
b. Total Paid Print Copies (Line 15c) + Paid Electronic Copies (Line 16a)	▸		
c. Total Print Distribution (Line 15f) + Paid Electronic Copies (Line 16a)	▸		
d. Percent Paid (Both Print & Electronic Copies) (16b divided by 16c × 100)	▸		

☒ I certify that 50% of all my distributed copies (electronic and print) are paid above a nominal price.

17. Publication of Statement of Ownership

☒ If the publication is a general publication, publication of this statement is required. Will be printed in the __NOVEMBER 2019__ issue of this publication.

☐ Publication not required.

18. Signature and Title of Editor, Publisher, Business Manager, or Owner

STEPHEN R. BUSHING, INVENTORY DISTRIBUTION CONTROL MANAGER

Date 9/18/2019

I certify that all information furnished on this form is true and complete. I understand that anyone who furnishes false or misleading information on this form or who omits material or information requested on the form may be subject to criminal sanctions (including fines and imprisonment) and/or civil sanctions (including civil penalties).

PS Form 3526, July 2014 *(Page 3 of 4)* PRIVACY NOTICE: See our privacy policy on www.usps.com

Moving?

Make sure your subscription moves with you!

To notify us of your new address, find your **Clinics Account Number** (located on your mailing label above your name), and contact customer service at:

Email: journalscustomerservice-usa@elsevier.com

800-654-2452 (subscribers in the U.S. & Canada)
314-447-8871 (subscribers outside of the U.S. & Canada)

Fax number: 314-447-8029

Elsevier Health Sciences Division
Subscription Customer Service
3251 Riverport Lane
Maryland Heights, MO 63043

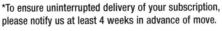

*To ensure uninterrupted delivery of your subscription, please notify us at least 4 weeks in advance of move.

ELSEVIER